MATH CALCULATIONS FOR PHARMACY TECHNICIANS

A WORKTEXT

FOURTH EDITION

MATH CALCULATIONS FOR PHARMACY TECHNICIANS

A WORKTEXT

Elaine Simmons Beale, RPh
Paul D. Camp Community College
Franklin, Virginia

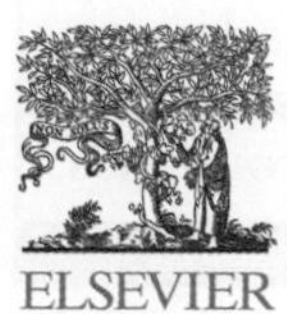

ELSEVIER

Elsevier
3251 Riverport Lane
St. Louis, Missouri 63043

MATH CALCULATIONS FOR PHARMACY TECHNICIANS, FOURTH EDITION ISBN: 978-0-323-76012-6

Publishing Director: Kristin Wilhelm
Senior Content Development Manager: Luke Held
Senior Content Development Specialist: Beck Rist
Publishing Services Manager: Deepthi Unni
Senior Project Manager: Umarani Natarajan
Design Direction: Ryan Cook

Printed in the United States of America

Last digit is the print number: 9 8 7 6 5 4 3 2 1

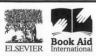

Dedication

In memory of my brother, Frank Simmons, RPh, who discussed pharmacy with me as long as I can remember.

To my students for helping me understand how people struggle with and eventually master mathematics, thank you for allowing me to share my love of the subject with you.

To the students who will use this text, I hope that it clarifies and makes the learning process easier for you. I wish you the best of luck in your chosen career.

Elaine Simmons Beale

Reviewers

Gae Carrol, MEd (c), HBPHE, RPhT
Provincial Coordinator of Pharmacy Technician Blended Program
CTS Canadian Career College
North Bay, Ontario, Canada

Lacey Crawford, CPhT
Pharmacy Technician Instructor of Health and Health Sciences
Kilgore College
Kilgore, Texas

David Harris, BA, MEd, CPhT
Allied Health—Pharmacy Technician Instructor
Manatee Technical College
Bradenton, Florida

Tetranetta Harris, CPhT, BA&Sc, MEd, MHA
Pharmacy Technician Department Chair
Remington College
Memphis, Tennessee

Kendra N. Johnson, CPhT
Allied Health Program Coordinator—Pharmacy Technician Program, Adult Education
Pickaway Ross Career & Technology Center
Chillicothe, Ohio

Kimberli Lopez, CPhT, AS, California Pharmacy Technician License
Adjunct Professor of Pharmacy Technology
Pharmacy Technology Department, Science Division
San Bernardino Valley College
San Bernardino, California

Mateo Lorico, BS, MH, CPhT, RPhT
CTT Pharmacy Technician Program
U.S. Department of Labor—Long Beach Job Corps
Long Beach, California

Marichu Parcasio, BS Pharmacy
Education
American Career College—Los Angeles
Los Angeles, California

Shamika Porcher, BS, CPhT
Pharmacy Technician Program Director
Remington College
Fort Worth, Texas

Tekia Rocker, MBA, BS, CPhT
Dean of Academics
Remington College
Mobile, Alabama

Meera Shah, PharmD, MBA
Product Development Manager
CVS Health
Austin, Texas

Preface

Patient safety depends on the ability of health care professionals, especially those responsible for the preparation, distribution, and administration of medication, to correctly calculate doses and dosages. Pharmacy technicians must learn this skill and use it throughout their careers. This text, which meets the guidelines prepared by the American Society of Health-System Pharmacists (ASHP) for accredited pharmacy technician programs, provides the basic mathematical concepts that are applied to pharmacy.

My goal with *Math Calculations for Pharmacy Technicians: A Worktext* is to assist pharmacy technician students in mastering the mathematical calculations necessary to prepare medications safely. It covers calculations used in inpatient settings, as well as outpatient settings, with a chapter covering basic business math for retail practice.

This text includes two basic methods of calculating medicinal doses and dosages: ratio/proportion and dimensional analysis. Even though I present both methods, you will learn that each one has its place in calculations, and you should complete the exercises using the method that is appropriate and most comfortable for you.

The book is organized from basic mathematical calculations (fractions, decimals, percentages) to basic medication calculations to more complicated dose and dosage calculations related to prescriptions and hospital orders. Each chapter builds upon the previous knowledge base to ensure that the student is competent in one skill before adding another. Some students may not need the very basic instructions, but I recommend at least working through the pretests and posttests to make certain you are confident enough to proceed to the next chapter. The final chapter presents routine retail accounting procedures and focuses on business calculations, as well as inventory control.

Because practice is so important, the text includes more than 1,800 practice problems covering a wide range of concepts. The concepts of pharmaceutical mathematics build from chapter to chapter, with reinforcement of previous material throughout the text. The worktext format allows students to work at a pace that is right for them and meets the needs of the instructor and course objectives. The time devoted to each chapter may vary depending on the student's mathematical level. For this reason, the student's prior mathematical competence is tested with each chapter. Be sure that calculations are shown for each problem; this allows for identifying and correcting errors.

ORGANIZATION OF MATERIAL

The text is divided into five sections: Section I, Introduction and Basic Math Skills, includes an assessment of math skills needed in the field, as well as a review of basic math skills; Section II, Measurements and Conversions Used in Health Care Occupations, explores the different measurement systems used in pharmacy; Section III, Calculations With Prescriptions and Medication Orders, focuses on calculations needed to fill common prescriptions and medication orders; Section IV, Special Medication Calculations, covers special population, compounding, and IV calculations; and Section V, Business Math, covers business math for retail pharmacy.

CHAPTER FEATURES

Learning Objectives and Key Words

Each chapter begins with a set of learning objectives and a list of key words.

OBJECTIVES

1. Introduce The Joint Commission (TJC) Official "Do Not Use" List and the Institute for Safe Medication Practices (ISMP) List of Error-Prone Abbreviations, Symbols, and Dose Designations.
2. Learn medical and pharmaceutical abbreviations.
3. Explain why proficiency in basic math skills is essential for pharmacy technicians, and assess level of basic mathematical skills necessary for pharmaceutical calculations.

KEY WORDS

Active ingredient The ingredient in a medication that has the desired effect on the body
Excipients Medicinally inactive substances that are added to medication formulations; fillers, binders, coloring agents, flavorings, preservatives
Pharmacology Study of drugs, their uses, and their interactions with living systems

Pretest and Posttest

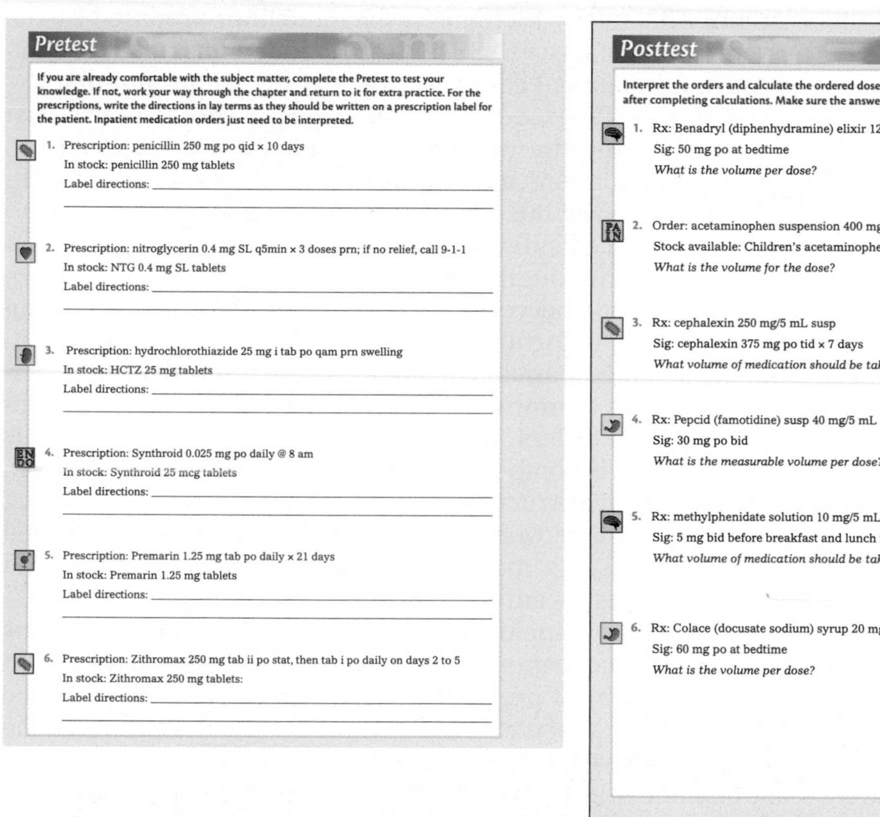

Pretest

If you are already comfortable with the subject matter, complete the Pretest to test your knowledge. If not, work your way through the chapter and return to it for extra practice. For the prescriptions, write the directions in lay terms as they should be written on a prescription label for the patient. Inpatient medication orders just need to be interpreted.

1. Prescription: penicillin 250 mg po qid × 10 days
   In stock: penicillin 250 mg tablets
   Label directions: ______
2. Prescription: nitroglycerin 0.4 mg SL q5min × 3 doses prn; if no relief, call 9-1-1
   In stock: NTG 0.4 mg SL tablets
   Label directions: ______
3. Prescription: hydrochlorothiazide 25 mg i tab po qam prn swelling
   In stock: HCTZ 25 mg tablets
   Label directions: ______
4. Prescription: Synthroid 0.025 mg po daily @ 8 am
   In stock: Synthroid 25 mcg tablets
   Label directions: ______
5. Prescription: Premarin 1.25 mg tab po daily × 21 days
   In stock: Premarin 1.25 mg tablets
   Label directions: ______
6. Prescription: Zithromax 250 mg tab ii po stat, then tab i po daily on days 2 to 5
   In stock: Zithromax 250 mg tablets:
   Label directions: ______

Posttest

Interpret the orders and calculate the ordered doses. Show your work. Round to the nearest tenth after completing calculations. Make sure the answer is a measurable volume.

1. Rx: Benadryl (diphenhydramine) elixir 12.5 mg/5 mL
   Sig: 50 mg po at bedtime
   What is the volume per dose?
2. Order: acetaminophen suspension 400 mg
   Stock available: Children's acetaminophen liquid suspension 160 mg/5 mL
   What is the volume for the dose?
3. Rx: cephalexin 250 mg/5 mL susp
   Sig: cephalexin 375 mg po tid × 7 days
   What volume of medication should be taken per dose?
4. Rx: Pepcid (famotidine) susp 40 mg/5 mL
   Sig: 30 mg po bid
   What is the measurable volume per dose?
5. Rx: methylphenidate solution 10 mg/5 mL
   Sig: 5 mg bid before breakfast and lunch for ADHD
   What volume of medication should be taken per dose?
6. Rx: Colace (docusate sodium) syrup 20 mg/5 mL
   Sig: 60 mg po at bedtime
   What is the volume per dose?

Each chapter includes a pretest that indicates the level of student understanding of the calculation principles to be presented. If the material presented is understood at a level upon which to build comprehension of future concepts, the student may find that only a brief review in that area is needed. Students should move on to the next chapter when they feel comfortable with the material presented and have demonstrated that they understand the subject matter.

Students who complete the exercises in each chapter may retake the pretest before taking the posttest at the end of the chapter to ensure that they have mastered the material. A student who continues to have problems with the posttest should study the chapter again. The importance of proper calculations cannot be overemphasized, and a working knowledge of accurate calculations is essential.

Practice Problems

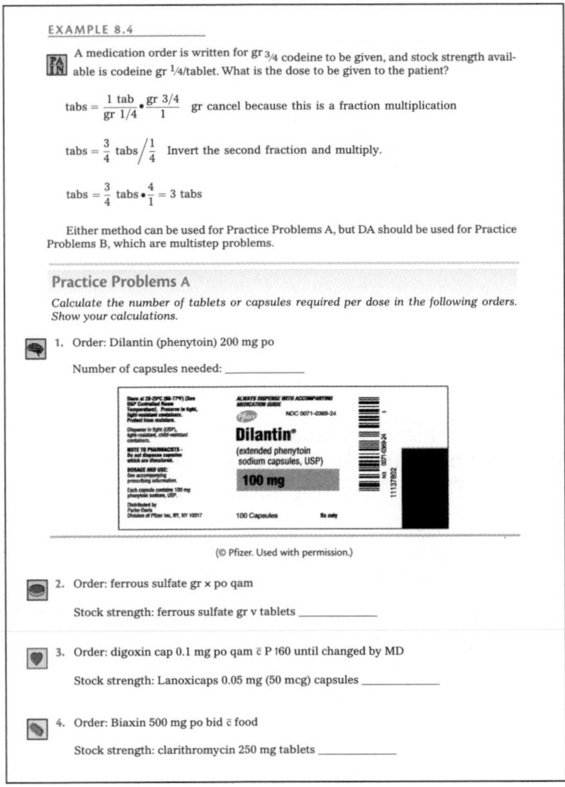

EXAMPLE 8.4

A medication order is written for gr 3/4 codeine to be given, and stock strength available is codeine gr 1/4/tablet. What is the dose to be given to the patient?

$$\text{tabs} = \frac{1\ \text{tab}}{\text{gr}\ 1/4} \bullet \frac{\text{gr}\ 3/4}{1}$$ gr cancel because this is a fraction multiplication

$$\text{tabs} = \frac{3}{4}\ \text{tabs} \Big/ \frac{1}{4}$$ Invert the second fraction and multiply.

$$\text{tabs} = \frac{3}{4}\ \text{tabs} \bullet \frac{4}{1} = 3\ \text{tabs}$$

Either method can be used for Practice Problems A, but DA should be used for Practice Problems B, which are multistep problems.

Practice Problems A

Calculate the number of tablets or capsules required per dose in the following orders. Show your calculations.

1. Order: Dilantin (phenytoin) 200 mg po

   Number of capsules needed: ____________

(© Pfizer. Used with permission.)

2. Order: ferrous sulfate gr x po qam

   Stock strength: ferrous sulfate gr v tablets ____________

3. Order: digoxin cap 0.1 mg po qam c̄ P ↑60 until changed by MD

   Stock strength: Lanoxicaps 0.05 mg (50 mcg) capsules ____________

4. Order: Biaxin 500 mg po bid c̄ food

   Stock strength: clarithromycin 250 mg tablets ____________

The practice problems may be used as in-class work, as well as homework. Be sure the knowledge base for each exercise is understood, so any previous mistakes are not made in subsequent calculations. Understanding the basis for pharmaceutical calculations is essential in preventing errors in actual practice. *Always look at your answer and ask yourself if it makes sense.* Then refigure for accuracy. Many errors can be prevented in this manner. Ask for assistance from the pharmacist if needed to ensure patients' safety.

Answer Key

The answers to every third problem are presented in the Partial Answer Key, so students can check their individual work and determine if they have completed the calculations correctly. If the answer is incorrect, the student has immediate feedback. Instructors should require students to show all mathematical calculations, so they can see the point at which mistakes occur and can correct the concept before students advance to more difficult calculations. The full Answer Key is available to instructors within the TEACH Instructor's Resource on Evolve.

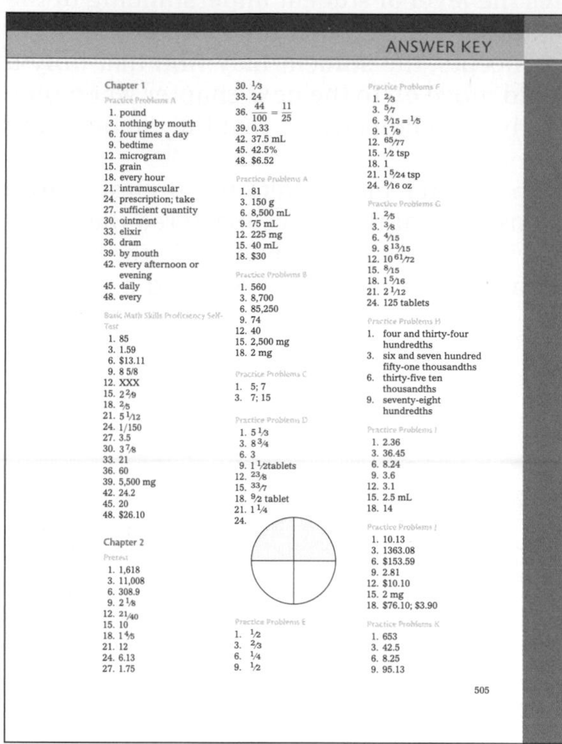

ANSWER KEY

Chapter 1

Practice Problems A

1. pound
3. nothing by mouth
6. four times a day
9. bedtime
12. microgram
15. grain
18. every hour
21. intramuscular
24. prescription; take
27. sufficient quantity
30. ointment
33. elixir
36. dram
39. by mouth
42. every afternoon or evening
45. daily
48. every

Basic Math Skills Proficiency Self-Test

1. 85
3. 1.59
6. $13.11
9. 8 5/8
12. XXX
15. 2 2/9
18. 2/5
21. 5 1/12
24. 1/150
27. 3.5
30. 3 7/8
33. 21
36. 60
39. 5,500 mg
42. 24.2
45. 20
48. $26.10

Chapter 2

Pretest

1. 1,618
3. 11,008
6. 308.9
9. 2 1/8
12. 21/40
15. 10
18. 1 4/5
21. 12
24. 6.13
27. 1.75
30. 1/3
33. 24
36. $\frac{44}{100} = \frac{11}{25}$
39. 0.33
42. 37.5 mL
45. 42.5%
48. $6.52

Practice Problems A

1. 81
3. 150 g
6. 8,500 mL
9. 75 mL
12. 225 mg
15. 40 mL
18. $30

Practice Problems B

1. 560
3. 8,700
6. 85,250
9. 74
12. 40
15. 2,500 mg
18. 2 mg

Practice Problems C

1. 5; 7
3. 7; 15

Practice Problems D

1. 5 1/3
3. 8 3/4
6. 3
9. 1 1/2tablets
12. 23/8
15. 33/7
18. 9/2 tablet
21. 1 1/4
24.

Practice Problems E

1. 1/2
3. 2/3
6. 1/4
9. 1/2

Practice Problems F

1. 2/3
3. 5/7
6. 3/15 = 1/5
9. 1 7/9
12. 65/77
15. 1/2 tsp
18. 1
21. 1 5/24 tsp
24. 9/16 oz

Practice Problems G

1. 2/5
3. 3/8
6. 4/15
9. 8 13/15
12. 10 61/72
15. 8/15
18. 1 5/16
21. 2 1/12
24. 125 tablets

Practice Problems H

1. four and thirty-four hundredths
3. six and seven hundred fifty-one thousandths
6. thirty-five ten thousandths
9. seventy-eight hundredths

Practice Problems I

1. 2.36
3. 36.45
6. 8.24
9. 3.6
12. 3.1
15. 2.5 mL
18. 14

Practice Problems J

1. 10.13
3. 1363.08
6. $153.59
9. 2.81
12. $10.10
15. 2 mg
18. $76.10; $3.90

Practice Problems K

1. 653
3. 42.5
6. 8.25
9. 95.13

505

Icons

Throughout the text, when medications are used in practice problems, icons indicate the general use for certain drugs. In this way, students learn mathematical calculations and are also exposed to the medications and their uses. The following icons are included in the text:

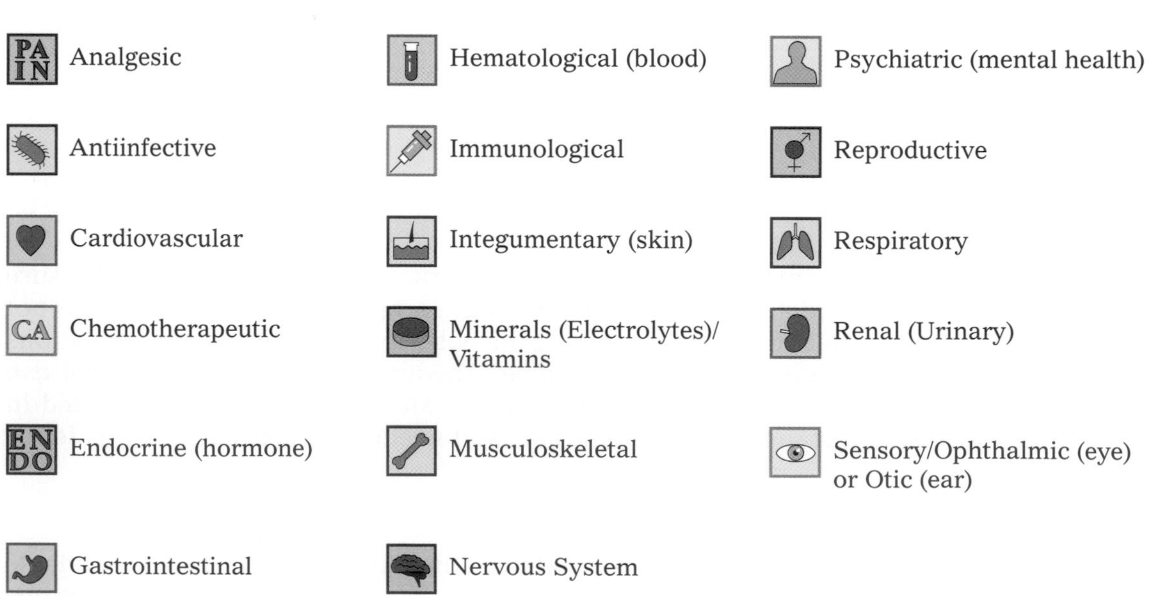

Tech Notes and Tech Alerts

Tech Notes boxes highlight important concepts. **Tech Alerts** assist students in focusing on areas where comprehension is *essential* to reduce errors and enhance patient safety.

> TECH NOTE
> Determining the appropriate place value when rounding medication doses depends on the potency, the amount, and the route of administration.

> ! TECH ALERT
> Only round the **final** answer when performing multiple step calculations.

ANCILLARIES

Instructor Ancillaries Available on Evolve

New and Improved TEACH Instructor's Resource: The TEACH Instructor's Resource provides instructors with customizable Lesson Plans, PowerPoint Slides, Student Handouts, and the full Answer Key. With these valuable resources, instructors will save valuable preparation time and create a learning environment that fully engages students in classroom preparation.

- **ExamView Test Bank:** Contains more than 1,100 multiple-choice questions.
- **Instructor Practice Problems:** Provide even more practice using these additional problems.
- **New! Mapping Guide** correlating content to ASHP accreditation standards and to certification blueprints.
- **Image Collection:** Includes images in the text so they can be used as teaching aids.

Student Ancillaries Available on Evolve

- **Student Practice Problems:** Enhance calculation skills with additional practice problems that correspond to every chapter in the text.
- **Comprehensive Posttest:** Interactively tests students' knowledge and mastery of all content.

SPECIAL NOTE

To comply with The Joint Commission (TJC) *Official "Do Not Use" List*, the following abbreviations and recommendations have been clearly identified in this text.

Official "Do Not Use" List[a]

DO NOT USE	POTENTIAL PROBLEM	USE INSTEAD
U, u (unit)	Mistaken for "0," the number "4" or "cc"	Write "unit"
IU (international unit)	Mistaken for IV (intravenous) or the number 10 (ten)	Write "International Unit"
QD, Q.D., qd, q.d. (daily)	Mistaken for each other	Write "daily"
Q.O.D., QOD, q.o.d, qod (every other day)	Period after the Q mistaken for "I" and the "O" mistaken for "I"	Write "every other day"
Trailing zero (X.0 mg)	Decimal point is missed	Write X mg
Lack of leading zero (.X mg)		Write 0.X mg
MS	Can mean morphine sulfate or magnesium sulfate	Write "morphine sulfate"
MSO_4 and $MgSO_4$	Confused for one another	Write "magnesium sulfate"

[a]Applies to all orders and all medication-related documentation.

In addition, please refer to the Institute for Safe Medication Practices (ISMP) *List of Error-Prone Abbreviations, Symbols, and Dose Designations* at https://www.ismp.org/tools/errorproneabbreviations.pdf and review this listing. This list is included on pages 2–6 of the text. To realistically teach pharmacy technicians, some of these abbreviations are included throughout this text since they are still frequently used with prescriptions and medication orders.

Elaine Simmons Beale, RPh

Acknowledgments

I would like to thank the following people from Elsevier: Beck Rist, Senior Content Development Specialist, Umarani Natarajan, Senior Project Manager, and Kristin Wilhelm, Content Director, for their continual help and guidance, as well as the numerous reviewers and editors.

Most of all, I would like to thank my family, who put up with my countless hours of work.

Elaine Simmons Beale

Table of Contents

IN SECTION I

SECTION I
Introduction and Basic Math Skills

CHAPTER 1

Abbreviations, Symbols, and Basic Mathematical Skills for Health Occupations

OBJECTIVES

1. Introduce The Joint Commission (TJC) Official "Do Not Use" List and the Institute for Safe Medication Practices (ISMP) List of Error-Prone Abbreviations, Symbols, and Dose Designations.
2. Learn medical and pharmaceutical abbreviations.
3. Explain why proficiency in basic math skills is essential for pharmacy technicians, and assess level of basic mathematical skills necessary for pharmaceutical calculations.

KEY WORDS

Active ingredient The ingredient in a medication that has the desired effect on the body

Excipients Medicinally inactive substances that are added to medication formulations; fillers, binders, coloring agents, flavorings, preservatives

Pharmacology Study of drugs, their uses, and their interactions with living systems

INTRODUCTION

Pharmacology is the study of the uses, mechanisms of action, and effects of medications on body systems. Chemicals used as medications, or drugs, are the basis of pharmacology. Medications used to treat conditions and diseases must be dosed, prepared, and administered correctly. Calculating doses correctly is essential for the safety of patients.

Different medicinal preparations contain different amounts of **active ingredients**. Preparations also contain a variety of **excipients**, which are medicinally inactive substances added to the formulation as fillers, binders, coloring agents, flavorings, and preservatives. Each drug has its own specific concentration of active ingredients in a formulation. For example, a tablet may be manufactured in 10 and 20 mg strengths and a liquid may be manufactured in 125 mg/5 mL and 250 mg/5 mL strengths. The safe and effective amount of medication has been tested and recognized as within acceptable limits by the U.S. Department of Health and Human Services' Food and Drug Administration (FDA). The *U.S. Pharmacopeia* and the *National Formulary (USP-NF)* are manuals that provide standards for medication ingredients, preparation, and storage, which are enforced by the FDA. Each medication has its own recommended dose and dosage range. The pharmacy technician must have a thorough understanding of both the mathematical skills and the terminology used in medicine in order to assist the pharmacist in providing excellent patient care.

INTERPRETING PHARMACEUTICAL ABBREVIATIONS AND SYMBOLS

Knowledge of medical terminology and abbreviations is necessary for properly interpreting and dispensing prescription and medication orders, as well as educating patients in taking medications at home. Abbreviations are used to refer to routes of administration, frequency of dosing, and units of measurement within systems, among others.

Some abbreviations that have been used for years have been found to lead to medication errors, which led to the development of The Joint Commission (TJC) *Official "Do Not Use" List* of abbreviations. To comply with this list, none of the included abbreviations have been used in this text.

Official "Do Not Use" List[a,b]

DO NOT USE	POTENTIAL PROBLEM	USE INSTEAD
U, u (unit)	Mistaken for "0," the number "4," or "cc"	Write "unit"
IU (international unit)	Mistaken for IV (intravenous) or the number 10 (ten)	Write "International Unit"
QD, Q.D., qd, q.d. (daily)	Mistaken for each other	Write "daily"
Q.O.D., QOD, q.o.d, qod (every other day)	Period after the Q mistaken for "I" and the "O" mistaken for "I"	Write "every other day"
Trailing zero (X.0 mg)	Decimal point is missed	Write X mg
Lack of leading zero (.X mg)		Write 0.X mg
MS	Can mean morphine sulfate or magnesium sulfate	Write "morphine sulfate"
MSO_4 and $MgSO_4$	Confused for one another	Write "magnesium sulfate"

[a]Applies to all orders and all medication-related documentation.

In addition, the Institute for Safe Medication Practices (ISMP) has compiled a List of Error-Prone Abbreviations, Symbols, and Dose Designations (https://www.ismp.org/tools/errorproneabbreviations.pdf).

List of Error-Prone Abbreviations, Symbols, and Dose Designations

ABBREVIATION	INTENDED MEANING	MISINTERPRETATION	CORRECTION
µg	Microgram	Mistaken as "mg"	Use "mcg"
AD, AS, AU	Right ear, left ear, each ear	Mistaken as "OD, OS, OU" (right eye, left eye, each eye)	Use "right ear," "left ear," or "each ear"
OD, OS, OU	Right eye, left eye, each eye	Mistaken as "AD, AS, AU" (right ear, left ear, each ear)	Use "right eye," "left eye," or "each eye"
BT	Bedtime	Mistaken as "BID" (twice daily)	Use "bedtime"
Cc	Cubic centimeters	Mistaken as "u" (units)	Use "mL" (milliliters)
D/C	Discharge or discontinue	Premature discontinuation of medications if D/C (intended to mean "discharge") has been misinterpreted as "discontinued" when followed by a list of discharge medications	Use "discharge" and "discontinue"
IJ	Injection	Mistaken as "IV" or "intrajugular"	Use "injection"

ABBREVIATION	INTENDED MEANING	MISINTERPRETATION	CORRECTION
IN	Intranasal	Mistaken as "IM" or "IV"	Use "intranasal" or "NAS"
HS	Half-strength	Mistaken as "bedtime"	Use "half-strength" or "bedtime"
hs	At bedtime, hours of sleep	Mistaken as "half-strength"	
IU[a]	International unit	Mistaken as "IV" (intravenous) or "10" (ten)	Use "units"
o.d. or OD	Once daily	Mistaken as "right eye" (OD-oculus dexter), leading to oral liquid medications administered in the eye	Use "daily"
OJ	Orange juice	Mistaken as "OD" or "OS" (right or left eye); drugs meant to be diluted in orange juice may be given in the eye	Use "orange juice"
Per os	By mouth, orally	The "os" can be mistaken as "left eye" (OS—oculus sinister)	Use "PO," "by mouth," or "orally"
q.d. or QD[a]	Every day	Mistaken as "q.i.d.," especially if the period after the "q" or the tail of the "q" is misunderstood as an "i"	Use "daily"
qhs	Nightly at bedtime	Mistaken as "qhr," or every hour	Use "nightly"
qn	Nightly or at bedtime	Mistaken as "qh" (every hour)	Use "nightly" or "at bedtime"
q.o.d. or QOD[a]	Every other day	Mistaken as "q.d." (daily) or "q.i.d." (four times daily) if the "o" is poorly written	Use "every other day"
q1d	Daily	Mistaken as "q.i.d." (four times daily)	Use "daily"
q6PM, etc.	Every evening at 6 PM	Mistaken as "every 6 hours"	Use "daily at 6 PM" or "6 PM daily"
SC, SQ, sub q	Subcutaneous	"SC" mistaken as "SL" (sublingual); "SQ" mistaken as "5 every"; the "q" in "sub q" has been mistaken as "every" (e.g., a heparin dose ordered "sub q 2 hours before surgery" misunderstood as "every 2 hours before surgery")	Use "subcut" or "subcutaneously"
ss	Sliding scale (insulin) or $\frac{1}{2}$ (apothecary)	Mistaken as "55"	Spell out "sliding scale"; use "one-half" or "$\frac{1}{2}$"
SSRI	Sliding scale regular insulin	Mistaken as "selective-serotonin reuptake inhibitor"	Spell out "sliding scale (insulin)"
SSI	Sliding scale insulin	Mistaken as "strong solution of iodine" (Lugol's)	
i/d	One daily	Mistaken as "tid"	Use "1 daily"
TIW or tiw	3 times a week	Mistaken as "3 times a day" or "twice in a week"	Use "3 times weekly"
U or u[a]	Unit	Mistaken as the number "0" or "4," causing a 10-fold overdose or greater (e.g., 4U seen as "40" or 4u seen as "44"); mistaken as "cc," so dose given in volume instead of units (e.g., "4u" seen as "4 cc")	Use "unit"

Continued

ABBREVIATION	INTENDED MEANING	MISINTERPRETATION	CORRECTION
UD	As directed ("ut dictum")	Mistaken as "unit dose" (e.g., diltiazem 125 mg IV infusion "UD" misinterpreted as meaning to give the entire infusion as a unit [bolus] dose)	Use "as directed"

DOSE DESIGNATIONS AND OTHER INFORMATION	INTENDED MEANING	MISINTERPRETATION	CORRECTION
Trailing zero after decimal point (e.g., 1.0 mg)[a]	1 mg	Mistaken as "10 mg" if the decimal point is not seen	Do not use trailing zeros for doses expressed in whole numbers
"Naked" decimal point (e.g., .5 mg)[a]	0.5 mg	Mistaken as "5 mg" if the decimal point is not seen	Use zero before a decimal point when the dose is less than a whole unit
Abbreviations such as mg. or mL. with a period following the abbreviation	mg mL	The period is unnecessary and could be mistaken as the number "1" if written poorly	Use "mg," "mL," etc. without a terminal period
Drug name and dose run together (especially problematic for drug names that end in "L" such as Inderal 40 mg; Tegretol 300 mg)	Inderal 40 mg Tegretol 300 mg	Mistaken as "Inderal 140 mg" Mistaken as "Tegretol 1300 mg"	Place adequate space between the drug name, dose, and unit of measure
Numerical dose and unit of measure run together (e.g., 10 mg, 100 mL)	10 mg 100 mL	The "m" is sometimes mistaken as a zero or two zeros, risking a 10- to 100-fold overdose	Place adequate space between the dose and unit of measure
Large doses without properly placed commas (e.g., 100000 units; 1000000 units)	100,000 units 1,000,000 units	100000 has been mistaken as 10,000 or 1,000,000; 1000000 has been mistaken as 100,000	Use commas for dosing units at or above 1,000, or use words such as 100 "thousand" or 1 "million" to improve readability

DRUG NAME ABBREVIATIONS	INTENDED MEANING	MISINTERPRETATION	CORRECTION
To avoid confusion, do not abbreviate drug names when communicating medical information. Examples of drug name abbreviations involved in medication errors include the following:			
APAP	acetaminophen	Not recognized as acetaminophen	Use complete drug name
ARA A	vidarabine	Mistaken as "cytarabine (ARA C)"	Use complete drug name
AZT	zidovudine (Retrovir)	Mistaken as "azathioprine" or "aztreonam"	Use complete drug name
CPZ	prochlorperazine (Compazine)	Mistaken as "chlorpromazine"	Use complete drug name
DPT	Demerol-Phenergan-Thorazine	Mistaken as "diphtheria-pertussis-tetanus" (vaccine)	Use complete drug name

DRUG NAME ABBREVIATIONS	INTENDED MEANING	MISINTERPRETATION	CORRECTION
DTO	Diluted tincture of opium, or deodorized tincture of opium (Paregoric)	Mistaken as "tincture of opium"	Use complete drug name
HCl	hydrochloric acid or hydrochloride	Mistaken as "potassium chloride" (the "H" is misinterpreted as "K")	Use complete drug name unless expressed as a salt of a drug
HCT	hydrocortisone	Mistaken as "hydrochlorothiazide"	Use complete drug name
HCTZ	hydrochloro-thiazide	Mistaken as "hydrocortisone" (seen as HCT 250 mg)	Use complete drug name
$MgSO_4$[a]	magnesium sulfate	Mistaken as "morphine sulfate"	Use complete drug name
MS, MSO_4[a]	morphine sulfate	Mistaken as "magnesium sulfate"	Use complete drug name
MTX	methotrexate	Mistaken as "mitoxantrone"	Use complete drug name
NoAc	Novel/new oral anticoagulant	No anticoagulant	Use complete drug name
PCA	procainamide	Mistaken as "patient-controlled analgesia (PCA)"	Use complete drug name
PTU	propylthiouracil	Mistaken as "mercaptopurine"	Use complete drug name
T3	Tylenol with codeine No. 3	Mistaken as "liothyronine"	Use complete drug name
TAC	triamcinolone	Mistaken as "tetracaine, Adrenalin, cocaine"	Use complete drug name
TNK	TNKase	Mistaken as "TPA"	Use complete drug name
TPA or tPA	Tissue plasminogen activator, alteplase (Activase)	Mistaken as "tenecteplase (TNKase)," or less often as another tissue plasminogen activator, "reteplase (Retavase)"	Use complete drug names
$ZnSO_4$	zinc sulfate	Mistaken as "morphine sulfate"	Use complete drug name

STEMMED DRUG NAMES	INTENDED MEANING	MISINTERPRETATION	CORRECTION
"Nitro" drip	nitroglycerin infusion	Mistaken as "sodium nitroprusside infusion"	Use complete drug name
"Norflox"	norfloxacin	Mistaken as "Norflex"	Use complete drug name
"IV Vanc"	intravenous vancomycin	Mistaken as "Invanz"	Use complete drug name

SYMBOLS	INTENDED MEANING	MISINTERPRETATION	CORRECTION
ʒ	Dram	Symbol for dram mistaken as "3"	Use the metric system
♏	Minim	Symbol for minim mistaken as "mL"	Use the metric system
x3d	For 3 days	Mistaken as "3 doses"	Use "for 3 days"

Continued

SYMBOLS	INTENDED MEANING	MISINTERPRETATION	CORRECTION
> and <	Greater than and less than	Mistaken as opposite of intended; mistakenly use incorrect symbol; "< 10" mistaken as "40"	Use "greater than" or "less than"
/ (slash mark)	Separates two doses or indicates "per"	Mistaken as the number "1" (e.g., "25 units/10 units" misread as "25 units and 110" units)	Use "per" rather than a slash mark to separate doses
@	At	Mistaken as "2"	Use "at"
&	And	Mistaken as "2"	Use "and"
+	Plus or and	Mistaken as "4"	Use "and"
°	Hour	Mistaken as a zero (e.g., q2° seen as q 20)	Use "hr," "h," or "hour"
Φ or ⊘	zero, null sign	Mistaken as numerals "4," "6," "8," and "9"	Use 0 or zero, or describe intent using whole words

[a]These abbreviations are included on The Joint Commission's "minimum list" of dangerous abbreviations, acronyms, and symbols that must be included on an organization's "Do Not Use" list, effective January 1, 2004. Visit www.jointcommission.org for more information about this Joint Commission requirement.

The following is a list of some common abbreviations and symbols that you should know. Although some of the following are included in one or both of the previous lists, you should still be aware of them and their preferred substitutes, which are bolded in the following list. Some may still be included on the PTCE—the national pharmacy technician certification examination.

ROUTES OF ADMINISTRATION

ID—intradermal
IM—intramuscular
IT—intrathecal
IV—intravenous
PO—by mouth
PR—rectal
PV—vaginal
*SC, SQ, sub q—subcutaneous—use ***"SUBCUT"***
SL—sublingual (under the tongue)
TOP—topical

FREQUENCY OF ADMINISTRATION

qh—every hour
q2h—every 2 hours
q4h—every 4 hours
q6h—every 6 hours
q8h—every 8 hours
q12h—every 12 hours
*†qd—once a day—use ***"daily"***
bid—twice a day
tid—three times a day
qid—four times a day
*†qod—every other day—use ***"every other day"***
q week—every week
q month—every month

TIMES OF ADMINISTRATION

ac—before meals
pc—after meals
am—morning
pm—evening
noc—night
*hs—hour of sleep—use ***"bedtime"***
prn—as needed
ASAP—as soon as possible
STAT—at once, immediately

DOSAGE FORMS

SOLIDS

cap—capsule
tab—tablet

LIQUIDS

fl, f—fluid
liq—liquid
susp—suspension
syr—syrup

SEMISOLIDS

cr—cream
lot—lotion
supp—suppository
ung/oint—ointment

MEASUREMENT SYSTEMS

METRIC SYSTEM

mcg—microgram
mg—milligram
g—gram
kg—kilogram
mL—milliliter
L—liter
m—meter

HOUSEHOLD SYSTEM

gtt—drop(s)
tsp, Tsp, t—teaspoon
tbsp, Tbsp, T—tablespoon
c, C—cup
oz—ounce
pt—pint
qt—quart
gal—gallon
#, lb—pound
″, in—inch
′, ft—foot

APOTHECARY SYSTEM—ABBREVIATIONS AND SYMBOLS

gr—grain
*ʒ/dr—dram—recommendation from ISMP is "use metric system"
℥/oz—ounce
*♏—minim—recommendation from ISMP is "use metric system"
*flʒ/fl dr—fluid dram
fl ℥/fl oz—fluid ounce

MISCELLANEOUS MEDICATION MEASUREMENTS

mEq—milliequivalent
*†IU/U—international unit/unit—use ***"international units"*** or ***"units"***

EARS AND EYES

*AD—right ear—use ***"right ear"***
*AS—left ear—use ***"left ear"***
*AU—each ear—use ***"each ear"***
*OD—right eye—use ***"right eye"***
*OS—left eye—use ***"left eye"***
*OU—each eye—use ***"each eye"***

GENERAL ABBREVIATIONS

$\bar{a}$—before
$\bar{p}$—after
$\bar{c}$—with
$\bar{s}$—without
=—equal to
≠—not equal to
*<—less than—use ***"less than"***
*>—greater than, more than—use ***"greater than"***
↑—higher than, increase
↓—lower than, decrease
$\overline{aa}$—of each
ad lib—as desired
DAW—dispense as written
NKA—no known allergies
NKDA—no known drug allergies
non rep—do not repeat
NPO, npo—nothing by mouth
OTC—over the counter
qs—sufficient quantity
rep—repeat
℞—prescription, treatment, take this drug
TO—telephone order
*UD—ut dict—use ***"as directed"***
VO—verbal order

*These abbreviations are found on the ISMP List of Error-Prone Abbreviations, Symbols, and Dose Designations due to medication safety issues. They should not be used but may still appear in the pharmacy setting.
*†Indicates terms on TJC Official "Do Not Use" list.

Practice Problems A

Interpret the following abbreviations.

1. #, lb ______________________
2. ↓ ______________________
3. npo ______________________
4. ↑ ______________________
5. gtt ______________________
6. qid ______________________
7. q4h ______________________
8. mL ______________________
[a]9. hs ______________________
10. fl ______________________
11. tbsp, T ______________________
12. mcg ______________________
[a]13. U ______________________
14. cap ______________________
15. gr ______________________
16. OTC ______________________
17. bid ______________________
18. qh ______________________
19. q2h ______________________
20. kg ______________________
21. IM ______________________
22. IV ______________________
23. ad lib ______________________
24. ℞ ______________________

25. tid ______________________ [a]26. qod ______________________

27. qs ______________________ 28. prn ______________________

29. tab ______________________ 30. ung ______________________

31. syr ______________________ 32. supp ______________________

33. elix ______________________ 34. $\overline{aa}$ ______________________

[a]35. ℥ ______________________ [a]36. ʒ ______________________

37. qam ______________________ 38. tsp, t ______________________

39. po ______________________ 40. $\overline{p}$ ______________________

41. ā ______________________ 42. qpm ______________________

43. stat ______________________ 44. q12h ______________________

45. qd ______________________ 46. $\overline{ss}$ ______________________

47. TO ______________________ 48. q ______________________

49. $\overline{s}$ ______________________ 50. $\overline{c}$ ______________________

[a]These abbreviations are found on the TJC *Official "Do Not Use" List* and ISMP *List of Error-Prone Abbreviations, Symbols, and Dose Designations* due to medication safety issues. They should not be used but may still appear in the pharmacy setting.

THE NEED FOR A PHARMACY TECHNICIAN TO MASTER MATHEMATICAL SKILLS

Pharmacy technicians are involved in the calculations of the amount of medication necessary to provide correct doses. They must also ensure that there are a sufficient number of doses for the desired length of therapy prescribed by the physician. Mathematics is used daily in the preparation of medications in both retail and institutional pharmacies. The responsibility that accompanies the preparation of medications is one that must be taken seriously so that effective drug levels are reached and dangerous drug levels are not reached. They must be familiar with acceptable limits—both minimums and maximums—of medications. They are responsible for the medications they prepare, although a pharmacist is required to double-check everything before it leaves the pharmacy.

Technicians are responsible for their actions, which are heavily dependent on mathematical skills. The course of pharmacology covers the skills required to master acceptable dosages and the expected results of medications. This text deals with the mathematical skills necessary for the safe preparation of the amount of medication prescribed for the patient.

The basic fundamental math skills necessary for pharmaceutical calculations include manipulation of fractions, decimals, and whole numbers to calculate the correct amount of medication needed. These skills are used for dose and dosage calculations in three measurement systems—household measurements such as teaspoons and tablespoons, which are used in the United States; metric system measurements such as grams, liters, and meters, which are commonly used throughout the rest of world; and apothecary system measurements such as grains, drams, and ounces, which were the basis of pharmacology but have now been mostly replaced by metric measurements. It is essential to understand these systems of measurement and be able to convert between them to prepare prescriptions for administration.

Additional mathematical conversions are also necessary, such as the conversion between 12-hour and 24-hour (military) time, because military time is used in inpatient settings for medication administration. The standard 12-hour time with AM and PM designations is used in most outpatient settings, so the ability to give the correct time in either situation is necessary. Conversions between Fahrenheit and Celsius temperatures and the use of Arabic and Roman numerals are also important in pharmacy.

BASIC MATH SKILLS USED IN PHARMACY

Basic math skills are necessary for safe and accurate dosage calculations. Understanding whole numbers, fractions, decimals, and percentages is crucial to pharmaceutical calculations. This knowledge is put to use in solving addition, subtraction, multiplication, and division problems on a basic algebra level. Many of the calculations will involve properly setting up and solving ratio and proportion equations. Knowing your multiplication tables *without* the use of a calculator is necessary for keeping up with the pace of work in a pharmacy. A calculator will be available, but most pharmacists will expect you to do simple calculations without one.

Practicing math skills without a calculator will increase your analytical math skills—skills that enable you to solve equations and take components of a whole to form relationships among its parts. Analysis of pharmacologic problems is an important step in ensuring accurate calculations with each medication order. *Always* ask yourself if your answer makes sense and check it.

The following is an assessment to help determine your strengths and weaknesses. It is also an indicator of your readiness to proceed through the text. Chapter 2 focuses on basic skills that you may need to review depending on your comfort level with this assessment. Proficiency in basic math skills is extremely important.

SELF-TEST OF BASIC MATH SKILLS

Directions

1. Figure decimals to three places, then **round** the answer to the hundredths place; for example, 1.454 would become 1.45 and 7.5685 would become 7.57.
2. Express fractions in their lowest possible terms; for example, $^4/_8$ should be reduced to $^1/_2$
3. Express ratios in their lowest possible terms; for example, 5:10 should be expressed as 1:2.
4. Do your work on paper, without a calculator, so that if you make an error, you can identify the mistake.

Basic Math Skills Proficiency Self-Test

1. Express the following sum in Arabic numerals: XXV + LX = __________
2. 156.90 + 368 = __________
3. 4.65 – 3.056 = __________
4. 3.50 × 43.5 = __________
5. \$12.56 + \$152.47 + \$4.98 + \$68.08 = __________
6. \$52.43 × 0.25 = __________
7. 0.7 ÷ 0.0035 = __________
8. 78 + 0.186 = __________
9. $\frac{3}{4} + 7\frac{7}{8} =$ __________
10. 25 – 13 = (express in Roman numerals) __________
11. \$15.43 × 25 = __________
12. 5,025 – 4,995 = (express in Roman numerals) __________
13. 1,932 ÷ 102 = __________
14. $\frac{1}{5} + \frac{4}{10} + \frac{3}{15} + \frac{5}{6} =$ __________
15. $\frac{5}{6} \div \frac{3}{8} =$ __________
16. $\frac{1}{200} \times 150 =$ __________
17. 6% of 36 = __________
18. Express 0.4 as a fraction. __________
19. Express 0.006 as a %. __________
20. 0.25% of 20 = __________
21. $1\frac{1}{3} + 3\frac{3}{4} =$ __________

22. $9\frac{1}{4} - 6\frac{3}{8} =$ ______

23. $1\frac{3}{8} \div \frac{1}{4} =$ ______

24. Which fraction has the greatest value? $\frac{1}{150}$, $\frac{1}{200}$, $\frac{1}{500}$ ______

25. Which decimal has the least value? 0.012, 0.12, 0.0125 ______

26. Change $\frac{3}{4}$ to a percentage. ______

27. Change $3\frac{1}{2}$ to a decimal. ______

28. $\frac{2.2}{4.4} \times 60 =$ ______

29. $\frac{12.75}{2.25} =$ ______

30. Which has the greatest value? 3.75, $3\frac{3}{4}$, $3\frac{7}{8}$ ______

31. One stock bottle of medication contains 20 tablets. How many tablets are in stock if the current inventory is $2\frac{1}{2}$ bottles? ______

32. A prescription is written for 150 tablets. How many 50-tablet containers will it take to fill the prescription? ______

33. A prescription is written for 3 capsules a day for 1 week. How many capsules are needed to fill the entire prescription? ______

34. 1 inch equals 2.54 cm. How many centimeters are in 10 inches? ______

35. Express 70:350 in its lowest terms. ______

36. Solve for x. $\frac{50}{25}x = 120$ ______

37. Solve for x. $\frac{1}{100} \times 350 = x$ ______

38. $7 \times -5 =$ ______

39. 1 g = 1,000 mg. How many milligrams are in 5.5 g? ______

40. 1 kg equals 2.2 lb. How many kg are in 88 lb? ______

41. There are 400 prescriptions to fill on one shift, and you have completed 25% of them. How many are left to fill? ______

42. 1 kg equals 2.2 lb. How many pounds are in 11 kg? ______

43. Express 4% as a ratio in its lowest term. ______

44. Solve for x. $\frac{25}{75} = \frac{x}{15}$ ______

45. A stock bottle of medicine contains 500 tablets. How many prescriptions of 25 tablets can be filled with that bottle of medication? ______

46. Subtract the following and express in Roman numerals.
    XIX – XIV = ______________

47. 3.6 ÷ 0.0005 = ______________

48. $4.28 + $5.65 + $0.78 + $15.39 = ______________

49. 195.46 – 35.86 = ______________

50. What is the least common multiple between 4, 6, and 8? ______________

Pharmaceutical calculations incorporate basic algebra skills that are easy to learn as long as one has a good understanding of basic math skills. Continue working on these basic skills in Chapter 2 if needed. Spending the time necessary to become comfortable with the basic skills and information in the first two chapters of the text will make progression through the following chapters much easier. It is exciting to see how these skills lead to an interesting career as a pharmacy technician!

Review of Basic Mathematical Skills

OBJECTIVES

1. Add, subtract, multiply, and divide whole numbers.
2. Add, subtract, multiply, and divide fractions, reduce fractions to the lowest terms, and discuss mixed numbers.
3. Add, subtract, multiply, and divide decimals, and round them to a specific place value.
4. Convert between fractions, decimals, and percentages.
5. Express numbers in ratio and proportion, and solve for unknowns.

KEY WORDS

Complex fractions Fractions in which the numerator, denominator, or both are fractional units

Convert Change from one form to another

Decimal Representation of a fraction where the denominator is a power of 10 and the numerator is a number placed to the right of a decimal point

Decimal place Place values found to the right of the decimal point

Denominator Bottom number of a fraction

Dividend Number being divided in division

Divisor Number by which another number is divided

Fraction Part of a whole number containing a numerator and denominator

Improper fraction Fraction in which the numerator is equal to or greater than the denominator; a fraction that is equal to or greater than 1

Invert To turn upside down or switch positions

Leading zero A zero placed before the decimal point in a number that is less than 1; necessary in pharmacy to reduce possible dosing errors

Least common denominator (LCD) The smallest whole number that can be divided evenly by all denominators of fractions within a problem; necessary for addition and subtraction of fractions; also known as least common multiple (LCM)

Lowest term Form of a fraction in which no common number will divide into both the numerator and denominator evenly

Mixed number Number containing a whole number and a fraction

Numerator Top number found in a fraction

Percent A means of expressing a portion of 100 parts

Product Number obtained by multiplying two numbers together

Proper fraction Fraction in which the numerator is less than the denominator; value is less than 1

Proportion Comparative relationship among the parts; one or more ratios that are compared

Quotient Answer to a division problem

Ratio A means of describing the relationship between two numbers; for example, 1:2

Remainder The amount left over after division

Round To express a number to its nearest place value such as ones, tenths, hundredths, etc.

Scored tablet Tablet containing an indentation for ease of breaking into equal parts

Trailing zero A zero in the farthest right place of a number following the decimal; not used in medication dosing due to the increased potential for errors

Whole number Numeral consisting of one or more digits; number that is not followed by a fraction or decimal

Pretest

Answer the following and show your work. Do not use a calculator. Round decimals to the nearest hundredth if necessary and reduce all fractions to the simplest form.

1. $154 + 1{,}063 + 25 + 376 =$ ____________
2. $163 - 69 =$ ____________
3. $256 \times 43 =$ ____________
4. $256 \div 16 =$ ____________
5. $25.6 + 456 + 35.67 =$ ____________
6. $354.29 - 45.390 =$ ____________
7. $12.56 \times 65.031 =$ ____________
8. $655.08 \div 1.2 =$ ____________
9. $\frac{1}{2} + \frac{3}{4} + \frac{7}{8} =$ ____________
10. $\frac{5}{8} - \frac{1}{6} =$ ____________
11. $\frac{1}{8} + \frac{5}{12} + \frac{5}{6} =$ ____________
12. $\frac{3}{5} \times \frac{7}{8} =$ ____________
13. $\frac{5}{8} \div \frac{1}{4} =$ ____________
14. $\frac{2}{3} \times \frac{14}{15} =$ ____________
15. $16 \times \frac{5}{8} =$ ____________
16. $36 \div \frac{4}{9} =$ ____________
17. $12\frac{1}{2} - 11\frac{5}{6} =$ ____________
18. $2\frac{3}{5} - 1\frac{1}{3} =$ ____________
19. $4\frac{1}{10} \times 2 =$ ____________
20. $\frac{2}{9} \times 3\frac{3}{5} \times \frac{5}{6} =$ ____________
21. $3 \div \frac{1}{4} =$ ____________

Pretest, cont.

Round the following decimals to the nearest hundredth.

22. 75.0023 ___________

23. 12.015 ___________

24. 6.12753 ___________

Change the following fractions to decimals.

25. $\frac{3}{5}$ ___________

26. $1\frac{3}{25}$ ___________

27. $1\frac{3}{4}$ ___________

28. $\frac{7}{20}$ ___________

Reduce to lowest terms.

29. $\frac{34}{68}$ ___________

30. $\frac{25}{75}$ ___________

31. $\frac{12}{96}$ ___________

Solve the following proportions.

32. $\frac{x}{3} = \frac{15}{30}$ $x =$ ___________

33. $\frac{5}{15} = \frac{8}{x}$ $x =$ ___________

34. $\frac{3}{x} = \frac{11}{33}$ $x =$ ___________

35. $\frac{1}{50} = \frac{x}{40}$ $x =$ ___________

Continued

Pretest, cont.

Write the following percents as fractions and simplify.

36. 44% ___________ **37.** 0.5% ___________

38. 125% ___________

Change the following percents to decimals.

39. 33% ___________ **40.** 0.04% ___________

41. 132% ___________

Solve the following.

42. A prescription calls for 15 mL of water to reconstitute a medication in a 20-mL vial. How many milliliters of water would be needed proportionally to reconstitute a 50-mL vial of the same medication?

43. A pharmacist is able to fill six prescriptions in 10 minutes with the assistance of a pharmacy technician. How many prescriptions can be completed in 1 hour?

44. A pharmacy offers a 10% discount for senior citizens. How much will a senior save off of a $25 prescription?

45. 85 is what percent of 200?

46. If 480 mL of medication is available in stock and a prescription calls for ¼ of this amount, how many milliliters of the medication are needed to fill the prescription?

47. A patient wants ½ of a prescription that costs $45. What is the cost to the patient?

Pretest, cont.

48. A customer buys front merchandise that costs $2.98, $5.36, $1.69, and $3.45. How much change should be given to the customer from a 20-dollar bill?

49. A patient is ordered to take three 75 mg tablets each morning. How many milligrams is this?

50. A patient is prescribed 16 oz of medication with instructions to use 1/16 of the bottle at bedtime every night. How many ounces should be taken each night?

INTRODUCTION

Accurate calculation of medication doses and dosages is extremely important for patient safety. The patient depends on your calculations and the pharmacist expects you to correctly make those calculations. Answers must be precise; partially correct answers are unacceptable and may endanger patient safety. Basic math skills are essential in pharmacy. Always look at your answer and ask, "Does it make sense?" Use estimation and your knowledge of normal medication doses to be sure your answer is within a normal range.

Review the following concepts and skills, paying close attention to the ones you have the most difficulty understanding. **Do not use a calculator** for this chapter so that you really learn the basic skills. Once you have performed the calculations, you can use a calculator to check your answers. These skills and concepts are the basis for pharmaceutical calculations.

WHOLE NUMBERS

A **whole number** is a numeral consisting of one or more digits that is not followed by a decimal or fraction. The digits used in math are 0, 1, 2, 3, 4, 5, 6, 7, 8, and 9. Numbers may also be written in words, such as one, two, ten, one hundred, one hundred thirty, and so on. Commas are recommended to be used on medication doses greater than 999, according to the Institute for Safe Medication Practices (ISMP) (see http://www.ismp.org/tools/guidelines/standardordersets.pdf). Therefore a dose of one thousand units of heparin should be written 1,000 units.

A whole number is always to the left of a decimal point. The numeral 0 is a whole number with the decimal understood to be at the right side of the zero. When adding, subtracting, or multiplying whole numbers, the answer will always be a whole number. This is not always the case when dividing whole numbers. Any number that remains when numbers are not exactly divisible is called a **remainder** and is expressed as a fraction or decimal. For example, 10 divided by 2 is 5, but 11 divided by 3 is $3\frac{2}{3}$ or $3.\overline{6}$; 11 and 3 are whole numbers, but they are not evenly divisible and the answer is expressed including a fraction or decimal.

Adding and Subtracting Whole Numbers

When adding or subtracting whole numbers, align the digits from the right and then add or subtract one set of digits at a time starting from the right (from ones to tens to hundreds, etc.).

Addition is finding a sum or total of numbers. Subtraction is finding the difference between two numbers.

EXAMPLE 2.1

$$\begin{array}{r} 25 \\ +\ 5 \\ \hline 30 \end{array} \qquad \begin{array}{r} 236 \\ -\ 24 \\ \hline 212 \end{array} \qquad \begin{array}{r} 1{,}302 \\ +\ 205 \\ \hline 1{,}507 \end{array} \qquad \begin{array}{r} 10{,}584 \\ -\ 10{,}263 \\ \hline 321 \end{array}$$

Practice Problems A

Add or subtract the following. Show your work. Include measurement units such as mg, g, and mL when needed.

1. 25 + 56 = __________
2. 105 + 235 = __________
3. 50 g + 100 g = __________
4. 25 mg + 90 mg = __________
5. 125,000 + 250,000 = __________
6. 7,500 mL + 1,000 mL = __________
7. 285 – 168 = __________
8. 1,549 – 1,374 = __________
9. 725 mL – 650 mL = __________
10. 525 g – 175 g = __________
11. 156# – 48# = __________
12. 350 mg – 125 mg = __________
13. 266 kg – 15 kg = __________
14. A bottle of antibiotic powder needs to be mixed with 100 mL of distilled water. You have a 50-mL graduated cylinder. How many times will you have to fill the graduated with water?
15. A vial of anesthetic contains 10 mL. The pharmacist asks that you add 30 mL of distilled water to prepare an anesthetic compound for mouth ulcers. How many milliliters will be in the bottle of prepared medication?

16. A bottle of cough medicine contains 120 mL. One dose is 5 mL. How much is left in the bottle after one dose?

17. A formula calls for 30 g of plain cream to be mixed with 15 g of a medicated cream. How much cream will be produced?

18. A customer buys 3 prescriptions costing $15, $10, and $5. Since there is no tax on these prescriptions, how much will you charge the customer?

19. If the customer from question 19 pays with a 50-dollar bill, what will you give him in change?

20. There are 600 tablets of a medication on the shelf. The reorder point is 350. How much can be dispensed before it needs to be reordered?

Multiplying Whole Numbers

When multiplying whole numbers, align the numbers or factors as you would for addition or subtraction. The use of "×" or "•" denotes that the numbers should be multiplied to find a **product**. Remember that a number multiplied by zero is zero.

First multiply the number on top of the problem by the number at the far right of the bottom of the equation. Place the ones digit of this answer under the line and carry the tens digit to the next place. Multiply the remaining numbers in the subsequent digits, moving from right to left, keeping the numbers in alignment. Move to the next number to the left in the bottom number and repeat the process. Remember that the second number is already in the tens place, so it must be placed one space to the left of the first answer. Sometimes it is helpful to place a zero in the ones place to keep the alignment (place holder shown in **bold** in the following examples). Finally, add the numbers that have been multiplied to obtain the product.

EXAMPLE 2.2

```
  125
  ×15
  625
+1250
1,875
```

EXAMPLE 2.3

```
   225
  × 10
   000
+ 2250
 2,250
```

Be sure to maintain the alignment!

Dividing Whole Numbers

Division is represented by either "÷" or "$\overline{)\ }$". The number being divided is called the **dividend**, and the number used to divide is the **divisor**. The result of division is the **quotient**.

$$\text{divisor}\overline{)\text{dividend}}^{\ \text{quotient}}$$

EXAMPLE 2.4

$$\begin{array}{r} 11 \\ 25\overline{)275} \\ -25 \\ \hline 25 \\ -25 \\ \hline 0 \end{array}$$

In this example, 25 cannot be divided into 2, so move to 27 to divide by 25. Be sure to place the 1 *directly above* the 7 and maintain the correct alignment.

General rules to remember with division:

Any number divided by itself equals 1: 7 ÷ 7 = 1
Any number divided by 1 equals that same number: 7 ÷ 1 = 7
Zero divided by any number remains zero: 0 ÷ 7 = 0
Zero can *never* be the divisor: 7 ÷ 0 is undefined

Practice Problems B

Multiply or divide the following. Show your work. Estimate first. Remember to include units for answers 14 and 15.

1. 56 × 10 = ___________

2. 76 • 11 = ___________

3. 100 × 87 = ___________

4. 3,500 × 265 = ___________

5. $\begin{array}{r} 653 \\ \times\ \ 30 \\ \hline \end{array}$ = ___________

6. $\begin{array}{r} 275 \\ \times\ 310 \\ \hline \end{array}$ = ___________

7. 105 ÷ 5 = ___________

8. 840 ÷ 40 = ___________

9. 296 ÷ 4 = ___________

10. 1125 ÷ 15 = ___________

11. 150 ÷ 15 = ___________

12. $15\overline{)600}$ = ___________

13. $12\overline{)276}$ = ___________

14. 150 mg × 4 = ___________

15. A prescription is written for ten 250 mg tablets. What is the weight of the medication in the total prescription?

16. The manufacturer's label states to add 375 mL of water to a medication for reconstitution. How many times do you need to fill a 125-mL graduated cylinder to reconstitute the medication?

17. The directions on a prescription read, "Take 1 capsule 3 times a day." How many mg will the patient take in one day if the capsules are 250 mg each?

18. A medication order reads, "Give 8 mg daily in 4 divided doses." How many mg should be given per dose?

19. The directions for mixing an antibiotic powder with water read, "Add 80 mL of water in two equal portions. Shake between each addition." How much water should be added each time?

20. A customer picks up 3 prescriptions, each with a cost of $15. How much should she be charged?

FRACTIONS

When a whole number or unit is divided into parts, the parts are called **fractions**. Fractions may be expressed in the form a/b or $\frac{a}{b}$, with the latter being preferred with pharmaceutical calculations for ease of keeping track of units and reducing numbers. The "*a*" is called the **numerator** (top number found in a fraction). The "*b*" is the **denominator** (bottom number of a fraction). Both numbers must be whole numbers, and the denominator can never be 0, as in $\frac{a}{0}$, which is undefined. The denominator tells how many times the whole unit has been divided.

The circle graph pictured shows a proper fraction. The shaded area shows the part of a whole. There are 3 (numerator) parts out of 4 (denominator) shaded, or ¾.

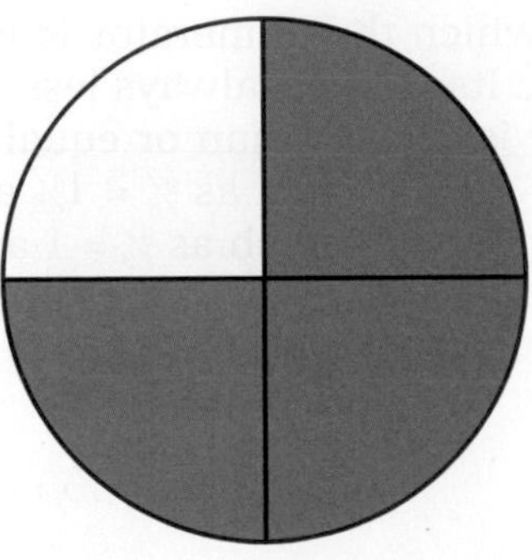

In the next picture, the numerator is 5 and the denominator is 6.

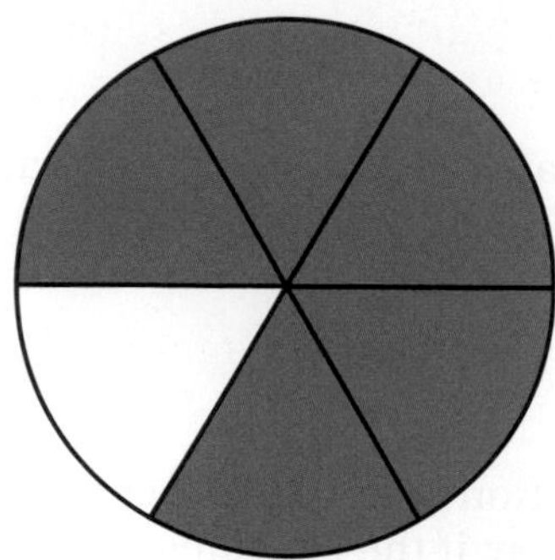

TECH NOTE

Fractions are used in pharmacy in both the household and apothecary systems, but not with the metric system.

Practice Problems C

In the following examples, indicate the numerator and the denominator.

1. $\frac{5}{7}$ Numerator ________ Denominator ________

2. $\frac{8}{11}$ Numerator ________ Denominator ________

3. $\frac{7}{15}$ Numerator ________ Denominator ________

4. $\frac{135}{356}$ Numerator ________ Denominator ________

5. $\frac{5}{6}$ Numerator ________ Denominator ________

TECH NOTE

Whole numbers are actually fractions in which the numerator is an exact multiple of the denominator. For instance the whole number 7 can be written $\frac{7}{1}, \frac{14}{2}, \frac{21}{3}$, etc.

A **proper fraction** is one in which the numerator is less than the denominator and is part of a whole, such as $\frac{2}{3}$ and $\frac{5}{8}$. Its value is always less than 1. An **improper fraction** is a fraction in which the numerator is greater than or equal to the denominator, making the fraction equivalent to or greater than 1, such as $\frac{9}{8} = 1\frac{1}{8}$ and $\frac{14}{7} = 2$. If the numerator and denominator are the same, the value is 1, such as $\frac{9}{9} = 1$ and $\frac{10}{10} = 1$.

An improper fraction can be changed into a **mixed number** (a whole number and a fraction). Because a fraction indicates division, the numerator divided by the denominator, when $\frac{a}{b}$ or $^{a}/_{b}$ is written, the fraction actually means a ÷ b. To **convert** or change an improper fraction to a mixed number, divide the numerator by the denominator. Any remainder is written over the denominator.

EXAMPLE 2.5

Convert the improper fraction $\frac{43}{8}$ to a mixed number.

$43 \div 8 = 5$ with a remainder of 3

$\frac{43}{8}$ as a mixed number is $5\frac{3}{8}$.

The remainder is the amount that is left over after the whole number has been divided into the numerator the maximum number of times.

To change a mixed number to an improper fraction, multiply the whole number by the denominator and add the amount found in the numerator.

EXAMPLE 2.6

Convert $4\frac{1}{8}$ to an improper fraction.

$4 \cdot 8 = 32$

Add the 1 found in the numerator of the fraction: 32 + 1 = 33

The denominator remains the same, so the improper fraction is $\frac{33}{8}$

Practice Problems D

Show your work. Indicate measurements as appropriate.

Convert the following improper fractions to mixed numbers or whole numbers.

1. $\frac{16}{3} =$ ____________
2. $\frac{24}{7} =$ ____________
3. $\frac{35}{4} =$ ____________
4. $\frac{223}{110} =$ ____________
5. $\frac{16}{15} =$ ____________
6. $\frac{21}{7} =$ ____________
7. gr $\frac{5}{4} =$ ____________
8. $\frac{9}{8}$ c = ____________

9. $\frac{3}{2}$ tab = ____________

10. $\frac{6}{6}$ tab = ____________

Convert the following mixed numbers to improper fractions.

11. $3\frac{1}{2}$ = ____________

12. $2\frac{7}{8}$ = ____________

13. $3\frac{1}{4}$ = ____________

14. $10\frac{9}{10}$ = ____________

15. $4\frac{5}{7}$ = ____________

16. $2\frac{1}{2}$ c = ____________

17. $6\frac{3}{4}$ qt = ____________

18. $4\frac{1}{2}$ tab = ____________

19. $3\frac{1}{3}$ c = ____________

20. $5\frac{1}{4}$ c = ____________

Indicate the fraction or mixed number for the following shaded areas.

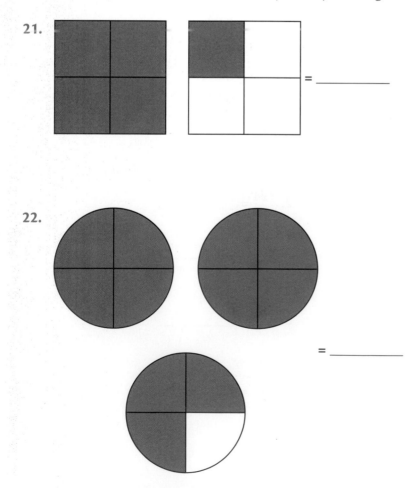

21.

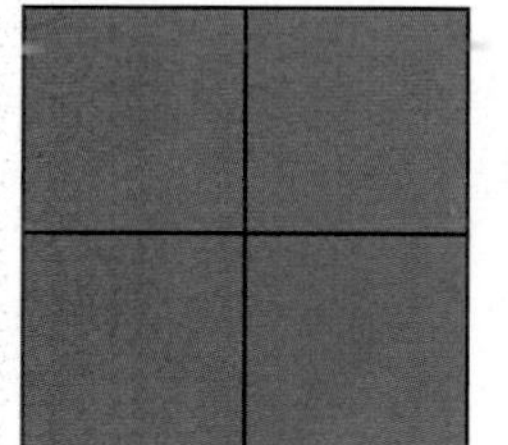

= ____________

22.

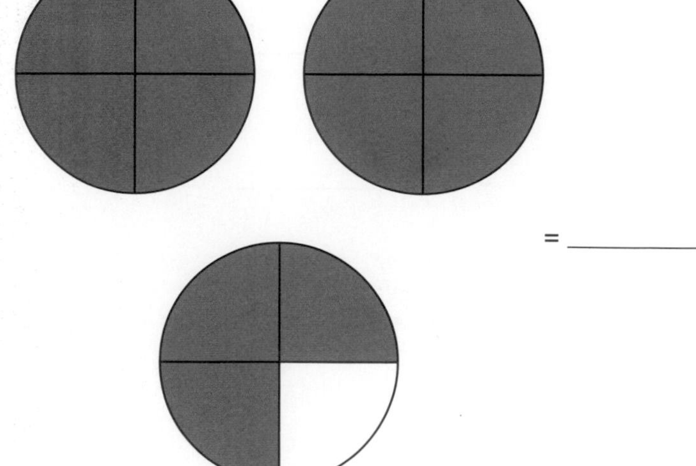

= ____________

23. A pharmacist has a medicine dropper that is divided into eight equal sections. She fills to the line to indicate five parts. What is the fractional amount that the pharmacist has filled?

24. A customer asks you to show him how to divide a tablet (i.e., a **scored tablet** that is divided into four equal parts) into one-half of a tablet. Fill in the following tablet to indicate this fraction.

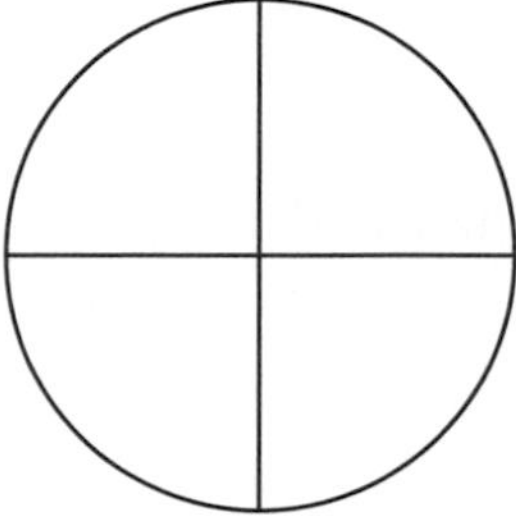

25. The pharmacy employees decide to share a pizza for dinner. It is sliced into 4 pieces. What is the fractional representation of the pizza before anyone takes a slice?

Reducing Fractions to the Lowest Term

Some fractions, called equivalent fractions, have the same value. The fraction $\frac{1}{2}$ is equivalent to $\frac{2}{4}$, $\frac{3}{6}$, or $\frac{50}{100}$. With $\frac{2}{4}$, the numerator and denominator can both be divided by 2 to give $\frac{1}{2}$; with $\frac{3}{6}$, both parts of the fraction can be divided by 3 to give $\frac{1}{2}$; with $\frac{50}{100}$, both components of the fraction can be divided by 50 to give $\frac{1}{2}$. Each of these fractions is actually one-half of the total number of equivalent parts of a whole.

When reducing fractions, the *numerator and the denominator* must be divided by the *same* nonzero number. For example, $\frac{3}{12}$ can be reduced to $\frac{1}{4}$ by dividing the numerator and denominator by 3. Dividing by $\frac{3}{3}$ is the same as dividing by 1, so it does not change the *value* of the fraction. A fraction is reduced to the **lowest term** when no common number will divide into both the numerator and denominator evenly.

Practice Problems E

Reduce the following fractions to the lowest terms. Show your calculations and indicate measurements as appropriate.

1. $\frac{3}{6} =$ ____________
2. $\frac{6}{9} =$ ____________
3. $\frac{8}{12} =$ ____________
4. $\frac{25}{125} =$ ____________

5. $\frac{7}{35}$ = ____________ 6. $\frac{27}{108}$ = ____________

7. $\frac{6}{48}$ = ____________ 8. $\frac{125}{750}$ = ____________

9. A pharmacist has a bottle of medication that contains 90 tablets. He dispenses 45 tablets. What is the fractional use?

10. A medication states to add the first 40 mL out of 60 mL of water and shake. What fraction of the water is added first?

Adding and Subtracting Fractions

When adding or subtracting fractions, the denominators must be the same. Once the denominators are the same number, the numerators may be either added or subtracted. The denominator remains the same.

EXAMPLE 2.7

$$\frac{3}{5}+\frac{1}{5}=\frac{4}{5}$$

EXAMPLE 2.8

$$\frac{3}{5}-\frac{1}{5}=\frac{2}{5}$$

Finding Common Denominators

If the denominators are not the same, the smallest whole number that can be divided evenly by both denominators within the problem is needed: the **least common denominator** (LCD). Sometimes the LCD is easily found because one denominator can be divided by the other. Since 15 is divisible by 5, it is a common denominator for $\frac{3}{5} + \frac{2}{15}$.

To change fractions to their equivalent fractions for adding or subtracting, first find the lowest common denominator. Then multiply the numerator and denominator of each fraction by the fraction *equaling 1* that will make the denominators equal to the LCD. Then add or subtract the fractions by adding or subtracting the numerators and leaving the denominator the same.

EXAMPLE 2.9

$$\frac{3}{10}-\frac{2}{15}$$

The smallest number that both 10 and 15 can divide into equally is 30—the LCD. 10 times 3 equals 30, so multiply the first fraction by $\frac{3}{3}$.

$$\frac{3}{10}\times\frac{3}{3}=\frac{9}{30}$$

15 times 2 equals 30, so multiply the second fraction by $\frac{2}{2}$.

$$\frac{2}{15} \times \frac{2}{2} = \frac{4}{30}$$

Remember that both $\frac{3}{3}$ and $\frac{2}{2}$ equal 1, so the *values* of the fractions are unchanged. Rewrite the equation and solve:

$$\frac{9}{30} - \frac{4}{30} = \frac{5}{30}$$

Reduce the answer by dividing the numerator and denominator by 5:

$$\frac{5}{30} \div \frac{5}{5} = \frac{1}{6}$$

$\frac{5}{5}$ equals 1, so the *value* of the answer is unchanged.

If a mixed number is in the expression, the mixed number should be converted to an improper fraction before finding the common denominator. Then convert both fractions to the LCD and add or subtract as indicated.

EXAMPLE 2.10

$$\frac{3}{4} \div 3\frac{5}{8}$$

3 times 8 is 24 plus 5 equals 29.

$$3\frac{5}{8} = \frac{29}{8}$$

Because 4 times 2 is 8, multiply the numerator and denominator of the first fraction by $\frac{2}{2}$:

$$\frac{3}{4} \times \frac{2}{2} = \frac{6}{8}$$

The problem becomes:

$$\frac{6}{8} + \frac{29}{8} = \frac{35}{8}$$

35 divided by 8 equals 4 with a remainder of 3, so the answer is $4\frac{3}{8}$.

If the LCD is not readily apparent, multiply the denominators and use that number as the common denominator (e.g., if the denominators are 5 and 7, one common denominator will always be 35 because 5 × 7 = 35). This method may not provide the LCD, but it can be used. It may require further reducing of the answer.

Practice Problems F

Add or subtract the following. Reduce to lowest terms. Show your calculations. Indicate measurements as appropriate.

1. $\frac{1}{3} + \frac{1}{3} =$ ____________

2. $\frac{3}{8} + \frac{4}{8} =$ ____________

3. $\frac{2}{7} + \frac{3}{7} =$ ____________

4. $\frac{5}{8} - \frac{1}{8} =$ ____________

5. $\frac{8}{9} - \frac{5}{9} =$ ____________

6. $\frac{13}{15} - \frac{10}{15} =$ ____________

7. $\frac{3}{8}c + \frac{2}{8}c =$ ____________

8. $\frac{5}{6}c - \frac{1}{6}c =$ ____________

9. $1\frac{1}{3} + \frac{4}{9} =$ ____________

10. $3\frac{2}{3} + 1\frac{3}{5} =$ ____________

11. $1\frac{3}{16} + 2\frac{3}{8} =$ ____________

12. $\frac{4}{7} + \frac{3}{11} =$ ____________

13. $\frac{5}{12} + \frac{3}{4} =$ ____________

14. $\frac{2}{3}c + \frac{1}{6}c =$ ____________

15. $\frac{1}{3}$ tsp + $\frac{1}{6}$ tsp = ____________

16. $2\frac{1}{2}$ qt + $\frac{1}{4}$ qt = ____________

17. $\frac{1}{8}$ qt + $\frac{3}{4}$ qt = ____________

18. $3\frac{1}{4} - 2\frac{1}{4} =$ ____________

19. $4\frac{1}{5} - 2\frac{9}{10} =$ ____________

20. $1\frac{7}{8}c - 1\frac{3}{16}c =$ ____________

21. $2\frac{3}{8}$ tsp − $1\frac{1}{6}$ tsp = ____________

22. $4\frac{3}{4}$ qt − $\frac{1}{16}$ qt = ____________

23. $3\frac{5}{16}$# − $1\frac{3}{8}$# = ____________

24. A bottle of medication granules contains $12\frac{1}{2}$ oz of the desired medication. A newer medication container holds $11\frac{15}{16}$ oz of the medication. What is the difference in the amount of medication in the two bottles?

25. You have $3\frac{3}{4}$ oz of a specific medication. In 1 day, you have used $2\frac{3}{16}$ oz of that medication. How much medication will you have left for use to fill prescriptions the next day?

Multiplying Fractions

To find the product of fractions, multiply the numerators *and* the denominators. The product should then be reduced to the lowest term. Multiplication of fractions *does not* require a common denominator.

EXAMPLE 2.11

$$\frac{5}{6} \bullet \frac{3}{5} = \frac{15}{30}$$

Both the numerator and denominator are divisible by 15, so divide the answer by $^{15}/_{15}$ to get $^{1}/_{2}$.

With multiplication of fractions, any number from either numerator can be reduced with any number in either denominator before multiplying, if possible. The previous example can be viewed as if the line extends over both fractions: $\frac{5 \bullet 3}{6 \bullet 5}$.

The 5 in the numerator of the first fraction could be reduced with the 5 in the denominator of the second fraction, both to 1. The 3 could also have been reduced to 1 and the 6 to 2 before doing any multiplying: $\frac{1 \bullet 1}{2 \bullet 1} = \frac{1}{2}$.

TECH NOTE

To multiply (or divide) mixed numbers, change the mixed number to an improper fraction first.

Dividing Fractions

Dividing fractions involves **inverting** the divisor (the *second* number in the expression, which is the number to the right of the division sign) so that the numerator becomes the denominator and the denominator becomes the numerator. In simpler terms, the numbers switch places. For example, if $^{4}/_{5}$ is inverted, the fraction would become $^{5}/_{4}$. This is also often called "taking the reciprocal" of the divisor. After inverting the numerator and denominator of the fraction to the *right* of the division sign, continue with the steps as for multiplication—multiply the numerators and multiply the denominators, placing the products with the numerators over the denominators. Finally, reduce the resultant fraction to the lowest possible terms.

EXAMPLE 2.12

$\frac{4}{5} \div \frac{5}{10}$ $\frac{5}{10}$ is the fraction to be inverted, so the problem becomes $\frac{4}{5} \bullet \frac{10}{5} = \frac{40}{25}$.

40 divided by 25 equals 1 with 15 left over, so the answer is changed to $1\frac{15}{25}$.

The fraction can be reduced by dividing the numerator and denominator by 5 for the quotient $1\frac{3}{5}$.

As with the previous example, once the multiplication problem has been set up, numbers may be reduced before multiplying. The 5 in the first fraction can be reduced with the 10 in the second fraction, resulting in $\frac{4}{1} \bullet \frac{2}{5} = \frac{8}{5}$. This can be converted to $1\frac{3}{5}$.

TECH NOTE

When dividing fractions, invert the fraction to the **right** of the division sign and multiply.

Practice Problems G

Perform the multiplication or division and then reduce the fractions to the lowest terms. Show calculations and indicate measurements as appropriate.

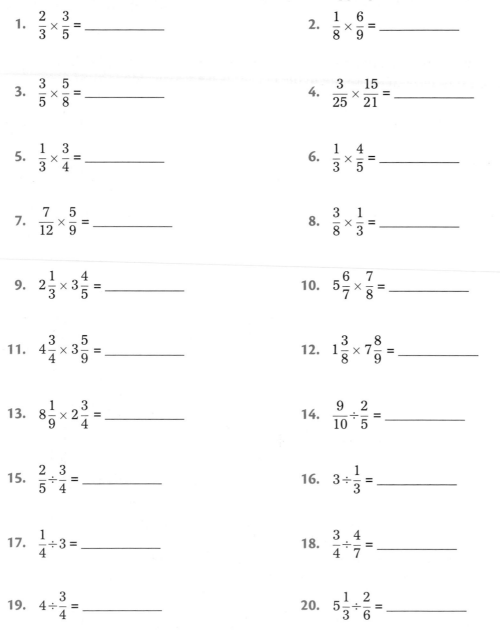

1. $\frac{2}{3} \times \frac{3}{5} =$ ____________

2. $\frac{1}{8} \times \frac{6}{9} =$ ____________

3. $\frac{3}{5} \times \frac{5}{8} =$ ____________

4. $\frac{3}{25} \times \frac{15}{21} =$ ____________

5. $\frac{1}{3} \times \frac{3}{4} =$ ____________

6. $\frac{1}{3} \times \frac{4}{5} =$ ____________

7. $\frac{7}{12} \times \frac{5}{9} =$ ____________

8. $\frac{3}{8} \times \frac{1}{3} =$ ____________

9. $2\frac{1}{3} \times 3\frac{4}{5} =$ ____________

10. $5\frac{6}{7} \times \frac{7}{8} =$ ____________

11. $4\frac{3}{4} \times 3\frac{5}{9} =$ ____________

12. $1\frac{3}{8} \times 7\frac{8}{9} =$ ____________

13. $8\frac{1}{9} \times 2\frac{3}{4} =$ ____________

14. $\frac{9}{10} \div \frac{2}{5} =$ ____________

15. $\frac{2}{5} \div \frac{3}{4} =$ ____________

16. $3 \div \frac{1}{3} =$ ____________

17. $\frac{1}{4} \div 3 =$ ____________

18. $\frac{3}{4} \div \frac{4}{7} =$ ____________

19. $4 \div \frac{3}{4} =$ ____________

20. $5\frac{1}{3} \div \frac{2}{6} =$ ____________

21. $4\frac{1}{3} \div 2\frac{2}{25} =$ __________

22. $7\frac{2}{3} \div 2\frac{2}{5} =$ __________

23. $4\frac{3}{4} \div 3\frac{1}{6} =$ __________

24. Your stock bottle of medication contains 500 tablets. You have used ¾ of the bottle. How many tablets do you have left in stock for filling future prescriptions?

25. A bottle of liquid antibiotic contains 150 mL of medication, or 30 teaspoons. If each dose is 1½ tsp, how many doses are in the bottle? If the medication is given four times a day, how many days will it last?

Complex Fractions

Complex fractions are fractional expressions in which the numerator, denominator, or both are expressed as fractions or decimals. This will be covered again in later chapters. Solving these fractions can be approached in a couple of different ways.

EXAMPLE 2.13

$\frac{1/4}{1/2}$ can be multiplied by $\frac{4}{4}$ to convert it to $\frac{1}{2}$.

$\frac{1/4}{1/2}$ can be written $\frac{1}{4} \div \frac{1}{2}$ and then inverted and multiplied: $\frac{1}{4} \times \frac{2}{1} = \frac{2}{4} = \frac{1}{2}$.

$\frac{0.4}{60}$ can be multiplied by $\frac{10}{10}$ to form the fraction $\frac{4}{600}$, which reduces to $\frac{1}{150}$.

$\frac{0.4}{60}$ can be written $\frac{4}{10} \div \frac{60}{1}$ and then inverted and multiplied: $\frac{4}{10} \times \frac{1}{60} = \frac{4}{600} = \frac{1}{150}$.

DECIMALS

Decimals are actually fractions with a denominator of 10, 100, 1,000, or any multiple of 10. Decimal numbers may include a whole number, a decimal point, and the decimal fraction. The metric system, the most frequently used measurement system in the medical field, uses decimals. Examples of decimals include 0.1 = $\frac{1}{10}$, 0.01 = $\frac{1}{100}$, or 0.001 = $\frac{1}{1,000}$.

To avoid errors in the medical field, a decimal less than 1 should always be written with a **leading zero**, a zero in front of the decimal point. For example, the decimal .25 should be written as 0.25, and .5 as 0.5. A medical professional should never write ".25" or ".5" because the decimal could be overlooked, leading to an overdose, which could be fatal.

To write decimals using word names, the number to the left will be a whole number and the decimal point becomes the word "and," with the number to the right of the **decimal place** followed by the place values of the decimal ending with "th."

Decimal Line

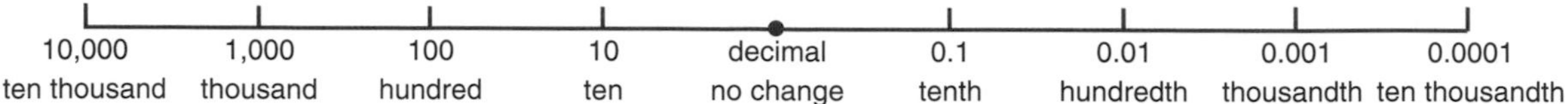

3.07 is three and seven hundredths.

Three	The number to the left of the decimal point
And	The decimal point
Seven	The number to the right of the decimal point
Hundredths	The place value of the decimal

AND

1.250 is one and two hundred fifty thousandths.

One	The number to the left of the decimal point
And	The decimal point
Two hundred fifty	The number to the right of the decimal point
Thousandths	The place value of the decimal

Zeros at the end of a decimal, **trailing zeros**, do not change the *value* of the number. Trailing zeros are on The Joint Commission's "Do Not Use" list and will *not* be used in pharmaceutical calculations because of possible interpretation errors.

1.250 has the same value as 1.25, so it can also be read as one and twenty-five hundredths.

Practice Problems H

Write the following decimal numbers in words.

1. 4.34 ______________________
2. 3.5 ______________________
3. 6.751 ______________________
4. 90.54 ______________________
5. 954.6 ______________________
6. 0.0035 ______________________
7. 4.02 ______________________
8. 0.26 ______________________

9. 0.78 ______

10. 0.175 ______

Comparing Decimals

To compare a decimal, the decimal amounts must be aligned at the decimal point and zeros should be added so that the numbers following the decimal point contain the same number of decimal places. This is important in the comparison of medications in the metric system of measurement.

EXAMPLE 2.14

Compare 0.125, 0.25, and 0.5.

0.125 may appear to be the largest number, but when the numbers are aligned and the proper zeros are added for numbers to have equal decimal places to the right of the decimal point, this proves to be incorrect.

0.125	One-hundred twenty-five thousandths
0.250	Two-hundred fifty thousandths
0.500	Five-hundred thousandths

Adding or removing trailing zeros does not change the value, but it makes the numbers easier to compare. The largest number is really 0.5 and not 0.125, which might not seem apparent without the added zeros. Note that the decimals are less than 1, so a leading zero was added to ensure that the decimal point was not overlooked.

Rounding Decimals

When calculating doses of medication, decimals may need to be rounded to a specific place value. Accuracy in calculating to a particular decimal place is necessary in some circumstances, whereas **rounding** or approximating is acceptable in others. For example, if 18 units of subcutaneous insulin U-100 are ordered, the volume given must be 0.18 mL. It cannot be rounded to 0.2 mL. If an oral medication dose is calculated to be 3.99 mg and a 4 mg tablet is available, the patient would receive one tablet by rounding to the whole number 4.

TECH NOTE

Determining the appropriate place value when rounding medication doses depends on the potency, the amount, and the route of administration.

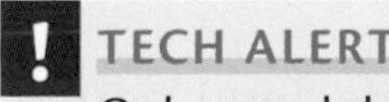

TECH ALERT

Only round the **final** answer when performing multiple step calculations.

Steps for Rounding

Step 1: Underline the digit in the place for rounding.
Step 2: Look at the digit to the right of the underlined digit:
If it is greater than or equal to 5, round the underlined digit to the next highest number and drop all digits to the right.
If it is less than 5, drop all digits to the right of the underlined digit and keep it the same.

EXAMPLE 2.15

Round 1.16 to the tenths place.

1.16: The 6 indicates that the number to its left should be rounded up to 1.2.

Round 1.14 to the tenths place.

1.14: The 4 indicates that the number to its left is to stay the same, or 1.1.

Practice Problems I

Round to the nearest hundredth.

1. 2.356 = ________
2. 5.652 = ________
3. 36.445 = ________
4. 2.984 = ________
5. 0.1245 = ________
6. 8.2374 = ________
7. 6.116 g = ________

Round to the nearest tenth.

8. 3.45 = ________
9. 3.64 = ________
10. 3.26 = ________
11. 12.14 = ________
12. 3.05 = ________
13. 12.49 mg = ________
14. 1.46 mg = ________
15. 2.54 mL = ________

Round to the nearest whole number.

16. 9.64 = ________
17. 10.08 = ________
18. 14.16 = ________
19. 125.3 mg = ________
20. 275.1 mL = ________

Estimating answers to addition, subtraction, multiplication, and division problems involving decimals can be done by rounding to whole numbers to get an approximate answer. This is a good way to check that the decimal is in the correct position in your final answer. For example, the problem 10.3578 divided by 2.15 can be estimated to be around 5 by dividing 10 by 2. Therefore if your final answer is near 0.5 or 50, you know that you have misplaced the decimal.

Adding and Subtracting Decimals

Adding and subtracting decimals requires aligning whole numbers and decimal points. After aligning the decimal points, add zeros at the end of the decimal fraction until all decimal numbers are to the same decimal place. Then just add or subtract as you would for whole numbers, remembering to correctly place the decimal point in the answer.

EXAMPLE 2.16

3.4678 − 2.34

$$\begin{array}{r} 3.4678 \\ -\,2.3400 \\ \hline 1.1278 \end{array}$$

Practice Problems J

Add or subtract as indicated. Show your work. Round final answers to the nearest hundredth and indicate measurements as appropriate.

1. 2.35 + 3.1 + 4.678 = __________

2. 5.7 + 18.25 + 95.37 = __________

3. 2.38 + 14.7 + 1,346 = __________

4. 6.002 + 3.23 + 9.1 = __________

5. 12.5 mg + 6.25 mg = __________

6. $12.50 + $0.42 + $140.67 = __________

7. $5.67 + $136.99 + $89.09 = __________

8. 2.76 – 1.98 = __________

9. 4.8 – 1.987 = __________

10. 75.3 – 16.95 = __________

11. 125 – 0.125 = __________

12. $15.75 – $5.65 = __________

13. $17.49 – $5.05 = __________

14. 0.2 g – 0.02 g = __________

15. 12.5 mg – 10.5 mg = __________

16. A prescription costs $25.50. The customer gives you two $20 bills. How much change do you owe the customer?

17. A stock bottle of medication contains 500 mg of drug used in compounding other medications. You used 125 mg for one prescription, 62.5 mg for a second prescription, and 25.25 mg for the third.

    What quantity of medication was used?

    What quantity of the original medication is left?

18. A customer has three prescriptions—one costing $35, the second costing $17.50, and the third costing $23.60.

What is the total cost of the prescriptions?

If the customer gives you four 20-dollar bills, how much should you return?

19. A patient is given two tablets per dose. One tablet is 2.5 mg and the other is 1.25 mg. What is the total dose?

20. A patient is taking 25 mg of medication per dose. The physician instructs him to reduce the dose by 12.5 mg. How much should the patient take per dose?

Multiplying Decimals

Multiplying decimals is similar to multiplying whole numbers. The alignment of the numbers is identical, without regard to the placement of the decimal. The difference is the proper placement of the decimal *after* the product has been calculated. After the product is calculated, count the number of places to the right of the decimal points in both of the numbers that were multiplied. Finally, place a decimal point in the product by counting from right to left the number of decimal places found in both elements of the problem.

EXAMPLE 2.17

37.25	(two decimal places)
$\times$ 1.5	(one decimal place)
18,625	(this is the product of 5 $\times$ 3,725)
+ 37,250	(this is the product of 10 $\times$ 3,725)
55,875	(count in three decimal places from the right)
55.875	Round to the nearest hundredth for 55.88 or tenth for 55.9

Because trailing zeros may be removed from a decimal number without changing the value, remove them and then multiply. This simplifies the multiplication. For example, if multiplying 7.350 × 0.20, drop the zeros at the ends so that the problem is 7.35 × 0.2 for an answer of 1.470. The trailing zero in the answer can then be dropped to give the final answer of 1.47.

If a number is multiplied by 10 or a multiple of 10, a shortcut in multiplying is to move the decimal of the number as many places to the right as there are zeros in the multiplier. With 12.2 × 10, move the decimal point one space to the *right* for the answer of 122. If the multiplier is 100, the decimal would be moved two places for the answer of 1,220; if the multiplier is 1,000, the decimal would be moved three places for the answer of 12,200; and so on.

Practice Problems K

Multiply the following. Show your work. Drop trailing zeros, round final answers to hundredths if necessary, and indicate measurements as needed.

1. 65.3 × 10 = ___________
2. 13.2 × 100 = ___________
3. 4.25 × 10 = ___________
4. 0.004 × 100 = ___________
5. 0.2 × 1000 = ___________
6. 16.5 × 0.5 = ___________
7. 23.52 × 0.5 = ___________
8. 0.35 × 0.45 = ___________
9. 45.3 × 2.1 = ___________
10. 101.3 × 6.3 = ___________
11. 0.75 mg × 3 = ___________
12. 64.8 mg × 2.5 = ___________
13. 12.5 mg × 4 = ___________
14. 1.25 mg × 6 = ___________
15. 2.5 mg × 2 = ___________
16. 250 mg × 3 = ___________
17. 500 mg × 4 = ___________
18. A physician orders 2.5 mg of medication taken daily for 10 days. What is the total amount of the medication the patient will take?
19. A mother gives her child 2.5 mL of an antipyretic *every 4 hours* for fever. How many milliliters of medication will the child receive in 1 day?
20. One bottle of medication contains 12.25 mg. Five bottles of the medication are in stock. How many total milligrams of medication are available for dispensing?

Dividing Decimals

Dividing decimals is much like dividing whole numbers. Write the problem as for long division. If a decimal appears in the divisor, move the decimal to the right until the divisor is a whole number. Then move the decimal point in the dividend the same number of places to the right.

EXAMPLE 2.18

Divide 2.5 by 1.25.

Add a terminal zero to 2.5, then move the decimal two places to the right on *both* terms.

$1.25\overline{)2.50}$

$125\overline{)250}$

Place a decimal point on the quotient (answer) line directly above the decimal point in the dividend and divide as usual. The answer is 2.

EXAMPLE 2.19

$1 \div 5$

$5\overline{)1}$

$5\overline{)1.0}$

By placing the decimal point directly above the decimal point in the dividend and then dividing, the answer is 0.2.

Remember, in medicine, if the decimal number is less than 1, a zero *must* be added in front of the decimal point to decrease the likelihood of medication errors.

EXAMPLE 2.20

$40.44 \div 0.4$

$0.4\overline{)40.44}$

Move the decimal in the divisor and the dividend one place to the right to make the divisor a whole number.

$4\overline{)404.4}$ The answer is 101.1.

In some cases division does not come out evenly, such as when 3 is divided into 1. The answer is $0.333\overline{3}$ to the number of places that zeros are added to the dividend. In these cases, the number may be shown as $0.\overline{3}$, with the line indicating that 3 is a repeating number.

If the divisor is 10 or a multiple of 10, a shortcut in dividing is to move the decimal as many places to the *left* as there are zeros in the divisor. With 122 ÷ 10, move the decimal point one space to the left to the answer of 12.2. If the divisor is 100, the decimal would be moved two places; 1,000, three places; and so on.

Practice Problems L

Divide the following. Show your work. Add a leading zero and round final answers to hundredths if necessary, and indicate measurements as appropriate.

1. 268.4 ÷ 4 = __________
2. 125 ÷ 0.25 = __________
3. 1.5 ÷ 0.3 = __________
4. 19.95 ÷ 10.5 = __________
5. 33.03 ÷ 0.03 = __________
6. 25.2 ÷ 100 = __________
7. 1,864.5 ÷ 6 = __________
8. 40.08 ÷ 3 = __________
9. 3.6 ÷ 0.3 = __________
10. 35.4 ÷ 10 = __________
11. 37.5 ÷ 3 = __________
12. 162 ÷ 64.8 = __________
13. 225.4 mg ÷ 4 = __________
14. 2.5 g ÷ 2 = __________
15. $124.80 ÷ 4 = __________
16. 1.25 g ÷ 5 = __________
17. 844.8 mg ÷ 4 = __________
18. 2,025 mL ÷ 100 = __________
19. A pharmacist needs to divide 1 mL of medication into five equal parts. How many milliliters will be in each?
20. A customer comes to the pharmacy to purchase an expensive medication, which costs $255.30 for a 90-day supply. She asks to purchase it as three separate prescriptions of 30 days each. How much will she pay for each prescription?

Converting Decimals to Fractions

A decimal point separates the whole number that appears to the left and the decimal fraction that is found on the right. To convert a decimal to a fraction, the numerator is the number following the decimal point and the denominator is a power of 10 dependent on the number of digits following the decimal. For example, 3.7 is $3\frac{7}{10}$. The 7 is placed over 10 because there is one place value after the decimal in 3.7. The decimal 0.71 would be $\frac{71}{100}$ because there are two place values after the decimal.

Whereas trailing zeros do not need to be counted as place values, zeros following the decimal point and zeros *between* two whole numbers of a decimal fraction must be counted as place values. For example, 0.05 has two place values, so the fractional equivalent is 5/100, and 0.505 has three place values, so the fractional equivalent is 505/1,000.

TECH NOTE

Decimals are used in medication calculations in the metric system and calculations of dollars and cents in business math. $1.25 actually means one dollar and twenty-five hundredths of a dollar, $10.50 is 10 dollars and fifty hundredths of a dollar, and so on.

Practice Problems M

Change the following decimals to fractions. Do not reduce 1 through 5. Reduce 6 through 10 to lowest terms.

1. 0.125 = ______
2. 0.55 = ______
3. 0.33 = ______
4. 0.525 = ______
5. 0.625 = ______
6. 0.05 = ______ ______
7. 0.150 = ______ ______
8. 0.95 = ______ ______
9. 0.1244 = ______ ______
10. 0.042 = ______ ______

Converting Fractions to Decimals

To convert fractions to decimals, divide the numerator by the denominator.

EXAMPLE 2.21

$\frac{1}{2}$ is 1 ÷ 2, which becomes 1.0 ÷ 2 because 2 cannot divide into 1, giving the answer of 0.5.

$\frac{3}{4}$ is 3 ÷ 4, which becomes 3.0 ÷ 4, giving the decimal answer of 0.75.

TECH NOTE

When converting a mixed number to a decimal, the whole number will stay the same and the fractional portion is added after the decimal point once it is converted to a decimal. For example, $1\frac{1}{2} = 1.5$.

Practice Problems N

Convert the following fractions to decimals. Round to the nearest hundredth if necessary.

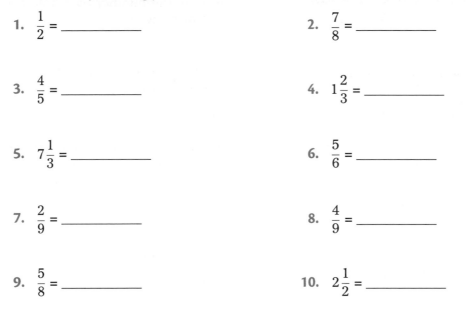

1. $\frac{1}{2}$ = __________
2. $\frac{7}{8}$ = __________
3. $\frac{4}{5}$ = __________
4. $1\frac{2}{3}$ = __________
5. $7\frac{1}{3}$ = __________
6. $\frac{5}{6}$ = __________
7. $\frac{2}{9}$ = __________
8. $\frac{4}{9}$ = __________
9. $\frac{5}{8}$ = __________
10. $2\frac{1}{2}$ = __________

POINTS TO REMEMBER

DECIMALS

- Always place a zero before a decimal if no whole number is present.
- When adding or subtracting decimals, align decimal points and add terminal zeros as necessary to make decimal places the same length.
- When multiplying decimals, multiply the numbers, count the number of decimal places in the numbers multiplied, and finally place the decimal point in the product.
- To divide decimal fractions, form a whole number in the divisor by moving the decimal point to the right, then move the decimal point in the dividend (number to be divided) the same number of decimal places to the right. Place the decimal point in the quotient (answer) directly over the decimal point in the dividend and divide as if the numbers are whole numbers.
- When multiplying by 10 or multiples of 10 (e.g., 100 or 1,000), the only step necessary is to move the decimal point in the other number to the right by the number of zeros in the multiplier.
- To divide by 10 or a multiple of 10, the decimal point in the dividend, the number being divided, may be moved to the left by the number of zeros in the divisor.

PERCENT

A **percent** is a part of 100 as a fraction (such as $\frac{1}{100}$) and hundredths as a decimal (such as 0.01). Percents are used to describe medication strengths, to determine the amount of solute in a solvent when preparing medications, to determine the amount of medication that has been administered over a given amount of time, and to determine discounts and markups in retail pharmacy.

Converting a Percent to a Fraction

To convert a percent to a fraction, drop the % sign and write the number over 100. The denominator will *always* be 100. Reduce the fraction to its lowest terms.

EXAMPLE 2.22

Change 16% to a fraction.

16% becomes $\frac{16}{100}$ and reduces to $\frac{4}{25}$.

If the percent is written as a mixed number, the mixed number becomes the numerator and 100 the denominator. The mixed number must be changed to an improper fraction first.

EXAMPLE 2.23

Change $2\frac{2}{5}\%$ to a fraction.

$2\frac{2}{5} = \frac{12}{5}$ Place the fraction over 100.

$$\frac{12/5}{100} \text{ or } \frac{12}{5} \div \frac{100}{1}$$

To divide fractions, invert and multiply.

$$\frac{12}{5} \times \frac{1}{100} = \frac{12}{500} = \frac{3}{125}$$

EXAMPLE 2.24

Change 0.5% to a fraction.

$$\frac{0.5}{100}$$

A decimal cannot be left in a numerator or denominator, so multiply by the smallest fraction that is equal to 1 that will remove the decimal:

$$\frac{0.5}{100} \times \frac{2}{2} = \frac{1}{200}$$

Another option for solving this is to move the decimal one place to the right in both the numerator and denominator: multiply by $\frac{10}{10}$.

$$\frac{0.5}{100} \times \frac{10}{10} = \frac{50}{1,000}$$

This would then reduce to $\frac{1}{200}$.

TECH NOTE

Any percent over 100 will include a whole number and a fraction.

Practice Problems O

Convert the following percents to fractions. On the first line, drop the percent sign and place the entire number over 100, then simplify. Show your calculations.

1. 50% = __________ __________
2. 10% = __________ __________
3. 76% = __________ __________
4. 320% = __________ __________
5. 0.1% = __________ __________
6. 12% = __________ __________
7. 60% = __________ __________
8. 125% = __________ __________
9. 33% = __________ __________
10. 75% = __________ __________
11. 80% = __________ __________
12. 0.25% = __________ __________
13. 0.45% = __________ __________
14. 12.5% = __________ __________
15. 0.05% = __________ __________
16. 4% = __________ __________
17. 0.025% = __________ __________

On the first line, show the multiplication equation that will be solved after dropping the percent sign and inverting 100 to multiply (i.e., multiply by $\frac{1}{100}$). Write your solution on the second line. Show your reduced answer on the third line if necessary.

18. $\frac{2}{3}\%$ = __________ __________, __________
19. $\frac{1}{4}\%$ = __________ __________, __________
20. $1\frac{1}{4}\%$ = __________ __________, __________

Converting a Fraction to a Percent

The denominator in a percent is always 100 (because any percent is a part of 100), and the number beside the % sign becomes the numerator. To convert a fraction to a percent multiply the fraction by 100 or by $^{100}/_{1}$ (the fraction for 100) and add the percent sign (%). This is the same as changing the fraction to a decimal and moving the decimal place to the right two places.

EXAMPLE 2.25

Convert to a percent.

$$\frac{1}{5} \cdot 100 = \frac{100}{5} = 20\%$$

If the fraction is a mixed number, change it to an improper fraction first, then multiply by 100.

EXAMPLE 2.26

$$2\frac{3}{5} = \_\_\_\_\%$$

$$2\frac{3}{5} = \frac{13}{5}$$

$$\frac{13}{5} \times \frac{100}{1} = \frac{1{,}300}{5} = 260\%$$

Practice Problems P

Convert the following fractions and mixed numbers to percents. First, write the fraction after multiplying by 100, and then show the percent. Round to hundredths if needed.

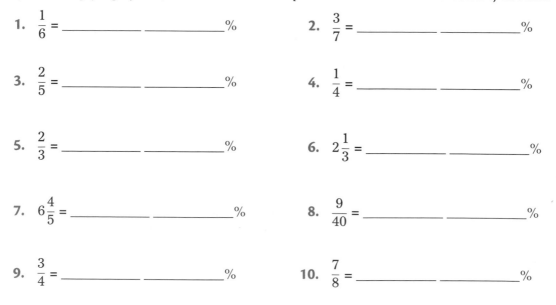

1. $\frac{1}{6}$ = ____________ ____________%

2. $\frac{3}{7}$ = ____________ ____________%

3. $\frac{2}{5}$ = ____________ ____________%

4. $\frac{1}{4}$ = ____________ ____________%

5. $\frac{2}{3}$ = ____________ ____________%

6. $2\frac{1}{3}$ = ____________ ____________%

7. $6\frac{4}{5}$ = ____________ ____________%

8. $\frac{9}{40}$ = ____________ ____________%

9. $\frac{3}{4}$ = ____________ ____________%

10. $\frac{7}{8}$ = ____________ ____________%

11. $1\frac{2}{3}$ = ____________ ____________%

12. $\frac{4}{5}$ = ____________ ____________%

13. $\frac{1}{2}$ = ____________ ____________%

14. $\frac{3}{4}$ = ____________ ____________%

15. $\frac{3}{10}$ = ____________ ____________%

Converting a Percent to a Decimal

To convert a percent to a decimal, drop the percent sign and divide the number by 100. Dividing by 100 is the same as moving the decimal point two places to the left.

EXAMPLE 2.27

25% = 25/100 25 divided by 100 = 0.25

25% becomes 0.25 by removing the % sign and moving the decimal two places to the left.

EXAMPLE 2.28

8% = 8/100 8 divided by 100 = 0.08

8% becomes 0.08 by removing the % sign and moving the decimal two places to the left. Zeros were added in front of the number so that two decimal places may be moved.

EXAMPLE 2.29

0.8% equals 0.8 divided by 100 = 0.008

0.8% becomes 0.008 by removing the % sign and moving the decimal two places to the left.

Zeros were added in front of the number here as well. If the percent is over 100, there will be a whole number before the decimal.

EXAMPLE 2.30

155% equals 155 divided by 100 = 1.55

EXAMPLE 2.31

Convert ½% to a decimal.

To change a fractional percent to a decimal, convert the fraction to a decimal and divide by 100.

$1 \div 2 = 0.5$

$0.5 \div 100 = 0.005$

Practice Problems Q

Convert the following percents to decimals. Do not round.

1. 60% = ________
2. 3% = ________
3. 78% = ________
4. 128% = ________
5. 1.3% = ________
6. 325% = ________
7. 0.05% = ________
8. 0.3% = ________
9. 32% = ________
10. 7% = ________
11. 8.2% = ________
12. 1,245% = ________
13. 56% = ________
14. 14.6% = ________
15. 0.06% = ________
16. $\frac{1}{4}\%$ = ________
17. $\frac{3}{4}\%$ = ________
18. $\frac{1}{8}\%$ = ________
19. $2\frac{1}{4}\%$ = ________
20. $\frac{4}{5}\%$ = ________

Converting a Decimal to a Percent

To convert a decimal to a percent, multiply by 100 and add a percent sign. Multiplying by 100 is the same as moving the decimal point two places to the right.

EXAMPLE 2.32

Express 0.50 as a percent.

0.50×100 moves the decimal two places to the right (50).

Add the % sign: 50%

If the number does not have two places to the right of the decimal point, add zeros so that the decimal point can be moved two places; 0.5 would need a zero added (0.50), and then the decimal point should be moved two places (0.50) so that 0.5 becomes 50%. If the number is a whole number such as 5, two zeros must be added to the number to find the percent. Thus 5 would require two added zeros, becoming 500%.

TECH NOTE

A number greater than 1 is always over 100% because one whole is 100%.

Practice Problems R

Convert the following decimals to percents.

1. 0.25 = __________ %
2. 0.68 = __________ %
3. 0.025 = __________ %
4. 0.6 = __________ %
5. 0.75 = __________ %
6. 5.5 = __________ %
7. 0.7 = __________ %
8. 6 = __________ %
9. 10.4 = __________ %
10. 0.05 = __________ %
11. 105 = __________ %
12. 0.15 = __________ %
13. 21.50 = __________ %
14. 1.025 = __________ %
15. 0.467 = __________ %
16. 0.75 = __________ %
17. 1.1 = __________ %
18. 0.01 = __________ %
19. 1 = __________ %
20. 0.4 = __________ %

The following table contains some common fractions, decimals, and percents for quick reference. Looking at them in this manner may help you see the pattern between the three.

FRACTION	DECIMAL	PERCENT
1/10	0.1	10%
1/4	0.25	25%
1/3	0.3333...	33.3%
1/2	0.5	50%
2/3	0.6666...	66.7%
3/4	0.75	75%
1	1	100%

RATIOS

Expressing Numbers as Ratios

A **ratio** indicates the relationship of one number to another *or* one number to a whole. A ratio expresses a numerator and denominator separated by a colon (:) rather than the division line found in fractions. Numerators are to the left of the colon, and denominators to the right, such as 1:2. The colon is the traditional way to write a division sign in a ratio and is representative of *of, per, to,* or *in*. For example, ¾ as a fractional expression would be 3:4 when written in ratio form. Like a fraction, a ratio may be reduced to lowest terms. Because of the relationship of the numbers in a ratio, the value of the ratio will not be changed if both the numerator and denominator are multiplied or divided by the same number. Multiplication and division are the only numeric operations that can be performed on a ratio without changing its value.

> **TECH NOTE**
> A ratio may be written as a fraction, and a fraction may be written as a ratio because each has a numerator and denominator (2:3 or $\frac{2}{3}$).

To change a percent to a ratio, express it as a fraction (the denominator will always be 100) and change the format.

30% = $^{30}/_{100}$ = 30:100

To change a decimal to a ratio, express it as a fraction and change the format.

0.09 is $\frac{9}{100}$ or 9:100

When numbers expressed in ratio form are used to compare quantities (one number related to another), they must be expressed in the same units of measure.

EXAMPLE 2.33

Establish a ratio of 3 inches to 1 foot.

1 foot must be changed to 12 inches (12″ = 1 foot).

3″:12″

Since both sides can be reduced by 3″, the unit of inches is canceled and no unit is required in the reduced ratio.

1:4

When numbers expressed in ratio form are used to describe one number as a part of a whole amount, they *may* have different units of measurements. In pharmacy, ratios are used in this manner. For example, mg is a measurement of weight or mass and mL is a measurement of volume, so one cannot be converted to the other. The relationship is the number of mg "in" or "per" mL.

EXAMPLE 2.34

Establish a ratio for 5 mg per 125 mL and reduce.

5 mg:125 mL (This is most often written as a fraction.)

1 mg:25 mL

Practice Problems S

Express the following as ratios and then reduce to lowest terms.

1. 2 is to 7 = ____________ ____________
2. 6 is to 9 = ____________ ____________
3. 5 is to 25 = ____________ ____________
4. 36% = ____________ ____________

5. 125% = ___________ ___________

6. 95% = ___________ ___________

7. $\frac{7}{8}$ = ___________ ___________

8. $\frac{75}{125}$ = ___________ ___________

9. $3\frac{1}{4}\%$ = ___________ ___________

10. 0.04% = ___________ ___________

11. 0.08 = ___________ ___________

12. 0.36 = ___________ ___________

13. 0.04 = ___________ ___________

14. 0.1 = ___________ ___________

15. 6 in:4 ft = ___________ ___________

16. 50¢:$3.50 = ___________ ___________

17. 0.25 in:25 in = ___________ ___________

18. 0.2 mL:5 mL = ___________ ___________

Include units on the following after reducing.

19. 50 mg:250 mL = ___________

20. 2 mg:8 mL = ___________

Expressing Ratios as Proportions

A true **proportion** is an expression of equality between two equivalent ratios, such as 4:8 and 6:12. Placing these in a proportional equation, 4:8::6:12, or a fractional equation, $\frac{4}{8} = \frac{6}{12}$, is read, 4 is to 8 as 6 is to 12. In these pairs of numbers, the relationship between 4 and 8 is that 8 is twice as much as 4 and the relationship between 6 and 12 is that 12 is twice as much as 6. Therefore these ratios are equally proportional to each other, although the numbers are not the same. Both can be reduced to 1:2.

When validating proportional equations such as 4:8::6:12, multiply the two outside numbers, the extremes, and the two inside numbers, the means, so 4 × 12 and 6 × 8. Because both answers are 48, it is a true proportion. The product of the means will equal the product of the extremes in a true proportion.

To verify this equality when written as fractions, cross-multiply $\frac{4}{8} \times \frac{6}{12}$. Because both answers are 48, it is a true proportion.

When writing the proportion in the form of $\frac{a}{b} = \frac{c}{d}$, like units of measure must be in positions "a and c" and in positions "b and d." When the proportion is designated in the following manner, $\frac{125\ \text{mg}}{5\ \text{mL}} = \frac{25\ \text{mg}}{1\ \text{mL}}$, positions "a and c" are in milligrams and "b and d" are in milliliters.

Practice Problems T

Which of the following are true proportions? Mark with either a yes or a no.

1. 3:9::9:27 ________
2. 5:25::10:250 ________
3. 4:12::6:18 ________
4. 10:90::1:9 ________
5. $\frac{15}{3} = \frac{5}{2}$ ________
6. $\frac{22}{88} = \frac{10}{40}$ ________
7. $\frac{1.5}{7.5} = \frac{0.25}{1.25}$ ________
8. $\frac{2 \text{ mg}}{4 \text{ mL}} = \frac{8 \text{ mg}}{16 \text{ mL}}$ ________
9. $\frac{2''}{12''} = \frac{6''}{24''}$ ________
10. $\frac{500 \text{ mg}}{5 \text{ mL}} = \frac{100 \text{ mg}}{10 \text{ mL}}$ ________

Solving for Unknowns Using Ratio and Proportion

In the health care field, the ratio and proportion method is often used to calculate different quantities of medication or to calculate doses. Knowing three of the four parts of the proportion is necessary to solve for the fourth. Proportional equations are used to find the missing or unknown amount, often represented by x. The relationship is set up using the fractional method and solved using cross-multiplication followed by division. This method will be used in this text when it comes to solving for the unknown value. Ratio and proportion calculations are one of the two main methods used in pharmaceutical calculations.

EXAMPLE 2.35

$\frac{5}{35} = \frac{x}{28}$ Cross-multiply.

$35x = 5 \bullet 28$

$35x = 140$ Divide each side by 35.

$x = 4$

A proportion may be verified by substituting the answer in the x position and cross-multiplying to verify that it is a true proportion: $5 \bullet 28 = 140$ and $4 \bullet 35 = 140$.

TECH NOTE

When three terms of a proportion are known, the sequence of cross-multiplication and division is used to find the unknown term.

Practice Problems U

Solve for the following unknown values. Write as fractions if needed and then cross-multiply and divide. Indicate measurements as appropriate. Show your work.

1. $x:2::14:7$

   $x =$ __________

2. $20:x::5:10$

   $x =$ __________

3. $\frac{7}{x} = \frac{35}{125}$

   $x =$ __________

4. $\frac{x}{11} = \frac{2}{2.2}$

   $x =$ __________

5. $\frac{2}{24} = \frac{x}{36}$

   $x =$ __________

6. $0.20:x::$1.00:$25

   $x =$ __________

7. $\frac{\$6.00}{8 \text{ capsules}} = \frac{x}{36 \text{ capsules}}$

   $x =$ __________

8. $\frac{\$75.00}{100 \text{ tablets}} = \frac{\$15.00}{x}$

   $x =$ __________

9. $\frac{3 \text{ capsules}}{1 \text{ day}} = \frac{x}{7 \text{ days}}$

   $x =$ __________

10. $\frac{0.4 \text{ g}}{0.15 \text{ g}} = \frac{0.16 \text{ g}}{x}$

    $x =$ __________

11. $\frac{14 \text{ mL}}{2 \text{ L}} = \frac{21 \text{ mL}}{x}$

    $x =$ __________

12. $\frac{20 \text{ mg}}{1 \text{ tab}} = \frac{60 \text{ mg}}{x}$

13. $\frac{250 \text{ mg}}{5 \text{ mL}} = \frac{750 \text{ mg}}{x}$

14. Mr. Smith needs 14 tablets for a week's supply of an antiinflammatory drug. He is going on vacation and needs a 4-week supply. How many tablets are needed to fill the prescription?

15. Periactin liquid is labeled as 5 mg/5 mL. How many mg would be in 25 mL?

16. A medication contains 5 mg per tablet. How many tablets are needed for a 35 mg dose?

17. A cough medication contains 50 mg of active ingredient per mL. The physician orders 100 mg per dose. How many milliliters are needed for one dose?

18. A physician orders a 250 mg dose of an antibiotic for a child. The pediatric liquid medication contains 125 mg per 5 mL. How many milliliters should the child be given for one dose?

19. There are 1,000 milligrams per 1 gram. How many milligrams are in 0.5 grams?

20. There are 0.9 grams of sodium chloride in 100 mL of fluid. How many grams are in 1,000 mL?

CALCULATIONS WITH PERCENTS

Determining the Percentage of a Quantity

Computation of a given percentage of a quantity may be determined in order to ascertain the part of a whole quantity that is in question. If a percentage of a whole quantity is in question, the known percent is changed to decimal form and multiplied by the whole quantity to provide the needed information. The equation for finding a percentage of a quantity follows:

$$\text{Amount} = \text{Percent required (written as a decimal)} \times \text{Whole amount}$$

EXAMPLE 2.36

What is 3% of 42?

Change the percent to a decimal by dividing by 100 or moving the decimal point two places to the left: 0.03.

$x = 0.03 \bullet 42$

$x = 1.26$

1.26 is 3% of 42.

A few tips on working with percentages of quantities:

- "what" is the unknown, or x
- "is" means "="
- % is the percent (written as a decimal when solving these equations)
- "of" translates to "times" (followed by the whole number)
- A question may be presented in three ways:

1. Find the percent: "What is 50% of 15?" $x = 0.5 \bullet 15$
   Note: remember to change the percent quantity to a decimal

2. Find the whole quantity: "7.5 is 50% of what number?" $7.5 = 0.5 \bullet x$
   Note: remember to change the percent quantity to a decimal
   Also: *"50% of what number is 7.5?"* $0.5 \bullet x = 7.5$

3. Find the percent: "7.5 is what percent of 15?" $7.5 = x \bullet 15$
   Note: remember to change the decimal answer to a percent
   Also: "What percent of 15 is 7.5?" $x \bullet 15 = 7.5$

Questions 2 and 3 may be asked in a reverse manner, which would result in the equation being written with the sides switched.

EXAMPLE 2.37

15 is 60% of what number?

$15 = 0.6 \bullet x$ Divide both sides by 0.6.

$x = 25$

15 is 60% of **25.**

EXAMPLE 2.38

15 is what percent of 45?

$15 = x \bullet 45$ Divide both sides by 45.

$x = 0.333$

15 is **33.3**% of 45.

Another method of working with percents is to use the knowledge that a percent is always an amount out of 100. One of the three known values will always be 100. A ratio and proportion equation can be set up to solve each of the previous questions as shown in Examples 2.39, 2.40, and 2.41:

EXAMPLE 2.39

What is 3% of 42?

$$\frac{3}{100} = \frac{x}{42} \quad 100x = 126 \quad x = 1.26$$

1.26 is 3% of 42.

EXAMPLE 2.40

15 is 60% of what number?

$$\frac{60}{100} = \frac{15}{x} \quad 60x = 1500 \quad x = 25$$

15 is 60% of **25.**

EXAMPLE 2.41

15 is what percent of 45?

$$\frac{x}{100} = \frac{15}{45} \quad 45x = 1,500 \quad x = 33.3$$

15 is **33.3**% of 45.

TECH NOTE

Percents are used to calculate the amount of active ingredients in a formulation, to compound medications, and to calculate markups and discounts in retail pharmacy.

Practice Problems V

Solve the following problems. Show your work. Indicate measurements as appropriate.

1. What percent of 105 is 35? (Round to tenths.)

2. 25 is what percent of 200?

3. 90% of 50 is what?

4. 105% of 0.9 is what?

5. What percent of 750 is 15?

6. What is 45% of 180?

7. 6 is what percent of 240?

8. What is 15% of $25.40?

9. What is 64% of 8 oz?

10. If you have 100 tablets, what is 5%?

11. What percent of 40 tablets is 22 tablets?

12. If a discount of 15% is applied to a purchase of $25, what is the amount of the discount?

13. If a patient wants 60% of a prescription that is written for 60 tablets, how many tablets will be dispensed to the patient?

14. A customer wants 50% of a prescription that is written for 300 mL. How many mL should be dispensed?

15. 35% of 70 tablets is what?

16. 40 tablets is what percent of 80 tablets?

17. 6 inches is what percent of 24 inches?

18. 120 tablets is what percent of 1,500 tablets?

19. 60% of 360 mL is what?

20. What is 3% of 1,200 mL?

Stop to Check Answers

Before continuing to another problem, ***always*** ask yourself the following question: "Does this answer make sense?" This is extremely important in pharmacy math. You will need to use your knowledge of specific medications when asking this question. When an answer is off by only one decimal point, the patient would receive either 10 times too much or 10 times too little medication. This is potentially very dangerous.

In addition to using your knowledge of drug doses, estimation is a good way to check mathematical calculations. To estimate a number, mentally round it to a slightly larger or smaller number containing fewer numerals. Then perform the calculation, mentally knowing that the answer will be slightly higher or lower than the actual calculation but will be close to the desired answer. For example, 12.2 times 3.8 could be thought of as 12 times 4, which equals 48. If your answer comes out closer to 5 or 500, you would know you made a decimal placement error. This process can help avoid many calculation errors.

Posttest

Solve the following problems.

1. 45 + 36 =

2. 35 – 17 =

3. 125 mg × 3 =

4. 975 mg ÷ 3 =

Solve the following fractional equations and then reduce to the lowest terms.

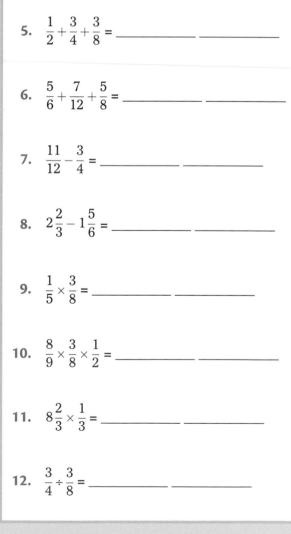

5. $\frac{1}{2}+\frac{3}{4}+\frac{3}{8}=$ __________ __________

6. $\frac{5}{6}+\frac{7}{12}+\frac{5}{8}=$ __________ __________

7. $\frac{11}{12}-\frac{3}{4}=$ __________ __________

8. $2\frac{2}{3}-1\frac{5}{6}=$ __________ __________

9. $\frac{1}{5}\times\frac{3}{8}=$ __________ __________

10. $\frac{8}{9}\times\frac{3}{8}\times\frac{1}{2}=$ __________ __________

11. $8\frac{2}{3}\times\frac{1}{3}=$ __________ __________

12. $\frac{3}{4}\div\frac{3}{8}=$ __________ __________

Posttest, cont.

13. $1\frac{1}{5} \div \frac{6}{7} =$ __________ __________

Solve the following problems. Round to the nearest hundredth if necessary.

14. 13 + 24.6 + 36.72 + 0.45 = __________

15. 15.87 – 5.2 = __________

16. 12.76 × 5.2 = __________

17. 25.01 × 10 = __________

18. 25 ÷ 0. 25 = __________

19. 16.82 ÷ 4.02 = __________

20. 2 – 1.75 = __________

21. 721 – 0.01 = __________

22. 1.06 + 3.871 = __________

23. 25.5 • 3.2 = __________

24. 12.02 ÷ 6.01 = __________

Continued

Posttest, cont.

Convert the following fractions to decimals. Round to the nearest hundredth.

25. $\frac{5}{9}$ = ___________

26. $2\frac{1}{3}$ = ___________

27. $\frac{16}{25}$ = ___________

28. $1\frac{5}{6}$ = ___________

Convert the following decimals to fractions. Reduce as appropriate.

29. 0.44 = ___________ ___________

30. 1.64 = ___________ ___________

31. 5.33 = ___________ ___________

32. 0.86 = ___________ ___________

33. 0.8 = ___________ ___________

Convert the following percents to decimals.

34. 33% = ___________

35. 1.5% = ___________

36. 100% = ___________

37. 14% = ___________

38. 230% = ___________

Convert the following percents to fractions and reduce to lowest terms.

39. 50% = ___________

40. 4% = ___________

41. 0.25% = ___________

42. 76% = ___________

43. 320% = ___________

Posttest, cont.

Convert the following decimals to percents.

44. 6.8 = __________

45. 0.3 = __________

46. 0.01 = __________

47. 0.75 = __________

48. 1.0 = __________

Convert the following fractions to percents.

49. $\frac{1}{2}$ = __________

50. $\frac{3}{4}$ = __________

51. $\frac{1}{8}$ = __________

52. $\frac{3}{10}$ = __________

53. $\frac{1}{3}$ = __________

Express the following as ratios and then reduce to lowest terms. Show your calculations.

54. $\frac{3}{5}$ __________ __________

55. 10% __________ __________

56. 500 mg in 10 mL __________ __________

57. An antibiotic contains 250 mg in 5 mL of medication. __________ __________

Continued

Posttest, cont.

Solve the following proportional equations.

58. 6 is to 12 as 5 is to x

59. 5 is to 15 as x is to 45

60. 13:39::1:x

61. One tablet contains 25 mg. How many mg are in three tablets?

62. Dr. Smith writes a prescription for a 3-month supply of medication for hypertension. A 1-month supply is 60 tablets. How many tablets are needed to fill the prescription?

Solve the following percent problems.

63. Three tablets are what percent of 90? (Round to hundredths.)

64. 45% of 1,500 mL is what?

65. What is 15% of 60 tablets?

66. 250 mg is what percent of 1,000 mg?

67. What is 40% of a prescription for 120 tablets?

68. 25 is 20% of how many capsules?

Posttest, cont.

69. 0.5% of 500 mL of a preparation must be cherry flavoring. How many mL of cherry flavoring are needed?

70. A patient wants 20% of their prescription of 180 capsules. How many capsules should you prepare?

IN SECTION II

SECTION II
Measurements and Conversions Used in Health Care Occupations

CHAPTER 3

Conversion of Clinical Measurements of Numbers, Time, and Temperature

OBJECTIVES

1. Convert between Arabic numerals and Roman numerals.
2. Convert time between standard time and military (or universal) time.
3. Convert temperature between Fahrenheit and Celsius.

KEY WORDS

Arabic numerals The numerals 1, 2, 3, etc.

Celsius (Centigrade) System of measuring temperature; 0° is the freezing point and 100° is the boiling point of water

Fahrenheit System of measuring temperature; 32° is the freezing point and 212° is the boiling point of water

Military time (International Standard Time) System of time that recognizes a 24-hour notation of hours and minutes

Roman numerals Letters from the Roman alphabet that are used to represent numbers, such as I for 1, V for 5, X for 10, etc.

Pretest

If you are already comfortable with the subject matter, perform the following calculations to test your knowledge. If not, work your way through the chapter and return to them for extra practice. Follow the directions below and show your calculations.

Change the following to Roman numerals.

1. 21 ________ **2.** 16 ________ **3.** 54 ________ **4.** 122 ________

5. 44 ________ **6.** 95 ________ **7.** 68 ________ **8.** 75 ________

Change the following to Arabic numerals.

9. viii ________ **10.** xix ________ **11.** lxiv ________ **12.** xcvii ________

13. ix$\overline{ss}$ ________ **14.** xvii$\overline{ss}$ ________ **15.** xxxvii$\overline{ss}$ ________ **16.** xxiv ________

17. xxiv$\overline{ss}$ ________ **18.** xliv$\overline{ss}$ ________

Change the following to universal, or 24-hour, time.

19. 7:30 AM ________ **20.** 5:32 PM ________ **21.** 12:01 AM ________ **22.** 11:59 AM ________

23. 1:59 PM ________ **24.** 1:46 AM ________ **25.** 8:42 PM ________ **26.** 9:08 PM ________

Change the following to 12-hour time.

27. 1102 ________ **28.** 0520 ________ **29.** 0052 ________ **30.** 2357 ________

31. 0001 ________ **32.** 0648 ________ **33.** 1645 ________ **34.** 1235 ________

Pretest, cont.

Convert the following temperatures as indicated. Round to the nearest tenth.

35. 98.6°F = __________ C **36.** 104.6°F = __________ C **37.** 38.6°C = __________ F

38. 29.6°C = __________ F **39.** 100.4°F = __________ C **40.** 41.8°C = __________ F

41. 41.8°F = __________ C **42.** 102.6°F = __________ C **43.** 0°F = __________ C

44. 10°C = __________ F **45.** 10°F = __________ C **46.** 95.6°F = __________ C

47. 32.2°C = __________ F **48.** 92.5°F = __________ C **49.** 212°F = __________ C

50. 100°C = __________ F

INTRODUCTION

It is important to be able to convert between time, temperature, and numerical systems when working in pharmacy. Many prescriptions include Roman numerals, medications must be stored at the correct temperatures, and the correct amount of medication must be prepared for the correct time. Pharmacy employees use both **Arabic numerals,** such as 1, 5, and 10, and **Roman numerals,** such as I, V, and X, when interpreting physicians' orders. Arabic numerals are commonly used in daily life, but Roman numerals are still occasionally used in the medical field and in literature. Similarly, we use the standard clock on a daily basis whereas institutional pharmacy settings use **military time** to prevent misinterpretation of order timing. Finally, temperature is read and recorded in **Fahrenheit** in daily lives in the United States, with 32° as the freezing point and 212° as the boiling point of water. The **Celsius** scale is the basic unit of temperature in the metric system and is used in most other parts of the world, with 0° as the freezing point and 100° as the boiling point of water. The Celsius scale is used in most clinical settings.

ARABIC AND ROMAN NUMERALS

Medication orders or prescriptions are written in both Arabic and Roman numerals, depending on the prescriber's preference. Arabic numerals, such as 2 for whole numbers, ½ for fractional numbers with the household system, and 0.5 for decimal numbers in the metric system, are used most often.

Roman numerals, which date back to the ancient Roman Empire, use letters to represent numerical amounts. The following equates Arabic numerals to Roman numerals.

ROMAN NUMERALS

½	$\overline{\text{SS}}$	10	X
1	I	50	L
2	II	100	C
3	III	500	D
4	IV	1,000	M
5	V		

Rules for Roman Numerals

1. When a numeral is repeated, its value is repeated.
   II = 2, XXX = 30

2. A numeral may not be repeated more than 3 times.
   40 = XL **not** XXXX

3. V, L, and D are *never* repeated.
   VV is **incorrect** because 10 = X
   LL is **incorrect** because 100 = C
   DD is **incorrect** because 1,000 = M

4. When a smaller numeral is placed after a larger numeral, it is added to the larger numeral.
   DC = 600 (500 + 100), LXVI = 66 (50 + 10 + 5 + 1)

5. When a smaller numeral is placed before a larger numeral, it is subtracted from the larger numeral.
   XL = 40 (50 – 10), XC = 90 (100 – 10)

6. *Never* subtract more than one numeral.
   8 = VIII **not** IIX

7. V, D, and L are *never* subtracted.
   LC is **not** correct because 50 = L

8. When subtracting, only use a numeral before the next *two* higher-value numerals.
   Only use: I before V or X
   X before L or C
   C before D or M

TECH NOTE

Roman numerals are often used when writing prescriptions because alphabetic symbols indicating quantity are more difficult to alter than Arabic numerals.

The most commonly used Roman numerals in pharmacy are combinations of I, V, and X. Medical notations of Roman numerals are often written in lower case with a line drawn over the numerals to prevent misinterpretation. Lowercase i's are frequently written with a line between the letter and the dot.

Converting Arabic Numerals to Roman Numerals

EXAMPLE 3.1

Change 24 to Roman numerals:

20 is 10 + 10, or xx

4 is (5 – 1), or iv (subtract 1 from 5)

So 24 is written as xxiv

Practice Problems A

Convert the following Arabic numerals to Roman numerals, using the correct medical notation to prevent misinterpretation.

1. 6 ____________ **2.** 11 ____________ **3.** 21 ____________

4. 56 ____________ **5.** $7\frac{1}{2}$ ____________ **6.** 9 ____________

7. $54\frac{1}{2}$ ____________ **8.** $17\frac{1}{2}$ ____________ **9.** 75 ____________

10. 101 ____________ **11.** 66 ____________ **12.** 35 ____________

13. $1\frac{1}{2}$ ____________ **14.** 49 ____________ **15.** $33\frac{1}{2}$ ____________

16. 93 ____________ **17.** 72 ____________ **18.** 59 ____________

19. 25 ____________ **20.** 2018 ____________

Converting Roman Numerals to Arabic Numerals

To change Roman numerals into Arabic numerals, divide the entire Roman numeral into the groups of letters that indicate a number, such as XIV where X = 10 and IV = 4. So the Roman numeral XIV = 14.

EXAMPLE 3.2

Change XLVII to an Arabic numeral.

Divide the numeral into XL and VII

XL means to subtract 10 (X) from 50 (L), which equals 40

VII is 5 (V) + 1(I) + 1 (I), or 7

When the numberals are placed together, XLVII (XL + VII) equals 47

EXAMPLE 3.3

Change xix$\overline{\text{ss}}$ into an Arabic numeral.

Divide the Roman numeral into separate parts

$x = 10$, $ix = (10 - 1) = 9$, $\overline{ss} = \frac{1}{2}$

$10 + 9 + \frac{1}{2} = 19\frac{1}{2}$

Practice Problems B

Convert the following Roman numerals to Arabic numerals.

1. viii ______ 2. ix ______ 3. xix ______

4. xxxix ______ 5. xliv ______ 6. lxvi ______

7. CXXV ______ 8. xxv$\overline{\text{ss}}$ ______ 9. xcv ______

10. vii$\overline{\text{ss}}$ ______ 11. ix$\overline{\text{ss}}$ ______ 12. xxxvii$\overline{\text{ss}}$ ______

13. xxv ______ 14. LXIII ______ 15. xcix ______

16. xli ______ 17. xlv ______ 18. cxxix ______

19. CD ______ 20. XCIX ______

CONVERSION BETWEEN 12-HOUR AND UNIVERSAL (MILITARY OR 24-HOUR) TIME

Because traditional time can be misinterpreted when using AM and PM with the same numbers to indicate the time of day for medication administration, most hospitals and other health care facilities use the 24-hour clock, also called military or universal time. The differentiation of time is not just dependent on the initials AM or PM but is actually a different number from 0001 to 2400. Orders are written 24 hours a day, and all medical-related caretakers must understand exactly when an order was written and when the medication or treatment is to take place. With this system, there is never any question as to when an order was written or which order supersedes another.

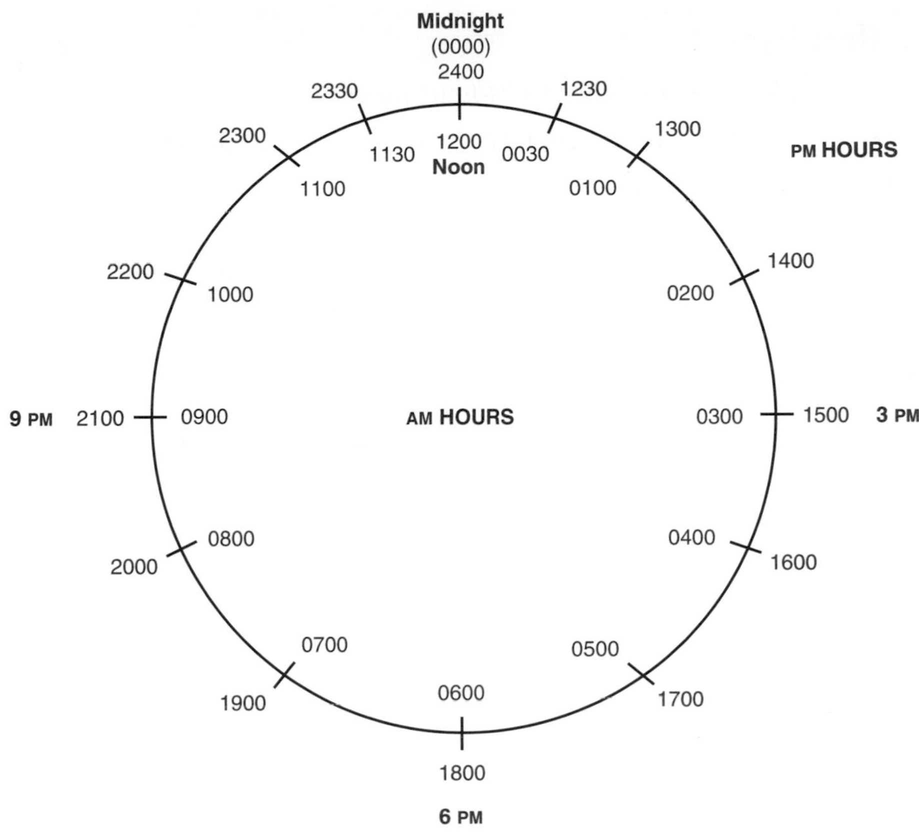

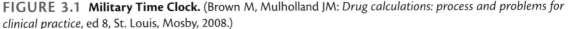

FIGURE 3.1 Military Time Clock. (Brown M, Mulholland JM: *Drug calculations: process and problems for clinical practice*, ed 8, St. Louis, Mosby, 2008.)

In universal time, all time is expressed in four-digit numbers beginning at 1 minute past midnight, or 0001. There is no colon between hours and minutes. The time is stated in hundreds of hours with 1 AM being 0100, "zero one-hundred hours." Ten in the morning, 1000, is "ten hundred hours." Noon is 1200, or "twelve hundred hours." One o'clock in the afternoon becomes 1300, or "thirteen hundred hours." Midnight is 2400, "twenty-four hundred hours," or 0000, "zero hundred hours." Fig. 3.1 shows an example of a military time clock. The AM (antemeridian, or before noon) readings are found on the inside of the clock face, and the PM (postmeridian, or after noon) readings are found on the outside of the clock face.

POINTS TO REMEMBER

CHANGING TO 24-HOUR, OR INTERNATIONAL, TIME

- Traditional and universal time use the same numbers from 1:00 AM (0100) to 12:59 PM (1259).
- Hours from 1:00 PM (1300) through 12:00 AM (2400 or 0000) are the 12-hour time plus 12; for instance, 5:00 PM would be 1700.
- Minutes are written in the third and fourth positions and are not separated by a colon, such as 1135 (11:35 AM). Minutes after midnight (0000) and before 1:00 AM (0100) are written as 00 with the number of minutes following, such as 0010 (12:10 AM).
- Midnight can be written as either 0000 or 2400 hours. In this text, we will use 0000 for midnight.

Practice Problems C

Convert the following 12-hour times to 24-hour times.

1. 12:35 AM ____________
2. 2:45 PM ____________
3. 6:15 AM ____________
4. 6:20 PM ____________
5. 12:05 AM ____________
6. 3:45 AM ____________
7. 12 AM ____________
8. 12 PM ____________
9. 6:55 AM ____________
10. 7:25 PM ____________
11. 2:15 PM ____________
12. 8:20 PM ____________
13. 9:05 AM ____________
14. 11 AM ____________
15. 11:59 PM ____________

Convert the following 24-hour times to 12-hour times. Be sure to indicate morning and evening.

16. 1130 ____________
17. 0354 ____________
18. 1201 ____________
19. 0030 ____________
20. 1425 ____________
21. 1615 ____________
22. 0830 ____________
23. 2345 ____________
24. 0705 ____________
25. 2145 ____________
26. 0404 ____________
27. 2020 ____________
28. 1020 ____________
29. 0330 ____________
30. 0945 ____________

CONVERSION BETWEEN FAHRENHEIT AND CELSIUS TEMPERATURE

In the United States, Fahrenheit (F) temperature is the measurement most commonly used. In countries where the metric system is used, Celsius (C) or centigrade temperature measurement is the most commonly used scale. In Fahrenheit, water boils at 212°, and in Celsius, water boils at 100°. Likewise, the freezing points are not the same; Fahrenheit is 32° and Celsius is 0°. Fig. 3.2 provides a comparison of the scales. As you can see, the Fahrenheit scale has 180° between the freezing and boiling points, whereas the Celsius

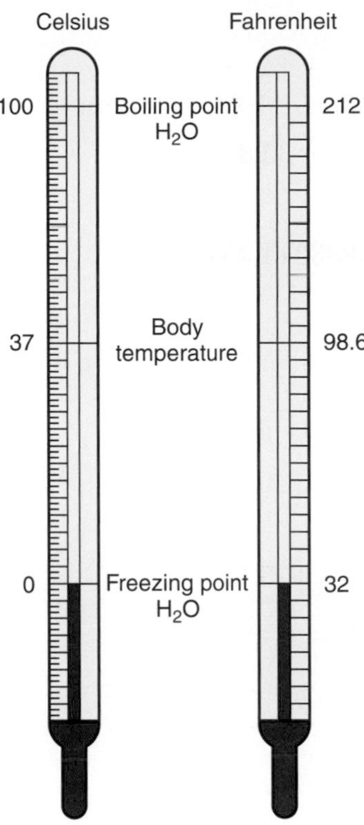

FIGURE 3.2 **Comparison of Celsius and Fahrenheit Thermometers.**

scale contains only 100°. The formulas for conversion between the two scales have been developed with these differences as the basis. The following conversion formulas may be used to change from one temperature scale to the other.

Converting Fahrenheit Temperature to Celsius Temperature

The equations can be written using decimals or fractions.

$$C = \frac{F - 32}{1.8} \quad \text{or} \quad C = (F - 32) \times \frac{5}{9}$$

In the first method, subtract 32 from the Fahrenheit temperature and then divide by 1.8. In the second method, subtract 32 from the Fahrenheit temperature, multiply that answer by 5, and then divide by 9. In either case, the remainder should be rounded to tenths.

Converting Celsius Temperature to Fahrenheit Temperature

To convert Celsius temperature to Fahrenheit temperature, you can also use two formulas:

$$F = 1.8\,C + 32 \quad \text{or} \quad F = \frac{9}{5}\,C + 32$$

In the first method, multiply the Celsius temperature by 1.8 and then add 32. In the second method, multiply the Celsius temperature by 9, divide that answer by 5, and then add 32 to that answer. In either case, the remainder should be rounded to tenths.

Alternate Formula for Converting Between Celsius and Fahrenheit

This one algebraic formula may be used for conversions for both systems: 9C = 5F – 160

Learn and use the formulas that are easiest for you.

EXAMPLE 3.4

Convert 96.5°F to C°.

$$C = (96.5^\circ - 32) \div 1.8 = 35.833 \text{ or } 35.8^\circ$$

OR

$$C = (96.5^\circ - 32) \times 5 \div 9 = 35.8333 \text{ or } 35.8^\circ$$

EXAMPLE 3.5

Convert 65°C to F°.

$$F = (65^\circ \times 1.8) + 32 = 149^\circ F$$

OR

$$F = (9 \times 65^\circ) \div 5 + 32 = 149^\circ F$$

EXAMPLE 3.6

Convert 65°C to F°.

$$9 \times 65^\circ = 5F - 160, \text{ add 160 to both sides}$$

$$9 \times 65^\circ + 160 = 5F, \text{ solve left side}$$

$$745^\circ = 5F, \text{ divide each side by 5}$$

$$149^\circ = F$$

EXAMPLE 3.7

Convert 96.5°F to C°.

$$9C = 96.5^\circ \times 5 - 160$$

$$9C = 482.5^\circ - 160$$

$$9C = 322.5^\circ, \text{ divide each side by 9}$$

$$C^\circ = 322.5^\circ \div 9$$

$$C^\circ = 35.8^\circ$$

TECH NOTE

When checking conversions for accuracy, the Celsius temperature will always be a lower number than the corresponding Fahrenheit temperature.

Practice Problems D

Convert the following temperatures using the appropriate formulas. Round to tenths as appropriate.

1. 1°F = __________ C
2. 35°C = __________ F
3. 35°F = __________ C
4. 19°C = __________ F
5. 112°F = __________ C
6. 34°C = __________ F
7. 36.5°C = __________ F
8. 102.6°F = __________ C
9. 98.6°F = __________ C
10. 99.2°F = __________ C
11. 37.2°C = __________ F
12. 100.2°F = __________ C
13. 10.2°C = __________ F
14. 130.6°F = __________ C
15. 48.2°C = __________ F
16. If a serum is to be stored at a temperature cooler than 40°F, what is the temperature for storage in a refrigerator on a Celsius thermometer? __________
17. Mrs. Jones is to receive an antibiotic if her temperature is above 103.8°F. What is the Celsius conversion? __________
18. A parenteral medication arrives through the mail. The label on the box states that the medication cannot be exposed to temperatures higher than 47.8°C. The current outdoor temperature is 100.2°F. What is the temperature in C? __________ Can the medication be safely used? __________
19. If a bottle of medication must be stored at a temperature cooler than 45°F, what is the Celsius temperature at which the medication must be stored? __________
20. A bag of fluids must be given at body temperature of 98.6°F. What is that temperature in the Celsius measurement? __________

REVIEW

This chapter covers the rules and equations used in time, temperature, and numerical system conversions, which will be important in your career as a pharmacy technician. Physicians use a combination of Arabic and Roman numerals when writing prescriptions and medication orders. Most clinical sites use the 24-hour clock, to avoid timing errors, as well as the Celsius temperature scale. Review these in the chapter and then proceed with the posttest to check your understanding.

Posttest

Complete the mathematical calculations as needed. Show your work.

Change the following to either Arabic or Roman numerals as appropriate.

1. xxvii$\overline{\text{ss}}$ ____________ **2.** xliv ____________ **3.** xciii$\overline{\text{ss}}$ ____________

4. ccl ____________ **5.** 45 ____________ **6.** $36\frac{1}{2}$ ____________

7. 46 ____________ **8.** 59 ____________ **9.** 75 ____________

10. viii$\overline{\text{ss}}$ ____________ **11.** lxviii ____________ **12.** cxxv ____________

13. xii ____________ **14.** 78 ____________ **15.** 165 ____________

Change the following to either 24-hour or 12-hour time as appropriate.

16. 0530 ____________ **17.** 8:30 AM ____________ **18.** 1625 ____________

19. 2:30 PM ____________ **20.** 1325 ____________ **21.** 0045 ____________

22. 12:05 AM ____________ **23.** 9:30 PM ____________ **24.** 12:10 PM ____________

Posttest, cont.

25. 0010 ____________ 26. 1755 ____________ 27. 3:26 PM ____________

28. 1455 ____________ 29. 5:30 PM ____________ 30. 0635 ____________

Convert the following temperatures. If Fahrenheit is listed, change to Celsius; if Celsius is given, change to Fahrenheit. Round to tenths.

31. 38.6°C ____________ 32. 86°F ____________ 33. 180°F ____________

34. 94.2°F ____________ 35. 103°F ____________ 36. 100°C ____________

37. 32°F ____________ 38. 2°F ____________ 39. 2°C ____________

Answer the following questions.

40. A medication cannot be frozen. The refrigerator is set for 5°C. What is the temperature in Fahrenheit? ________ Will the medication freeze? ________

41. A patient has a temperature of 38.6°C. What is the temperature in Fahrenheit? ________ Should the medical professional be concerned about this body temperature? ________

42. A refrigerator in the pharmacy department shows a temperature of 35.2°C. What is the temperature in Fahrenheit? ________ Should the pharmacy technician be concerned about any medications that must be stored below 50°F? ________

43. A physician writes an order for xxiv tablets. How many tablets should be dispensed? ________

Continued

Posttest, cont.

44. An order shows to dispense xc tablets. How many tablets will be dispensed? ________

45. A physician wants medication to be given every 6 hours beginning at 6:00 AM. Write the universal time for every 6 hours. ________ ________ ________ ________

46. A chart reads that the patient had pain medication at 5:35 PM. The medication can be taken every 6 hours. At what time in universal time could the next dose of medicine be given? ________

47. A medication order is to dispense xlviii tablets. How many tablets is this in Arabic numerals? ________

48. You supply a medication to the floor at 4:30 PM. You must chart the supply in universal time. What is the time of delivery? ________

49. If a medication is to be stored below 45°F, what would be the temperature on a Celsius thermometer in a refrigerator? ________

50. If a medication must be frozen at all times and the label states that it should be stored below 27°F, what would the refrigerator temperature need to be in Celsius? ________

Measurement Systems, Units, and Equivalencies

OBJECTIVES

1. Know the standard abbreviations, rules for expressing measurements, and basic equivalencies for the household system of measurement.
2. Know the standard abbreviations, rules for expressing measurements, and basic equivalencies for the metric system of measurement.
3. Know the standard abbreviations, rules for expressing measurements, and basic equivalencies for the apothecary system of measurement.

KEYWORDS

Apothecary system One of the oldest measurement systems used to calculate drug orders using measurements such as grains and minims

Biologics Substances made from natural sources such as human, animal, or microorganism that are used as drug treatments or to prevent or diagnose diseases; tested for potency in a biologic system

Electrolytes Elements such as sodium (Na), potassium (K), magnesium (Mg), and calcium (Ca) that are necessary for normal body functions

International System of Units (metric system) Internationally accepted system of measurement of mass, length, and time

International unit/Unit A *specific unit* of measurement used for biologicals; describes a standard amount of an *individual* drug that can produce a given biological effect; a measurement of a medication's action as opposed to its weight (as with the units mcg, mg, g); units of one substance are *not* equivalent to the same number of units of another substance (specific to each particular medication)

Milliequivalents (mEq) A type of unit used to express the concentration of electrolytes

Specific gravity The ratio of the density of a substance to the density of water when dealing with liquids in pharmacy

Standards An exact quantity agreed on for use in comparing measurements

Unit A general term covering any quantity chosen as a standard; for a measurement to make sense, it must include a number and a unit; examples of units: mg, mL, teaspoon

U.S. customary system (household system) System of measurement based on U.S. common kitchen measuring devices

Viscosity Thickness of a substance

Pretest

If you are already comfortable with the material, answer the following to test your knowledge. If not, work your way through the chapter and return to them for extra practice.

Items marked with an asterisk (*) are apothecary symbols, which are included in the Institute for Safe Medication Practices (ISMP) *List of Error-Prone Abbreviations, Symbols, and Dose Designations*. Technicians must still be familiar with them.

Continued

Pretest, cont.

Write the meaning of the following abbreviations or symbols.

1. mg ________________
2. mcg ________________
3. g ________________
4. gr ________________
5. kg ________________
6. ″ ________________
7. oz ________________
8. *fl℥ ________________
9. mEq ________________
10. *flʒ ________________
11. gtt ________________
12. tsp ________________
13. Tbsp ________________
14. *♏ ________________
15. lb., # ________________
16. mL ________________
17. L ________________
18. How should one and one-half teaspoons be written? ____________
19. How should two and five-tenths milliliters be written? ____________
20. How should nine and one-half grains be written? ____________
21. How should one thousand units be written? ____________

Pretest, cont.

22. *How should twenty apothecary fluid drams be written? ____________

23. How many teaspoons are in one tablespoon? ____________

24. How many milliliters are in one liter? ____________

25. How many ounces are in one cup? ____________

26. How many micrograms are in one milligram? ____________

27. How many apothecary drams are in one ounce ____________

28. How many household ounces are in a pound? ____________

29. How many tablespoons are in one ounce? ____________

30. How many quarts are in one gallon? ____________

*On the Institute for Safe Medication Practices (ISMP) *List of Error-Prone Abbreviations, Symbols, and Dose Designations.*

INTRODUCTION

Three measurement systems are presently used in the medical field to calculate length, volume, or weight, although length is not as commonly used in the pharmaceutical field as in other medical disciplines. Each system has a unique set of measurement units that have been chosen as **standards.** Numbers without units are meaningless. Consider telling someone that you will be gone for 3. Without the unit designating minutes, hours, days, months, or years, there is no meaning to the 3.

The **U.S. customary system**, or **household system**, uses measurements such as inches, teaspoons, and pounds. The **International System of Units**, or the **metric system**, which is used in most of the remaining world, uses meters, liters, and grams. The **apothecary system**, which uses grains and drams, is an older system used in pharmacy for many years, but less frequently today. All three systems—household, metric, and apothecary—have units of measure for weight and volume that are used in pharmacy, but only household and metric systems have commonly used units for length. Knowledge of the units for weight and volume in the three systems and length in the household and metric systems is necessary to interpret medication orders and prescriptions.

In pharmacy, length is used to measure medications that require application to the body that must be measured in inches, centimeters, or millimeters. In these instances, the means of application is usually premarked on a dispensing paper for ease in ensuring that the correct amount of medication is administered, such as with nitroglycerin ointment. Another pharmaceutical use of length is in finding body surface area (BSA) where height and weight are used for dose calculations, which will be covered in Chapter 12.

Mass is the measurement of the amount of matter in an object and is commonly referred to as weight. Metric weight is the measurement used most often in pharmacy to express doses. Most medications are ordered and supplied by the weight of a drug in solid or liquid amounts. Most solid medications are supplied in micrograms, milligrams, or grams. A few older medications are still supplied in grains from the apothecary system. Household measurements of weight are not used in medication strengths.

Volume is the amount of space something occupies and is used to measure amounts of liquids. A derived unit that is used to describe liquid medication strengths is density, which is weight divided by volume. Most liquid medications are described in terms of mg/mL. Occasionally some products, such as milk of magnesia, are still labeled with the amount of active ingredient per tablespoon (15 mL).

Some other specific types of medications are dosed in **milliequivalents (mEq)** and **International units**, or **units** (not to be confused with the generic term *unit* that applies to a quantity chosen as a standard measurement). Milliequivalents are used to express concentrations of **electrolytes** that are needed for normal body functions. For example, K-Dur 20 tablets contain 20 mEq of potassium per tablet. Units, as a measurement, are assigned to various **biologics**, which are substances made from living organisms that are used therapeutically as medications. The *unit* measurement is actually assigned according to a medication's *activity* in the body. Units are specific to each individual medication and do not relate to one another. For example, Units of insulin cannot be compared with Units of heparin. Measurements of these two medications are covered in detail in Chapter 10.

Most measurements need a unit to have meaning. The one exception to this is **specific gravity**, which is the density of a substance in g/mL, divided by the density of water, which is 1 g/mL. In this calculation, the units cancel, leaving specific gravity without a unit. If the density of a substance is x g/mL, once it is divided by the density of water or 1 g/mL, the units cancel and the specific gravity of the substance is x. Specific gravity is used occasionally in pharmacy to calculate the weight or volume of a solution.

TECH NOTE

The Joint Commission's *Official "Do Not Use" List* includes the use of the abbreviations u or U, which should be written "unit," and IU, which should be written "International unit."

Some of the previously mentioned measurements are used daily, whereas others may be foreign and need explanation. This chapter covers the basic measurements per system, which are essential for applying the conversion methods used in Chapters 5 and 6.

HOUSEHOLD OR U.S. CUSTOMARY SYSTEM

Household measurements and abbreviations of weight can be found in Table 4.1, length in Table 4.2, and volume in Table 4.3. Learn the equivalents presented, because an equivalency table may not be available when you need to make a conversion.

TABLE 4.1 Household Measurements of Weight

MEASUREMENT UNIT	ABBREVIATION	EQUIVALENTS
Ounce	Oz	—
Pound	lb, #	16 oz
Ton	T	2,000 #

TABLE 4.2 Household Measurements of Length

MEASUREMENT UNIT	ABBREVIATION	EQUIVALENTS
Inch	in, ″	—
Foot	ft, ′	12 inches
Yard	Yd	36 inches, 3 feet

TABLE 4.3 Household Measurements of Volume*

MEASUREMENT UNIT	ABBREVIATION[a]	EQUIVALENTS
Drops	**gtt**	—
Teaspoon	**tsp**, Tsp, t	60 drops (depending on the size of the dropper and the viscosity of the medication)
Tablespoon	**Tbsp**, tbsp, tbs, T	3 teaspoons
Ounce	**oz**	2 Tbsp or 6 tsp
Cup	c, C	8 oz
Pint	**pt**	2 c, 16 oz
Quart	**qt**	2 pt, 4 c, 32 oz
Gallon	**gal**	4 qt, 8 pt, 16 c, 128 oz

*Preferred abbreviations used in this text are **bolded.**

Household measurements are expressed in Arabic numerals with fractions for expressing parts of a whole, such as ½, ⅔, or ¾. The abbreviation for each measurement follows the number, such as 5 tsp or 2 ½ pt.

Household measurements are often used in the home setting for administration of medication, although they are *not* optimal and should be considered approximations. Some use their flatware for table use instead of actual teaspoon and tablespoon measuring spoons, which greatly increases the likelihood of a significant error.

The use of a measurement device provided with the medication by the pharmacy increases the accuracy of dosing and therefore patient safety. The household system is *not* used in hospital settings.

TECH NOTE

The smallest measurement of volume, a drop in any system, is totally dependent on the size of the opening in the dropper and the **viscosity** (thickness) of the liquid; therefore the 60 drops per teaspoon equivalence often found in tables of household measurements is only an approximation. Drops should not be used for measuring drugs unless there is a specific dropper calibrated for the medication.

TECH NOTE

Pharmacy technicians should commit the following basic household equivalencies to memory and can use methods presented in Chapter 5 to calculate any of the others.

VOLUME		WEIGHT
2 Tbsp = 1 oz	3 TSP = 1 TBSP	16 OZ = 1 LB
8 oz = 1 c		
2 c = 1 pt		
2 pt = 1 qt		
4 qt = 1 gal		

POINTS TO REMEMBER

THE HOUSEHOLD SYSTEM

- The household system uses fractions and Arabic numerals.
- Teaspoon and tablespoon are common household measurements.
- For patient safety, household flatware *should not* be used.
- For correct dosing, use the measuring device provided with the medication.

Practice Problems A

1. 1 c = ________ oz

2. 1 Tbsp = ________ tsp

3. 1 qt = ________ pt

4. 1 gal = ________ qt

5. 1 pt = ________ c

6. 1 oz = ________ Tbsp

7. 1 lb = ________ oz

Write the meaning of the following abbreviations.

8. c ________________

9. Tbsp ________________

10. tsp ________________

11. oz ________________

12. gal ________________

13. pt ________________

14. qt ________________

Rewrite the following using appropriate numerals and abbreviations.

15. two hundred pounds = ____________

16. six pints = ____________

17. ten drops = ____________

18. two and one-half cups = ____________

19. one and three-fourths quarts = ______

20. 6 gallons = ____________

METRIC SYSTEM OF MEASUREMENT

The metric system of measurement is the most widely used system in the world and the most commonly used system for measuring medications and doses because of its accuracy. Most prescriptions are written in the metric system, and most liquid drugs are administered using this system. The *U.S. Pharmacopeia* considers the metric system the appropriate system for use on drug labels.

Medication labels should be written in the appropriate metric units. Some medication labels include household measurements as well as metric measurements, as seen with the label for zidovudine (Retrovir) in Fig. 4.1. Additionally, some labels still contain nonrecommended abbreviations, such as µg (microgram) found on the labels for digoxin (Lanoxin), Fig. 4.2, and cc (cubic centimeter), which is equivalent to mL (milliliter).

The metric system is based on units of 10. The basic measurements are the gram for weight, liter for volume, and meter for length. Prefixes for the base measurements are used to indicate the multiple or submultiple of the base that is being described. Fig. 4.3 illustrates the following prefixes: Deka (10 base units), hecto (100 base units), and kilo (1,000 base units) indicate multiples. Deci (one-tenth of the base), centi (one-hundredth of the base), milli (one-thousandth of the base), and micro (one-millionth of the base) are submultiples. Table 4.4 applies these prefixes to weight, volume, and length. Table 4.5 lists the equivalents between the measurements.

TECH NOTE

The prefixes most commonly used in pharmacy are micro, milli, and kilo.

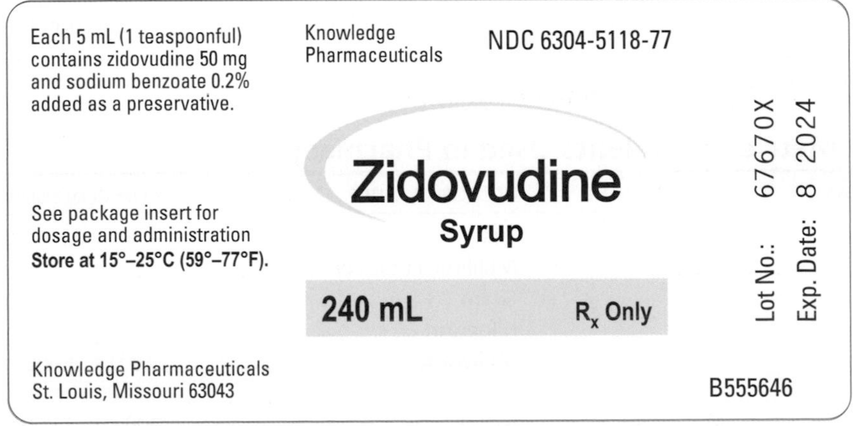

FIGURE 4.1 Label for Zidovudine Syrup.

100 Tablets
NCD 6304-7733-66
DIGOXIN
Each scored tablet contains
125 µg (0.125 mg)
Rx Only.
Knowledge Pharmaceuticals
St. Louis, MO 63043
Caution: Federal law prohibits dispensing without prescription.
For indications, dosage, precautions, etc., see package insert.
Store at 15°–25°C (59°–77°F) in a dry place.
Dispense in tight, light-resistant container as defined in the U.S.P.
Lot No.: 77037E
Exp. Date: 10 2024
100 Tablets
NCD 6304-7742-66
DIGOXIN
Each scored tablet contains
500 µg (0.5 mg)
Rx Only.
Knowledge Pharmaceuticals
St. Louis, MO 63043
Caution: Federal law prohibits dispensing without prescription.
For indications, dosage, precautions, etc., see package insert.
Store at 15°–30°C (59°–86°F) in a dry place.
Dispense in tight, light-resistant container as defined in the U.S.P.

FIGURE 4.2 **Labels for Digoxin Tablets.**

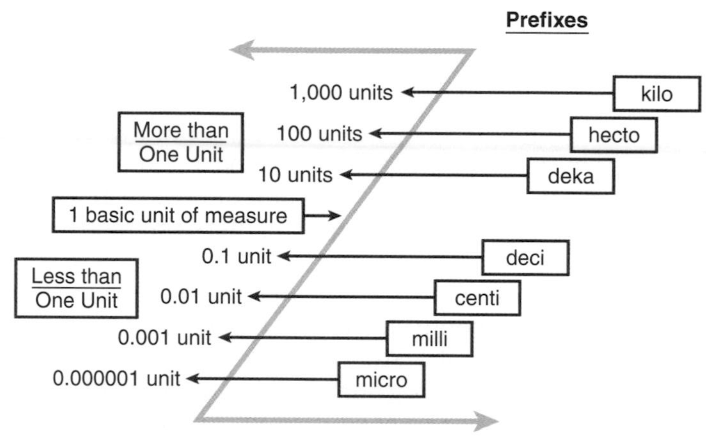

FIGURE 4.3 **The Basic Units of Measure—Gram, Liter, and Meter—With Prefixes Indicating Larger or Smaller Measures. (Modified from Fulcher EM, Soto CD, Fulcher RM: *Pharmacology: principles and applications*, ed 3, St. Louis, Saunders, 2012.)**

TABLE 4.4 Metric System of Measurements*

UNIT	WEIGHT	VOLUME	LENGTH
1,000 units	**kilogram**	kiloliter	kilometer
100 units	hectogram	hectoliter	hectometer
10 units	dekagram	dekaliter	dekameter
Base Unit	**gram**	**liter**	**meter**
1/10th unit	decigram	deciliter	decimeter
1/100th unit	centigram	centiliter	centimeter
1/1,000th unit	**milligram**	**milliliter**	millimeter
1/1,000,000th unit	**microgram**	microliter	micrometer

*__Bolded__ measurements are commonly used in pharmacy.

TABLE 4.5 Metric Equivalents Used in Pharmacy*

TYPE OF SUBSTANCE	ABBREVIATION	UNIT OF MEASURE	COMMON EQUIVALENTS
Volume/liquid	L, l	Liter	1,000 mL, 1,000 cc**
	mL, cc**	Milliliter, cubic centimeter*	0.001 L
Weight	**g**	Gram	1,000 mg, 0.001 kg
	kg	Kilogram	1,000 g
	mg	Milligram	0.001 g, 1,000 mcg
	mcg, µg**	Microgram	0.000001 g, 0.001 mg
Length	**M**	Meter	100 cm, 1,000 mm

*Preferred abbreviations used in this text are **bolded**.
**On the ISMP *List of Error-Prone Abbreviations, Symbols, and Dose Designations.*

A cubic centimeter is another way to express a milliliter. One cubic centimeter is the amount of space that is required to hold one milliliter of liquid. The abbreviation "cc" is *not recommended* because of the danger of misreading it as "00" (double zeros), but it is occasionally still found on prescriptions and medication orders. The preferred abbreviation is **mL.** The abbreviation "μg" for microgram may be misinterpreted as mg, causing a 1,000-fold error. The preferred abbreviation is **mcg**.

It is important to have a general idea of the weight, volume, or length of a unit. Most people in the United States are familiar with household but not metric units. The following comparisons may be helpful.

A gram is about the weight of two large-sized paper clips.

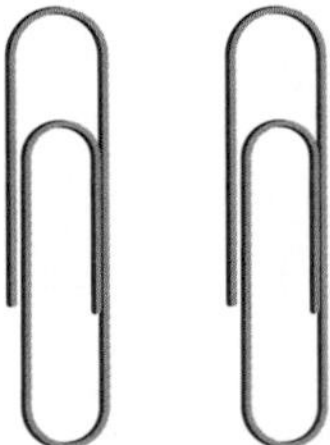

A liter is about the size of a quart container.

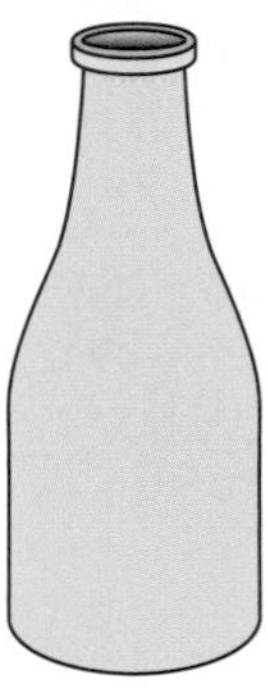

A meter is a little longer than a yardstick.

Inches

Centimeters

Fractional parts of numbers in the metric system are indicated with decimals. A zero, called a *leading zero*, should always be placed before a decimal when the number is less than 1 to prevent confusion and a possible error in interpretation. For instance, .25 mg might be misread as 25 mg if the measurement is not written as 0.25 mg. The potential error would be 100 times too much medication being administered to a patient. Also *no* zeros, called *trailing zeros*, should be added at the end of a fractional portion following a decimal point. For instance, to prevent errors, 2.50 mg should be written 2.5 mg, and 1.500 L should be written 1.5 L. Zeros found at the *end* of a number to the right of the decimal point may be removed without changing the value of the number.

The following depicts the weight measurements used in pharmacy from largest to smallest. There is a 1,000-unit difference between each of the following measurements of mass.

Metric Measurements of Mass in Pharmacy

kg ________ g ________ mg ________ mcg

(1 kg = 1,000 g) (1 g = 1,000 mg) (1 mg = 1,000 mcg)

Metric Measurements of Volume in Pharmacy

L ________ mL

1 L = 1,000 mL

TECH NOTE

Pharmacy technicians should commit the following basic metric equivalencies to memory and use methods presented in Chapter 5 to calculate any of the others needed.

Weight:	1,000 mcg = 1 mg	1,000 mg = 1 g	1,000 g = 1 kg
Volume:		1,000 mL = 1 L	

POINTS TO REMEMBER

THE METRIC SYSTEM

- A system of "place values" with the *base* being the unit from which all place values are measured. The gram, meter, and liter are at place 1, or the base site; kilo is at place 10^3 (the thousands place); milli is 10^{-3} (the one-thousandths place); and micro is 10^{-6} (the one-millionths place).
- The numeral is written before the abbreviation for the quantity, with a full space between the number and abbreviation (e.g., 10 mg, 2.5 mm, 1.5 L).
- All fractional parts are written as *decimal* numbers (e.g., 1.5 mL, 2.5 g, or 2.75 m).
- Any number with a value less than zero needs a "0" preceding the decimal point, a leading zero.
- Do not use trailing zeros.

Practice Problems B

1. 1 mg = 1,000 ________
2. 1 kg = 1,000 ________
3. 1 L = 1,000 ________
4. 1 g = 1,000 ________

Write the meanings of the following abbreviations.

5. kg ________
6. g ________
7. mg ________
8. L ________
9. mL ________
10. mcg ________

Rewrite the following using appropriate numerals and abbreviations.

11. two hundred fifty micrograms = ____

12. three and five-tenths liters = ______

13. ten and five-tenths milliliters = _____

14. five kilograms = __________

15. one hundred grams = __________

16. one and seventy-five hundredths milliliters = __________

17. five-tenths grams = __________

18. eight-tenths milligrams = _________

19. twenty-five micrograms = _________

20. twenty-five hundredths milligrams = __________

APOTHECARY SYSTEM OF MEASUREMENT

The apothecary system is one of the oldest systems of measurement. First used by an apothecary (early pharmacist), this system is gradually being replaced with the metric system. In ancient times, a minim (drop) of water was considered to weigh the same as a grain of wheat. Therefore the basic unit of liquid in the apothecary system is a minim (♏) and the basic unit of weight is a grain (gr). Apothecary measurements of volume such as minims (♏), fluid drams (flʒ), and fluid ounces (fl℥) are still found on some pharmacy bottles and medication dispensing cups even though the use of these measurements is discouraged. These apothecary symbols are found on the ISMP *List of Error-Prone Abbreviations, Symbols, and Dose Designations.* Although the metric system is preferred, the apothecary grain is still used with some older medications, such as nitroglycerin sublingual tablets (Nitrostat) (Fig. 4.4).

In the apothecary system, lowercase Roman numerals are used for expression of numbers 10 and below, rather than Arabic numerals as found in the metric and household systems. The Roman numerals should be expressed with lines placed over them to tie them together, such as $\overline{\text{i}}$, $\overline{\text{ii}}$, $\overline{\text{iii}}$, $\overline{\text{iv}}$, $\overline{\text{v}}$and $\overline{\text{x}}$, and lowercase i's are often expressed with the dots above that line. Arabic numerals may be used for numbers higher than 10, except for 20 ($\overline{\text{xx}}$) and 30 ($\overline{\text{xxx}}$), for which Roman numerals are required. Over the years the use of the line over the Roman numeral has gradually diminished, but using it is correct. Fractions other than ½, which is $\overline{\text{ss}}$, are expressed using Arabic numerals. Roman numerals and Arabic numerals are never used together in one measurement, so when using a fraction other than $\overline{\text{ss}}$, use Arabic numerals for the whole number as well. Therefore seven and three-fourths would be 7 ¾, not vii ¾. Decimals are *not* used with the apothecary system. The unit abbreviation is written first with Roman numerals placed to the right of the unit of measure. For example, 5 ounces is written ℥ v and 10 drams is ʒ x. See Table 4.6 for equivalents in the apothecary system.

TECH NOTE

The household pound (#) is 16 ounces; the apothecary pound is 12 ounces. The household pound (16 oz) will be used for conversions with body weight in pharmacy.

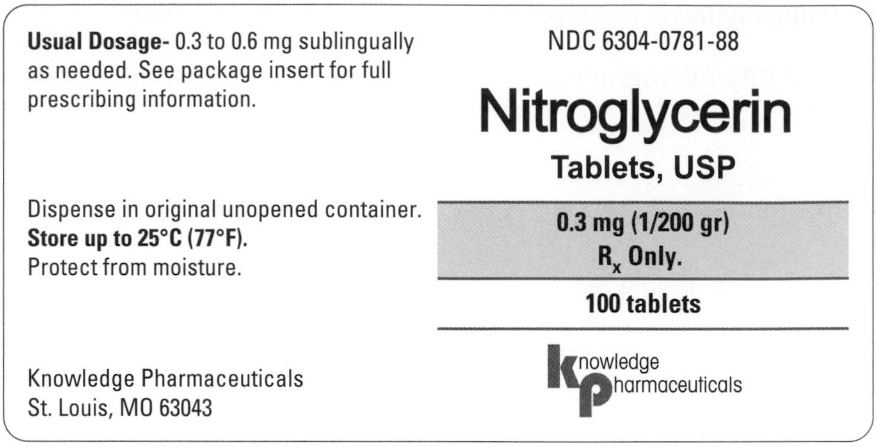

Usual Dosage- 0.3 to 0.6 mg sublingually as needed. See package insert for full prescribing information.

NDC 6304-0781-88

Nitroglycerin

Tablets, USP

Dispense in original unopened container.
Store up to 25°C (77°F).
Protect from moisture.

0.3 mg (1/200 gr)
R_x Only.

100 tablets

Knowledge Pharmaceuticals
St. Louis, MO 63043

knowledge pharmaceuticals

FIGURE 4.4 **Label for Nitroglycerin Sublingual Tablets.**

TABLE 4.6 Equivalents in the Apothecary System

TYPE OF SUBSTANCE	ABBREVIATION	UNIT OF MEASURE	COMMON EQUIVALENTS
Volume/liquid	♏	Minim	—
	flʒ*	Fluid dram	♏ lx (60)
	fl℥*	Fluid ounce	ʒ viii (8)
Mass/weight	Gr	Grain	—
	ʒ	Dram	gr lx (60)
	℥	Ounce	ʒ viii (8)
	#	Pound	℥ xii (12)

*On the ISMP *List of Error-Prone Abbreviations, Symbols, and Dose Designations.* An ounce is larger than a dram; the ounce symbol has one more loop than the dram symbol.

TECH NOTE

Although they are not used often, pharmacy technicians should be familiar with the following apothecary equivalencies.

Weight: ℥ i = ʒ viii

Volume: fl ℥ i = fl ʒ viii

POINTS TO REMEMBER

THE APOTHECARY SYSTEM

- The quantity should be expressed in lowercase Roman numerals, frequently with a line placed over the entire numeral and a dot above the line with the numeral i.
- Amounts greater than 10, other than 20 and 30, *may* be written in Arabic numerals.
- Numbers less than 1 are written as fractions, except ½, which is written $\overline{\text{ss}}$.
- Do not combine Roman and Arabic numerals in the same measurement.
- The symbol or abbreviation is written before the quantity.

Practice Problems C

Identify the following symbols and abbreviations.

1. fl ℥ i = fl ℥ ________________ 2. fl ℥ ________________

3. ♏ ________________ 4. # ________________

5. fl ʒ ________________ 6. gr ________________

7. ʒ ________________ 8. ℥ ________________

Rewrite the following using appropriate numerals and abbreviations.

5. 8 fluid drams = ________________ 6. six and one-half drams = ________________

7. three and one-fourth drams = ________ 8. nine minims = ________________

9. one hundredth grains = ________ 10. four fluid ounces = ________________

11. ten grains = ________________ 12. sixteen fluid ounces = ________________

13. twenty-five grains = ________ 14. twenty grains = ________________

15. fifty grains = ________________ 16. thirty grains = ________________

REVIEW

Three measurement systems are used in the field of medicine in the United States. The household system is used on a daily basis in homes. However, using the household system for medication dosing provides only approximate measurements. The use of actual measuring spoons as opposed to individual flatware can help decrease the variation. The metric system is the standard unit of measure throughout the rest of the world. Most medications are designated in the metric system today. The use of the apothecary system is discouraged; this system is used occasionally for some medications. The measurements for length, weight, and volume must be learned for conversions within and between the systems.

Posttest

Rewrite the following using the appropriate numerals and abbreviations (or numerals and symbols with the apothecary system).

1. thirty-six kilograms = __________
2. five and four-tenths grams = __________
3. three teaspoons = __________
4. nine tablespoons = __________
5. five grains = __________
6. ten fluid drams = __________
7. six pints = __________
8. one hundred twenty-five micrograms = __________
9. twelve and five-tenths milligrams = __________
10. five-tenths milliliters = __________
11. one and seventy-five hundredths liters = __________
12. two and one-half quarts = __________
13. three drops = __________
14. two ounces = __________
15. four cups = __________
16. six apothecary fluid ounces = __________
17. four minims = __________
18. one hundred ten pounds = __________

Posttest, cont.

19. sixty-five grains = ___________

20. three and one-half fluid drams = ___

21. forty milliequivalents = ___________

22. one thousand units = ___________

Complete the following equivalencies.

23. one Apothecary fluid ounce = _____ Apothecary fluid drams

24. 1 c = ___________ oz

25. 1 kg = 1,000 ___________

26. 1 L = 1,000 ___________

27. 3 tsp = 1 ___________

28. 2 pt = 1 ___________

29. 1 gal = ___________ qt

30. 1,000 mcg = 1 ___________

REVIEW OF RULES

Household System

- Uses fractions and Arabic numerals.

Metric System

- Uses decimals and Arabic numerals.

Apothecary System

- Uses lowercase Roman numerals, frequently with a line placed over the entire numeral and a dot above the line for the numeral i for some amounts.
- Amounts greater than 10, other than 20 and 30, *may* be written in Arabic numerals.
- Numbers less than 1 are written as fractions, except ½, which is written $\overline{\text{ss}}$.
- Never combine Roman and Arabic numerals in the same measurement.
- The symbol or abbreviation is written before the quantity.

CHAPTER 5

Conversions Within Measurement Systems

OBJECTIVES

1. Identify, convert, and calculate within household system measurements of weight and volume using both the ratio and proportion method and dimensional analysis.
2. Identify, convert, and calculate within metric system measurements of weight and volume using both the ratio and proportion method and dimensional analysis.
3. Identify, convert, and calculate within apothecary system measurements of weight and volume.

KEY WORDS

Conversion factor A ratio equal to 1 that is used to change one *unit* to another without changing the *value* of the answer

Dimensional analysis (DA) A method used for converting between units and calculating medication doses and dosages that involves multiplying a series of fractions in an order whereby all unnecessary units are sequentially canceled until the desired unit is reached

Ratio and proportion (R&P) A method used for *single-step* conversions between units and for calculating medication doses and dosages; involves solving for two equivalent fractions using cross-multiplication and division

Pretest

If you are comfortable with the subject matter, answer the following to test your knowledge. If not, work your way through the chapter and return to them for extra practice. Show your calculations. Perform ounce and pound weight conversions in the household system. Do not round your answers.

1. 15 gtt = ____________ tsp
2. 6 Tbsp = ____________ oz
3. 15 tsp = ____________ Tbsp
4. 2 mcg = ____________ mg
5. 6 kg = ____________ mg
6. ʒ viii = ℥ ____________
7. 4 c = ____________ oz
8. 6 pt = ____________ qt

Pretest, cont.

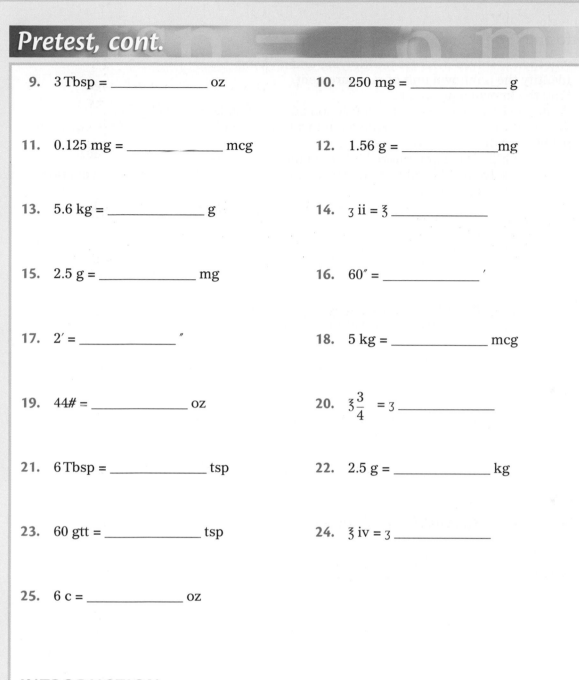

9. 3 Tbsp = ____________ oz

10. 250 mg = ____________ g

11. 0.125 mg = ____________ mcg

12. 1.56 g = ____________ mg

13. 5.6 kg = ____________ g

14. ʒ ii = ℥ ____________

15. 2.5 g = ____________ mg

16. 60″ = ____________ ′

17. 2′ = ____________ ″

18. 5 kg = ____________ mcg

19. 44# = ____________ oz

20. ℥ $\frac{3}{4}$ = ʒ ____________

21. 6 Tbsp = ____________ tsp

22. 2.5 g = ____________ kg

23. 60 gtt = ____________ tsp

24. ℥ iv = ʒ ____________

25. 6 c = ____________ oz

INTRODUCTION

This chapter focuses on converting from one unit to another within the household, metric, and apothecary systems. All conversions, and most pharmaceutical calculations, can be completed using one of two basic calculation methods: **dimensional analysis (DA) or ratio and proportion (R&P)**. You will use all of the basic equivalencies from Chapter 4.

HOUSEHOLD OR U.S. CUSTOMARY SYSTEM

How many inches are in 2 feet? That is fairly simple for people in the United States because it is used in everyday life. We know that 1 foot equals 12 inches, so 2 feet will equal 24 inches. This is actually an example of the R&P method of solving a conversion.

Ratio and Proportion

This method is solved by cross-multiplying and dividing.

1. Identify the unknown unit of measurement.
2. Find the known equivalent.
3. Write the known equivalent in a fraction on the left side of the equation.
4. Write the unknown desired equivalent in a fraction on the right side of the equation, using x for the unknown value.
5. Cross-multiply the numerators and denominators.
6. Divide to solve for the value of x. (The unit that is repeated in the original equation cancels when dividing.)

EXAMPLE 5.1

How many inches are in 2 feet? We know that there are 12 inches in 1 foot.

$$\frac{12''}{1'} = \frac{x}{2'}$$

$$1' \bullet x = 2' \bullet 12''$$ (Note that when dividing both sides by 1 foot, the units of feet cancel leaving the answer in inches.)

$$x = 24''$$

! TECH ALERT

The units in the numerators of equivalent fractions must be the same and the units in the denominators of equivalent fractions must be the same!

EXAMPLE 5.2

How many tablespoons are equivalent to 7 tsp?

From Table 4.3: 3 tsp equals 1 Tbsp; therefore:

$$\frac{1 \text{ Tbsp}}{3 \text{ tsp}} = \frac{x}{7 \text{ tsp}} \qquad 3x = 7 \text{ Tbsp}$$

Divide each side by 3.

$$x = \frac{7}{3} \text{ Tbsp}$$

Simplify the answer to $2\frac{1}{3}$ Tbsp.

TECH NOTE

Leave your answer as a whole number and a fraction when using the household measurement system.

Dimensional analysis is another method for converting between units. Some students prefer using this method since it is easier for them to keep track of units. For this reason, we will use DA exclusively when dealing with multistep calculations.

A **conversion factor** is a ratio that is equal to 1 and is used to change one *unit* to another. Because it is equivalent to 1, it does not change the *value* of the answer, only the unit. $\frac{12''}{1'}$ is a conversion factor; 12″ divided by 1′ has a value of 1 because they are equivalent amounts.

Dimensional Analysis

1. Identify the unit of the *answer* needed and follow it with an equal sign.
2. Set up a fraction such that the unit of the *desired* answer is in the numerator of the first fraction of the DA equation—this unit will *never* be cancelled.
3. Set up the next fraction in the equation so the unit of its numerator is the same as the unit of the denominator of the first fraction (so they will cancel when the fractions are multiplied).
4. Continue this pattern when dealing with multistep conversions.

EXAMPLE 5.3

How many inches are in 2 feet?

The conversion factor is $\frac{12''}{1'}$, which equals the *value* of 1.

$$'' = \frac{12''}{1'} \bullet \frac{2'}{1} = 24''$$

The unit of feet cancels, and inches is left.

! TECH ALERT

DA involves multiplication of fractions—NOT cross-multiplication as with R&P!

EXAMPLE 5.4

How many Tbsp are equivalent to 7 tsp?

The conversion factor is $\frac{1\text{ Tbsp}}{3\text{ tsp}}$, which has a value of 1.

$$\text{Tbsp} = \frac{1\text{ Tbsp}}{3\text{ tsp}} \times \frac{7\text{ tsp}}{1} = \frac{7\text{ Tbsp}}{3} = 2\frac{1}{3}\text{ Tbsp}$$

The unit *tsp* cancels, leaving *Tbsp*.

EXAMPLE 5.5

24 Tbsp is equivalent to how many cups?

If you do not remember how many tablespoons are in 1 cup, use the basic equivalencies 2 Tbsp equals 1 oz and 8 oz equals 1 cup, to set up a multistep DA equation:

$$\text{cups} = \frac{1\text{ c}}{8\text{ oz}} \times \frac{1\text{ oz}}{2\text{ Tbsp}} \times \frac{24\text{ Tbsp}}{1} = \frac{24\text{ c}}{16} = 1\frac{1}{2}\text{ c}$$

As long as you know the basic equivalencies in Table 5.1, you can solve any conversion within the household system.

TECH NOTE

The use of R&P is *only* appropriate with single-step conversions. DA can be used for single-step or multistep conversions.

TABLE 5.1 Household Equivalencies/Conversions

LIQUID MEASUREMENTS (VOLUME)

MEASUREMENT	ABBREVIATION	EQUIVALENT
1 drop	gtt	
1 teaspoon	tsp	60 gtt (varies with viscosity and dropper size)
1 tablespoon	Tbsp	3 tsp
1 ounce	oz	2 Tbsp
1 cup	c	8 oz
1 pint	pt	2 c
1 quart	qt	2 pt
1 gallon	gal	4 qt

DRY WEIGHT MEASUREMENT

MEASUREMENT	ABBREVIATION	EQUIVALENT
1 pound	lb or #	16 oz

Practice Problems A

Calculate the following conversions using your preferred method. Show your calculations.

1. 9 tsp = ____________ Tbsp
2. 2 qt = ____________ gal
3. 3 Tbsp = ____________ oz
4. 6 oz = ____________ c
5. 5 c = ____________ oz
6. 15 tsp = ____________ Tbsp
7. 4 ½ oz = ____________ tsp
8. 4 c = ____________ pt
9. 20 oz = ____________ #
10. 4′ 6″ = ___ ″ (Hint: convert 4′ to inches and then add 6″)
11. 3 ½ # = ____________ oz
12. ½ Tbsp = ____________ tsp
13. 3 pt = ____________ qt
14. 6 qt = ____________ gal

15. 3 tsp = ____________ gtt

16. 45 gtt = ____________ tsp

17. 24 oz = ____________ c

18. 10 c = ____________ oz

19. 32 oz = ____________ #

20. 8 Tbsp = ____________ oz

Patients should use calibrated medication cups or oral syringes at home to take medications; however, the pharmacy technician must have an understanding of conversions within household measurements. Convert the following orders to the requested household measurements.

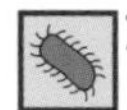

21. A physician orders 4 ½ tsp of amoxicillin.

How many tablespoons should the patient take? ____________

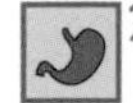

22. A physician orders 1 oz of milk of magnesia.

How many tablespoons should the patient take? ____________

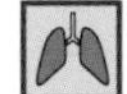

23. A physician orders ⅓ tablespoonful of Rondec DM (chlorpheniramine, dextromethorphan, and phenylephrine) for a child.

How many teaspoons would you give the child? ____________

24. A patient is to drink 1 quart of GoLytely in preparation for x-rays.

How many cups should the patient drink? ____________

25. A physician tells the patient to drink at least 24 additional ounces of water a day.

How many additional cups of water would the patient need to drink? ____________

METRIC SYSTEM CONVERSIONS

Because the metric system is based on units of 10, conversions can be made within the system by moving decimal places. This is a quick method, but a thorough understanding of the relationship between units is needed to master it. DA and R&P can always be used as well.

Metric Measurements of Mass Used in Pharmacy

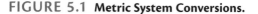

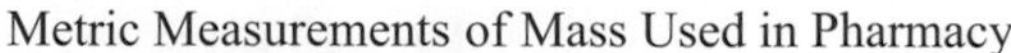

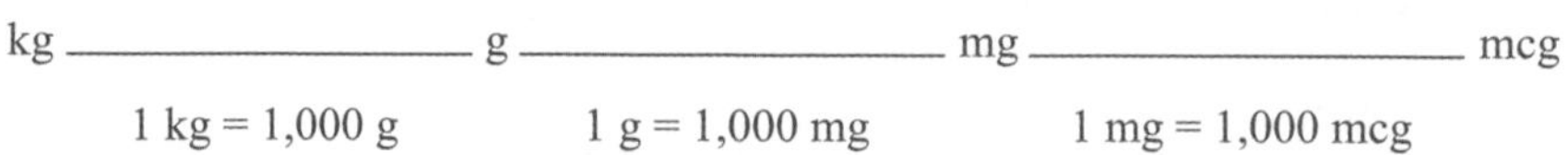

There is a 1,000-fold (3 decimal place) difference between *(kg & g)*, *(g & mg)*, & *(mg & mcg)*
There is a 1,000,000-fold (6 decimal place) difference between (kg & mg) & (g & mcg)
There is a 1,000,000,000-fold (9 decimal place) difference between (kg & mcg)

FIGURE 5.1 **Metric System Conversions.**

TABLE 5.2 Metric Conversions Used in Pharmacy

WEIGHT
1 kg = 1,000 g
1 g = 1,000 mg
1 mg = 1,000 mcg
VOLUME
1 L = 1,000 mL

! TECH ALERT

Be careful to distinguish between mcg, mg, g, and kg (weight) and mL and L (volume) to prevent medication errors. The abbreviation µg (mcg) is on the "Do Not Use" list but is still found on some medication labels.

The units used for weight in pharmacy are, from largest to smallest, kilogram, gram, milligram, and microgram, with a 1,000-fold or 3-decimal-place difference between each closest measurement. Fig. 5.1 is helpful for remembering this.

The units used for volume in pharmacy are, from largest to smallest, liter and milliliter, with a 1,000-fold or 3-decimal-place difference between each. The main conversion factor that is used in pharmacy for volume is 1 L = 1,000 mL (Table 5.2).

TECH NOTE

When numbers in an answer are 1,000 or more, add commas to avoid mistakes.

CONVERTING FROM LARGER METRIC NUMBERS TO SMALLER METRIC NUMBERS

The placement of the decimal point is based on moving through powers of 10 by moving the decimal point. First, determine the number of the decimal place difference between the two numbers. When converting from a larger metric unit to a smaller one, move the decimal point to the right by the number of the decimal place difference between the two *or* multiply by 1 plus the number of zeros in the equivalent (large unit to smaller unit → multiply). This method can be verified or checked by using R&P or DA as well. The following examples depict moving the decimal point, multiplying by 1 plus the number of zeros difference, R&P, and DA.

EXAMPLE 5.6

Moving the decimal or multiplying

1.2 L = ______ mL

A liter is larger than a milliliter by three place values, so move the decimal three places to the right or multiply by 1,000.

1.2 L becomes 1.2 0 0. or 1,200 mL

$$\begin{array}{r} 1.2 \\ \times \quad 1{,}000 \\ \hline 1{,}200.\not{0} \end{array}$$

$1.2\,\text{L} = 1{,}200\,\text{mL}$

Ratio and proportion

$$\frac{1\,\text{L}}{1{,}000\,\text{mL}} = \frac{1.2\,\text{L}}{x}$$

$$x = 1{,}200\,\text{mL}$$

Dimensional analysis

$$\text{mL} = \frac{1{,}000\,\text{mL}}{1\,\text{L}} \bullet \frac{1.2\,\text{L}}{1} = 1{,}200\,\text{mL}$$

EXAMPLE 5.7

Moving the decimal or multiplying

5.4 kg = ______ mg

A kilogram is larger than a milligram by six place values, so move the decimal six places to the right or multiply by 1,000,000.

5.4 kg becomes 5.4 0 0 0 0 0.

$$\begin{array}{r} 5.4 \\ \times \quad 1{,}000{,}000 \\ \hline 5{,}400{,}000.\not{0} \end{array}$$

$5.4\,\text{kg} = 5{,}400{,}000\,\text{mg}$

Ratio and proportion

$$\frac{1\,\text{kg}}{1{,}000{,}000\,\text{mg}} = \frac{5.4\,\text{kg}}{x} \quad x = 5{,}400{,}000\,\text{mg}$$

Dimensional analysis

If you are more comfortable moving from the closest unit in steps, DA analysis can be used.

$$\text{mg} = \frac{1{,}000\,\text{mg}}{1\,\text{g}} \bullet \frac{1{,}000\,\text{g}}{1\,\text{kg}} \bullet \frac{5.4\,\text{kg}}{1} = 5{,}400{,}000\,\text{mg}$$

TECH NOTE

To convert a **L**arger unit to a **S**maller unit, move the decimal to the **R**ight: **"L to S go R."**

CONVERTING FROM A SMALLER METRIC NUMBER TO A LARGER METRIC NUMBER

First, determine the number of the decimal place difference between the two numbers. When converting from a smaller metric unit to a larger one, move the decimal point to the left by the number of the decimal place difference between the two *or* divide by 1 plus the number of zeros in the equivalent (small unit to large unit → divide).

EXAMPLE 5.8

Moving the decimal or dividing

5 mg = ______ g

A milligram is smaller than a gram by three place values, so move the decimal three places to the left or divide by 1,000.

5 mg is the same as 0.0 0 5 g or 5 ÷ 1,000

$$5 \text{ mg} = 0.005 \text{ g}$$

Ratio and proportion

$$\frac{1,000 \text{ mg}}{1 \text{ g}} = \frac{5 \text{ mg}}{x}$$

$$1,000x = 5 \text{ g}$$

Divide both sides by 1,000.

$$x = 0.005 \text{ g}$$

Dimensional analysis

$$\text{g} = \frac{1 \text{ g}}{1,000 \text{ mg}} \bullet \frac{5 \text{ mg}}{1} = 0.005 \text{ g}$$

TECH NOTE

Always place a leading zero before the decimal point if the number is less than 1.

EXAMPLE 5.9

500 g = ______ kg

A gram is smaller than a kilogram by three place values, so move the decimal three places to the left or divide by 1,000.

500 g is the same as 0.5 0 0 kg or 500 ÷ 1,000

Because zeros at the end of a decimal (trailing zeros) can be dropped, the answer is 0.5 kg.

TECH NOTE

To convert from a **S**maller unit to a **L**arger unit, move the decimal to the **L**eft: **"S to L go L."**

Practice Problems B

Complete the following problems.

1. 2 L = ____________ mL
2. 2.5 mg = ____________ mcg
3. 4 kg = ____________ g
4. 450 g = ____________ kg
5. 0.5 L = ____________ mL
6. 0.5 mg = ____________ mcg
7. 0.5 mg = ____________ g
8. 2.5 mL = ____________ L
9. 50 mL = ____________ L
10. 5.5 L = ____________ mL
11. 1.5 g = ____________ mg
12. 6.54 kg = ____________ mg
13. 450 mg = ____________ g
14. 25 mcg = ____________ mg
15. 50.6 kg = ____________ g
16. 10 L = ____________ mL
17. 500 mL = ____________ L
18. 3,500 mL = ____________ L
19. 0.0045 kg = ____________ g
20. 0.3 mg = ____________ mcg
21. 5 mL = ____________ L
22. 58,400 mL = ____________ L

23. 510 mL = ____________ L

24. 300 mg = ____________ mcg

25. A container of IV fluids contains 0.5 L.

How many milliliters is this? ____________

26. Amoxicillin is available as 250 mg/capsule.

How many grams of amoxicillin does each capsule contain? ____________

27. A tablet of digoxin contains 250 mcg.

How would this be written in mg? ____________

28. A physician orders 1 g of Cipro (ciprofloxacin).

How many mg should be administered to the patient? ____________

29. A physician orders a thyroid replacement, Synthroid 0.175 mg.

How many micrograms would be given to the patient? ____________

30. A physician orders 1,500 mg of Keflex (cephalexin).

How many grams of cephalexin are in a 1,500 mg dose? ____________

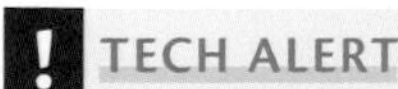

TECH ALERT

The abbreviation "cc" is on the ISMP *List of Error-Prone Abbreviations, Symbols, and Dose Designations* because of the danger of reading the abbreviation as "00" (zeros); the unit mL should be used instead.

APOTHECARY SYSTEM OF MEASUREMENT

The measurement of grains is still found on labels of nitroglycerin, codeine, phenobarbital, Armour Thyroid, aspirin, and ferrous sulfate (iron). Some physicians will order these medications, as well as acetaminophen, in grains, which is the apothecary unit used most in pharmacy. Apothecary symbols are found on the ISMP *List of Error-Prone Abbreviations, Symbols, and Dose Designations*. They will be used in Chapters 5 and 6 *only*. Apothecary equivalents that will be used as conversion factors in Practice Problems C are found in Table 5.3.

! TECH ALERT

Care should be taken that gr (grain) and g or gm (which is sometimes still seen used for gram) are not confused. These measurements have different weights and are in two separate measurement systems.

TABLE 5.3 Apothecary System Symbols and Equivalencies

MEASUREMENT	ABBREVIATION	EQUIVALENT
Volume		
1 minim	♏	
1 fluid dram	fl ʒ	♏ 60
1 fluid ounce	fl ℥	fl ʒ viii (8)
Weight		
1 grain[a]	gr	
1 dram	ʒ	gr 60
1 ounce	℥	ʒ viii (8)
1 pound	#	℥ xii (12)

[a]The only weight measurement frequently used in pharmacy is the grain.

TECH NOTE

Although symbols used for the apothecary system may be unfamiliar, they cancel just like units for the metric and household systems. Set these problems up the same as with those systems.

EXAMPLE 5.10

How many fluid drams are in 2 apothecary fluid ounces?

Ratio and proportion

Known Unknown

$$\frac{\text{℥ i}}{\text{ʒ viii}} \times \frac{\text{℥ ii}}{x}$$

1 • x = ʒ viii • ii (The math may be easier to perform if it is changed to 1 • x = ʒ 8 • 2

$$x = \text{ʒ } 16, \quad \text{so} \quad \frac{\text{℥ i}}{\text{ʒ viii}} = \frac{\text{℥ ii}}{\text{ʒ xvi}} \quad \text{or} \quad \text{℥ ii} = \text{ʒ xvi}$$

Single-step and multistep conversions can be solved using DA.

TECH NOTE

It may be easier to change your numbers to Arabic numerals while performing calculations. Just be sure to change your answer back into Roman numerals if necessary. This is especially helpful with multistep conversions using DA. Remember that apothecary symbols cancel the same as metric and household units.

Practice Problems C

Practice your skills in the apothecary system, using Roman numerals in your answers when required. Show your calculations.

1. flʒ vi = fl℥ ____________
2. fl℥ xii = flʒ ____________
3. gr iv = ʒ ____________
4. gr xxx = ʒ ____________
5. gr x = ʒ ____________
6. fl℥ v = flʒ ____________
7. fl℥ ii = flʒ ____________
8. flʒ iii = fl℥ ____________
9. ♏30 = flʒ ____________
10. ♏90 = flʒ ____________

REVIEW

Three measurement systems are used in medicine. The household system, used most commonly on a daily basis in the United States, is sometimes used for administration of liquid medications at home if an appropriate dispenser is not provided. Using the household system for volume provides only approximate measurements because of the differences in flatware and measuring spoons; it may lead to an inaccurate dose when used for administering medication. The metric system is used as a standard unit of measure throughout the world. Most medications are labeled and dosed in the metric system. The final system, rarely used today but still found with some medications, is the apothecary system. Although this system is not popular and its use is being discouraged, these measurements are still seen occasionally with some medications.

R&P and DA may be used for the calculation of conversions within a system. With the metric system, the decimal may be moved as a shortcut to make the necessary conversion.

Posttest

Using the appropriate system of measurement, figure the equivalents found in this posttest. Show your calculations.

1. 36 kg = ____________ g
2. 5.4 g = ____________ mg
3. 2 tsp = ____________ gtt
4. 4 Tbsp = ____________ tsp

Posttest, cont.

5. gr v = ʒ __________

6. flʒ x = fl℥ __________

7. 6 pt = __________ qt

8. 125 mcg = __________ mg

9. 12.5 mg = __________ g

10. 0.5 mL = __________ cc (on ISMP *List of Error-Prone Abbreviations*)

11. 1.75 L = __________ mL

12. 2 qt = __________ gal

13. 2 Tbsp = __________ oz

14. 4 oz = __________ c

15. 4 c = __________ pt

16. 0.4 mg = __________ mcg

17. 1.3 kg = __________ mg

18. 1 Tbsp = __________ oz

19. 4 oz = __________ tsp

20. flʒ xvi = fl℥ __________

21. 40.5 mg = __________ g

22. 40.5 mg = __________ mcg

23. 3.75 L = __________ mL

24. 12 c = __________ qt

25. 250 mg = __________ g

26. 0.25 g = __________ mg

27. 75 mL = __________ L

28. 250 mL = __________ L

Continued

Posttest, cont.

29. 2 tsp = ____________ Tbsp

30. 8 Tbsp = ____________ oz

31. 32 oz = ____________ c

32. 64 oz = ____________ pt

33. 24 tsp = ____________ oz

34. 1.2 mg = ____________ mcg

35. ʒ xxiv = ℥ ____________

36. 4 c = ____________ oz

37. 9 tsp = ____________ Tbsp

38. 55 mg = ____________ g

39. 600 mg = ____________ g

40. 650 mcg = ____________ mg

41. 15 Tbsp = ____________ oz

42. 15 tsp = ____________ oz

43. 0.05 g = ____________ mg

44. 0.0025 g = ____________ mg

45. 2.5 kg = ____________ g

46. A physician orders 1 Lanoxin (digoxin) 0.125-mg tablet. How many micrograms of medication is this?

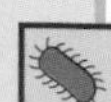

47. An order is given for amoxicillin 250 mg. How many grams is this?

Posttest, cont.

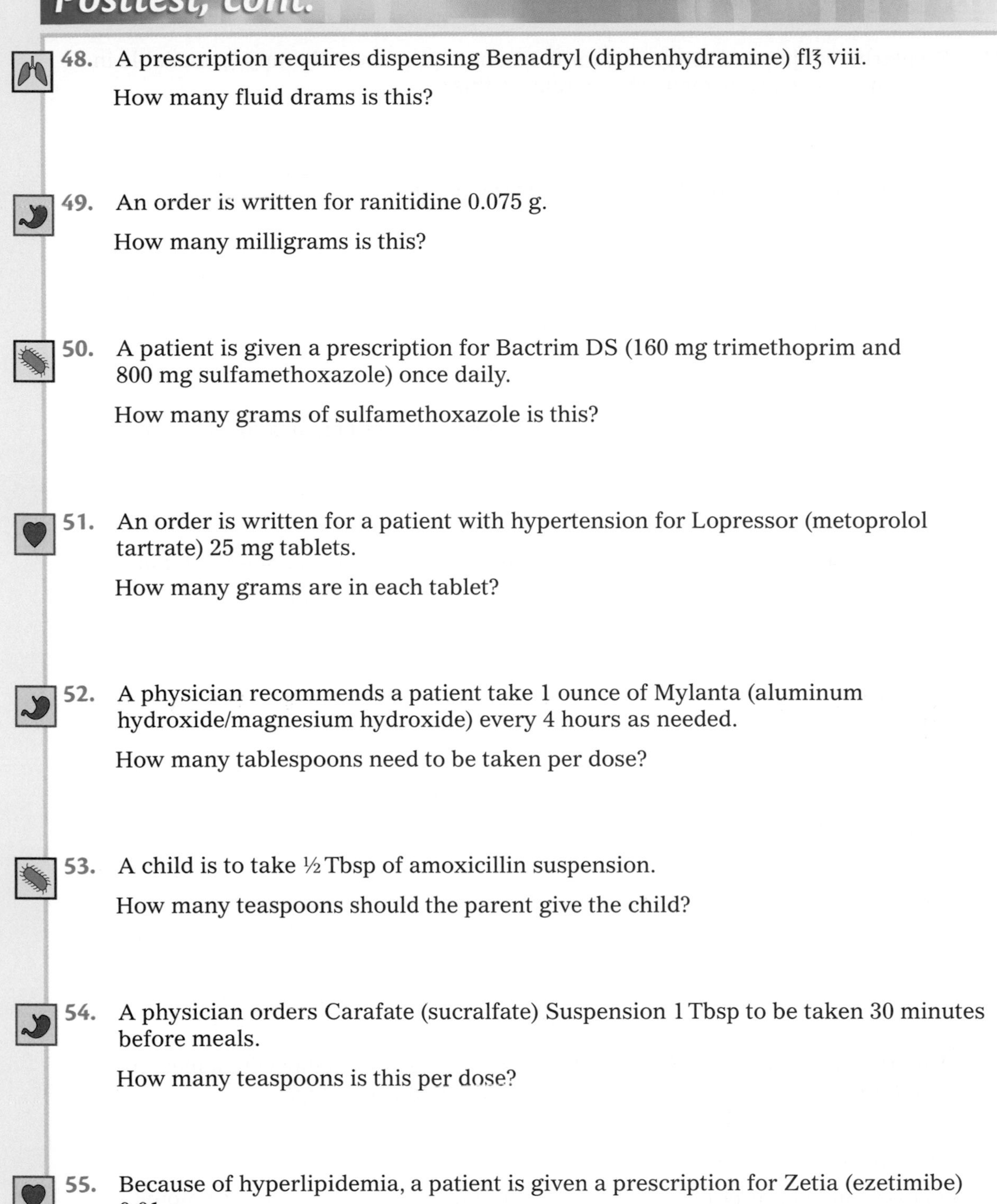

48. A prescription requires dispensing Benadryl (diphenhydramine) fl℥ viii.

How many fluid drams is this?

49. An order is written for ranitidine 0.075 g.

How many milligrams is this?

50. A patient is given a prescription for Bactrim DS (160 mg trimethoprim and 800 mg sulfamethoxazole) once daily.

How many grams of sulfamethoxazole is this?

51. An order is written for a patient with hypertension for Lopressor (metoprolol tartrate) 25 mg tablets.

How many grams are in each tablet?

52. A physician recommends a patient take 1 ounce of Mylanta (aluminum hydroxide/magnesium hydroxide) every 4 hours as needed.

How many tablespoons need to be taken per dose?

53. A child is to take ½ Tbsp of amoxicillin suspension.

How many teaspoons should the parent give the child?

54. A physician orders Carafate (sucralfate) Suspension 1 Tbsp to be taken 30 minutes before meals.

How many teaspoons is this per dose?

55. Because of hyperlipidemia, a patient is given a prescription for Zetia (ezetimibe) 0.01 g.

How many milligrams is this?

Continued

Posttest, cont.

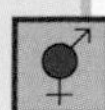

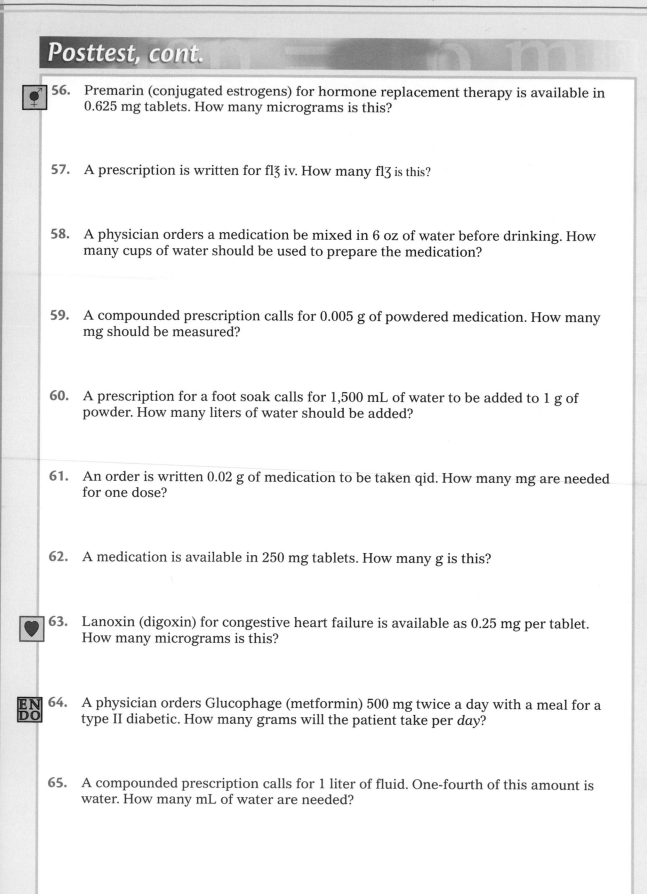

56. Premarin (conjugated estrogens) for hormone replacement therapy is available in 0.625 mg tablets. How many micrograms is this?

57. A prescription is written for fl℥ iv. How many flʒ is this?

58. A physician orders a medication be mixed in 6 oz of water before drinking. How many cups of water should be used to prepare the medication?

59. A compounded prescription calls for 0.005 g of powdered medication. How many mg should be measured?

60. A prescription for a foot soak calls for 1,500 mL of water to be added to 1 g of powder. How many liters of water should be added?

61. An order is written 0.02 g of medication to be taken qid. How many mg are needed for one dose?

62. A medication is available in 250 mg tablets. How many g is this?

63. Lanoxin (digoxin) for congestive heart failure is available as 0.25 mg per tablet. How many micrograms is this?

64. A physician orders Glucophage (metformin) 500 mg twice a day with a meal for a type II diabetic. How many grams will the patient take per *day*?

65. A compounded prescription calls for 1 liter of fluid. One-fourth of this amount is water. How many mL of water are needed?

Posttest, cont.

66. A patient is 6 1/4 feet tall. How many inches is he?

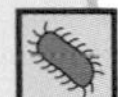

67. A patient is taking 500 mg of amoxicillin *every 8 hours* for bronchitis. How many grams is the patient receiving per *day*?

68. A patient is prescribed 1 g of antibiotic per day in *4 divided doses*. How many milligrams is the patient to receive per *dose*?

69. A doctor recommends drinking eight 8-ounce glasses of water per day. How many gallons is this?

70. A formulation for a batch of antiseptic calls for 14 quarts of water. How many gallons is this?

Conversions Between Measurement Systems

OBJECTIVES

1. Discuss conversions and conversion factors, including the rules for using ratio and proportion and dimensional analysis.
2. Describe how to perform conversions between household, apothecary, and metric systems of measurement.

KEY WORDS

Measurable amount The quantity of medication that can be most accurately measured with the device available

> **! TECH ALERT**
> When converting between two measurement systems, the answers will not be exact due to the differences between the measurement systems. Other factors include the viscosity of the medication and the size of the devices used to provide the medication.

Pretest

If you are already comfortable with the subject matter, answer the following to test your knowledge. If not, work your way through the chapter and return to them for extra practice. Show your calculations and round to the nearest tenth.

1. 1 oz = ____________ mL
2. 1 gal = ____________ mL
3. 2 kg = ____________#
4. 1 Tbsp = ____________ mL
5. 1# = ____________ g
6. 2 tsp = ____________ mL
7. 2 pt = ____________ mL
8. 4 oz = ____________ mL
9. 4 tsp = ʒ ____________
10. gr $\frac{1}{4}$ = ____________ mg

Pretest, cont.

11. 88# = ____________ kg

12. 120 mg = gr ____________

13. 180 mL = ____________ oz

14. 15 mL = ____________ tsp

15. 325 mg aspirin = gr ____________

16. 1 ½ tsp = ____________ mL

17. 15 tsp = ʒ ____________

18. nitroglycerin gr 1/150 = ____________ mg

19. nitroglycerin 0.6 mg = gr ____________

20. 60 g = ____________ oz

21. 2.5 mL = ____________ tsp

22. 3.84 L = ____________ gal

23. 4 Tbsp = ℥ ____________

24. 6″ = ____________ cm

25. 1 c = ____________ mL

26. 2 Tbsp = ____________ mL

27. codeine gr i = ____________ mg

28. 5 kg = ____________#

29. 44# = ____________ kg

30. flʒ vi = ____________ Tbsp

INTRODUCTION

The previous chapter covered conversions within the household, metric, and apothecary systems of measurement. The metric system is the most common and accurate. Because all three systems are used in the United States, conversions between the systems must be covered in detail. The two other units used in dosage calculations—milliequivalents and units—are rarely converted because they are unique to individual medications.

If a physician writes an order using one system and the medication is labeled using another, you need to convert the dose to an approximate equivalent to ensure that the patient receives the correct amount. Conversions between systems are approximations and may incur dosing variability. As the metric system becomes more widely accepted, the need for conversion will decrease, although the need to calculate a dose in household measurements will remain as long as the United States continues using the household system. Household measurements are more accurate when using actual measuring spoons as opposed to flatware; however, it is more appropriate to dispense a measuring device to ensure accurate dosing in the home environment because people may use their own flatware, which varies greatly in measurements.

CONVERSION FACTORS

Conversion factors are equivalents between two measurements, whether within the same system or between different systems. Each part of a conversion factor includes a value (number) and a label (unit of measurement).

TECH NOTE

The **value** of a conversion factor is always 1. It is used to *change one unit to another* **without** changing the value of the original measurement. For example, 5 mL = 1 tsp has a numerical *value* of 1.

Table 6.1 lists necessary equivalents between the three systems of measurement that are used as conversion factors. The **bolded** conversion factors used most often in pharmaceutical calculations should be committed to memory.

TABLE 6.1 Common Conversions: Metric, Apothecary, and Household Systems of Measurement

PARAMETER	APOTHECARY UNITS	HOUSEHOLD UNITS	METRIC UNITS
VOLUME	♏ i	1 gtt	
		20 gtt	1 mL
	flʒ i	1 tsp	5 mL
	fl℥ $\overline{ss}$	1 Tbsp	15 mL
	fl℥ i	1 oz	30 mL
	fl℥ viii	1 c	240 mL
	1 pt	1 pt	473.2 mL/480 mL[a]
	1 qt	1 qt	960 mL
	1 gal	1 gal	3,840 mL
MASS/WEIGHT	gr i	N/A	60–65 mg
	℥ i	1 oz	30 g
	[b]	1# or 1 lb	454 g
		2.2#	1 kg
LENGTH		1″	2.54 cm

[a]The exact conversion is 1 pt = 473.2 mL. The approximate value of 1 pt = 480 mL is often used in conversions because 1 pt = 16 oz and 1 oz = 30 mL. **1 pt = 480 mL** will be used in this text.

[b]An apothecary pound contains only 12 oz, whereas a household pound contains 16 oz, which is considered to be equivalent to 454 g. The apothecary pound is not used in this text.

TECH NOTE

Remember that equivalents between systems are approximate, not exact; therefore, when converting between two measurement systems, the conversion is approximate. The final answer should always be one that is measurable in the system; 1.7 tsp would be 1 ¾ tsp in household measurements, because 0.7 tsp cannot be measured.

As you can see from Table 6.1, the apothecary grain has a range of equivalencies. The conversion between grains and milligrams actually varies between different medications. Table 6.2 illustrates some of the more common medications that are still dosed in both grains and milligrams. *Any* conversion with grains is an approximation. Another approximation is that a dram is sometimes considered equivalent to a teaspoon, which is equivalent to 5 mL, when a dram is actually given a range from 4 to 5 mL in the metric system.

The conversion of 20 drops per 1 mL is based on a viscosity close to that of water. Remember that the number of drops varies according to drop size and thickness of the liquid. This conversion is *not used* in dosing because medications dosed in drops come with a specific dropper for administration. It is mostly used for determining day's supply with eyedrops or eardrops for submission to insurance companies.

TECH ALERT

Medicine droppers provided by the manufacturer with specific medications are the only ones that are guaranteed to deliver the correct dose. Random droppers may not deliver the correct amount.

TABLE 6.2 Common Medications Dosed in Grains and Milligrams

MEDICATION	CONVERSION FACTOR
codeine NTG SL—sublingual nitroglycerin Armour Thyroid phenobarbital*	**60 mg/gr**
ASA—aspirin APAP—acetaminophen ferrous sulfate—iron	**65 mg/gr**

*Phenobarbital also comes in strengths based on 64.8 mg/gr.

Practice Problems A

After reviewing Tables 6.1 and 6.2, complete the following.

1. 1 oz = ____________ g
2. gr i aspirin = ____________ mg
3. 1 tsp = ____________ mL
4. 1 pt = ____________ mL
5. 1 gal = ____________ mL
6. 1 Tbsp = ____________ mL

7. fl3 i = ______________ tsp

8. 1# = ______________ g

9. 1 kg = ______________ #

10. 1 oz = ______________ mL

11. gr i codeine = ______________ mg

12. 1 mL = ______________ gtt

CONVERSIONS

If one factor is in one system, such as the metric system, and the other factor is in another system, such as the household system, either ratio and proportion (R&P) or dimensional analysis (DA) may be used for conversion. *Always* use DA with multistep problems to keep track of units.

POINTS TO REMEMBER

RULES FOR USING RATIO AND PROPORTION

- Set up the conversion ratio with the known conversion units on the left of the equation.
- Set up the second ratio of the proportion with the conversion units for the unknowns.
- Label the units so that the like unit is placed in the same position within each R&P. This sets the ratios so that they are equivalent to each other.
- Cross-multiply and divide to solve for the unknown.

EXAMPLE 6.1

A physician orders a 10-mL dose of antibiotic tid. How many teaspoons constitute one dose? This is a single-step conversion, so it is performed easily with R&P.

R&P $\frac{1 \text{ tsp}}{5 \text{ mL}} = \frac{x}{10 \text{ mL}}$

$5x = 10$ tsp   Divide both sides by 5.

$x = 2$ tsp

POINTS TO REMEMBER

RULES FOR USING DIMENSIONAL ANALYSIS

- Identify the unit of the *answer* needed followed by an equal sign.
- Set up a fraction such that the unit of the *desired* answer is in the numerator of the first fraction of the DA equation—this unit will *never* be canceled.
- Set up the next fraction in the equation so the unit in its numerator is the same as the unit in the denominator of the first fraction (so these units will cancel when the fractions are multiplied).
- Continue this process when dealing with multistep problems.
- Cancel units to ensure proper setup of the fractions.
- Multiply the numerators and denominators.
- Complete the problem by reducing if necessary.

EXAMPLE 6.2

A physician orders a 10-mL dose of antibiotic tid. How many teaspoons constitute one dose?

$$\textbf{DA}\quad \text{tsp} = \frac{1\ \text{tsp}}{5\ \text{mL}} \times \frac{10\ \text{mL}}{1} = 2\ \text{tsp}$$

! TECH ALERT

When using DA, be sure to place the unit desired for the answer in the numerator of the first fraction and follow with the additional information in the sequence needed to cancel all unnecessary units.

CONVERSIONS BETWEEN HOUSEHOLD AND APOTHECARY SYSTEMS

The apothecary system has only a few measurements that, although not commonly used, do convert into household measurements. Of note are minims to drops, drams to teaspoons, and ounces to tablespoons (Fig. 6.1). Cups, pints, quarts, and gallons are used by both systems. Length is not measured in the apothecary system.

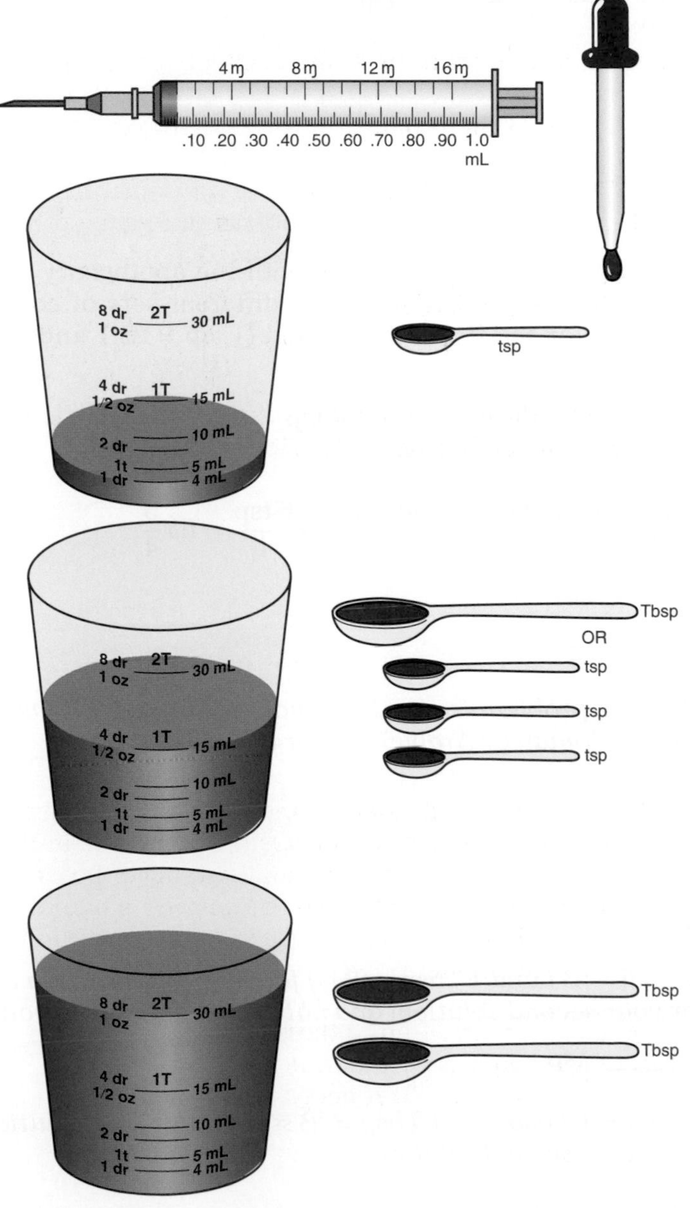

FIGURE 6.1 **Equivalents Between Apothecary and Household Measurements.**

Although the single-step conversions can be performed using ratio and proportion or dimensional analysis, use DA when converting with the apothecary system to keep better track of the units. It is easier to write out the words and convert all numbers to Arabic when performing the math and then change the answer back to Roman numerals and symbols. Remember, this is a learning experience only, as the apothecary symbols are prone to misinterpretation and the recommendation is to use the metric system.

> **! TECH ALERT**
> Do not confuse the symbols for ʒ (dram) and ℥ (ounce). If it is difficult to work with the symbols, use the words in your R&P or DA setup. Just remember to change the answer back to symbols if it is an apothecary measurement.

EXAMPLE 6.3

flʒ iii = ________ tsp

Use the conversion factor 1 tsp = flʒ i

$$\text{tsp} = \frac{1\ \text{tsp}}{1\ \text{fluid dram}} \bullet \frac{3\ \text{fluid dram}}{1} = 3\ \text{tsp}$$

D DAS

EXAMPLE 6.4

6 tsp = fl℥ ____________

To illustrate just how approximate conversion with the apothecary system can be, solve this multistep question using the following two different *sets* of conversions: (3 tsp = 1 Tbsp and 1 Tbsp = fl℥ $\overline{\text{ss}}$) for the first solution and (1 tsp = flʒ 1 and flʒ viii = fl℥ i) for the second solution.

$$\text{fluid ounce} = \frac{1/2\ \text{fluid ounce}}{1\ \text{Tbsp}} \bullet \frac{1\ \text{Tbsp}}{3\ \text{tsp}} \bullet \frac{6\ \text{tsp}}{1} = \text{fl℥ i}$$

$$\text{fluid ounce} = \frac{1\ \text{fluid ounce}}{8\ \text{fluid dram}} \bullet \frac{1\ \text{fluid dram}}{1\ \text{tsp}} \bullet \frac{6\ \text{tsp}}{1} = \text{fl℥}\ \frac{3}{4}$$

Practice Problems B

Calculate the following problems using DA. Show your calculations. Be sure to use the correct numeral form (Roman or Arabic) in your answers.

1. 2 tsp = flʒ ____________

2. 16 gtt = ♏ ____________

3. 4 Tbsp = flʒ ____________

Solve #3 using: (flʒ viii = fl℥ i and 1 Tbsp = fl℥ $\overline{\text{ss}}$) for your first solution and (1 tsp = flʒ i and 3 tsp = 1 Tbsp) for your second solution, and note the difference in your answers.

4. fl℥ $\overline{\text{ss}}$= ____________ tsp

Solve #4 using: (3 tsp = 1 Tbsp and 1 Tbsp = fl℥ $\overline{\text{ss}}$) for your first solution and (1 tsp = flʒ i and flʒ viii = fl℥ i) for your second solution.

5. 24 gtt = ♏ ______________

6. flʒ v = ______________ tsp

7. 3 Tbsp = fl℥ ______________

8. 8 c = fl℥ ______________

9. fl℥ xxiv = ______________ c

10. 4 tsp = fl℥ ______________

Solve #10 using: (3 tsp = 1 Tbsp and 1 Tbsp = fl℥ $\overline{\text{ss}}$) for your first solution and (1 tsp = flʒ i and flʒ viii = fl℥ i) for your second solution.

11. 30 tsp = fl℥ ______________

Solve #11 using: (3 tsp = 1 Tbsp and 1 Tbsp = fl℥ $\overline{\text{ss}}$) for your first solution and (1 tsp = flʒ i and flʒ viii = fl℥ i) for your second solution.

12. flʒ xxx = ______________ Tbsp

13. A physician writes a prescription for ʒ ii of Robitussin cough medication q4h.

How much is this in household measurements? ______________

How often will the person take the medication? ______________

14. The directions on the bottle of Maalox read fl℥ i$\overline{\text{ss}}$ q3–4h prn indigestion.

How many tablespoons are equivalent to one dose? ______________

How often can a dose be taken? ______________

15. A physician writes a prescription for MiraLAX one capful in H_2O fl℥ viii.

How could you tell the patient to easily measure the water? *(Hint: convert to household measurement.)* ______________

CONVERSIONS BETWEEN HOUSEHOLD AND METRIC UNITS

Most conversions from metric to household, such as milliliters to teaspoons or ounces, are volume conversions, although length from inches to centimeters is sometimes used in the medical field. Fig. 6.2 illustrates some of the conversions from Table 6.1.

EXAMPLE 6.5

60 mL = _______________ oz

$$\frac{1\text{ oz}}{30\text{ mL}} = \frac{x}{60\text{ mL}}$$

$30x = 60$ oz Divide both sides by 30.

$x = 2$ oz

EXAMPLE 6.6

4′ = _______________ cm

Because most of us do not know how many centimeters are in 1 foot, this is calculated more easily as a multistep DA equation using two familiar conversion factors.

$$\text{cm} = \frac{2.54\text{ cm}}{1\text{ in}} \times \frac{12\text{ in}}{1\text{ ft}} \times \frac{4\text{ ft}}{1} = 121.92\text{ cm}$$

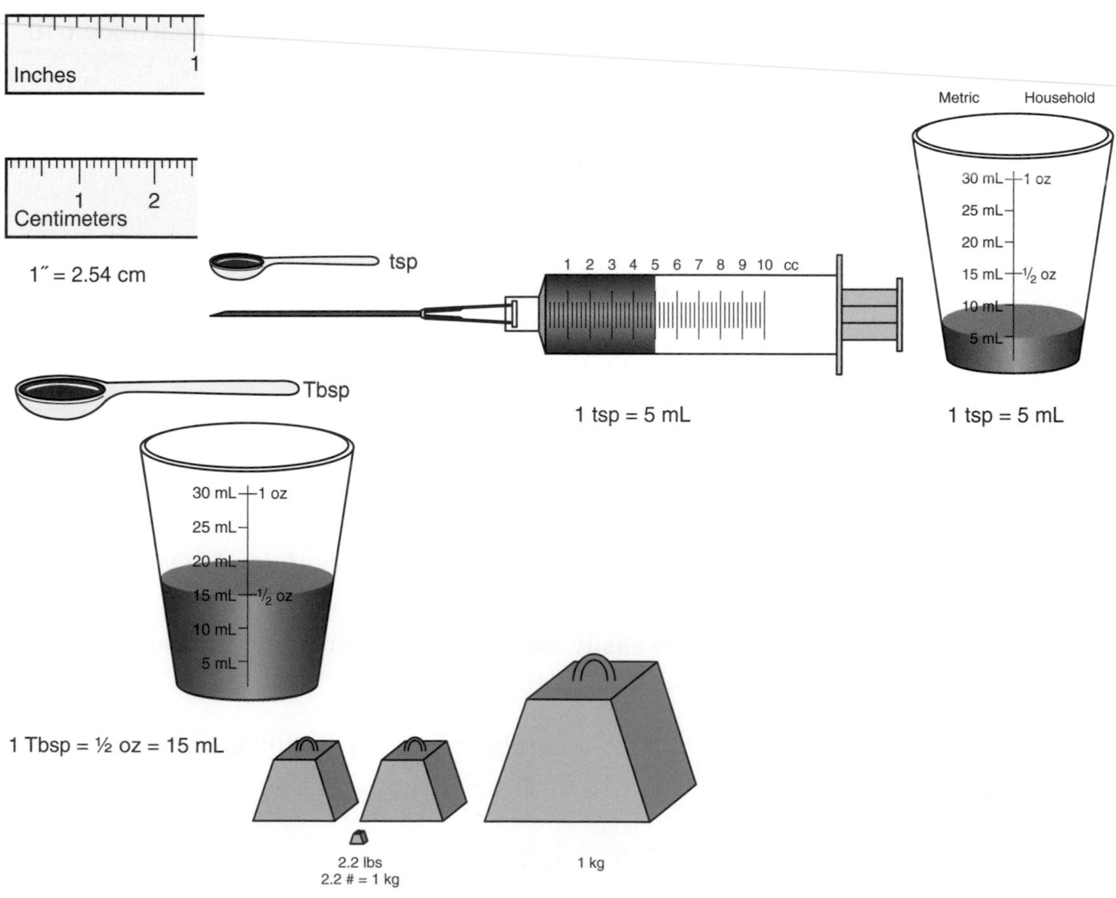

FIGURE 6.2 **Equivalents Between Household and Metric Measurements.**

TECH NOTE

When converting between systems, make sure the answer is a **measurable amount**. For example, an answer of 0.9 tsp should be rounded to 1 tsp.

Practice Problems C

Calculate the following conversions. Use fractions with the household system and decimals with the metric system. Use DA with multistep problems. Round to the nearest tenth. Show your calculations.

1. 16 oz = ______________ mL

2. 8 kg = ______________#

3. 3 tsp = ______________ mL

4. 2 pt = ______________ mL

5. 5″ = ______________ cm

6. 3 c = ______________ mL

7. 90 mL = ______________ oz

8. 10.2 cm = ______________

9. 75 mL = ______________ oz

10. 10 kg = ______________#

11. 720 mL = ______________ pt

12. 720 mL = ______________ qt

13. 10 tsp = ______________ mL

14. 500 mL = ______________ qt

15. 6 tsp = ______________ mL

16. 1.5 L = ______________ pt

17. 10 c = ______________ L

18. 5 ft = ______________ cm

19. A physician writes an order for an anthelmintic for a child weighing 35#. The dosage must be calculated in mg/kg body weight.

How many kilograms does the child weigh?

20. 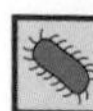 A physician writes a prescription for 5 mL of Zithromax (azithromycin) liquid for a child.

How many teaspoons would you tell the parent to give the child?

CONVERSIONS BETWEEN METRIC AND APOTHECARY SYSTEMS

The metric system uses grams, liters, and meters, whereas the apothecary system uses grains, minims, drams, and ounces.

The following important conversions to remember are approximations, as stated earlier in the chapter:

MASS	VOLUME
gr i = 60–65 mg	flʒ i = 5 mL
1 g = gr xv	fl℥ i = 30 mL

TECH NOTE

The conversions are approximate, NOT EXACT, so use the conversion that will give you a measurable answer.

An interesting way to remember the strengths of medications based on the conversion gr i = 60 mg is to think of a clock. There are 60 minutes in 1 hour, just as there are 60 mg in 1 grain. Therefore, if you think of $\frac{1}{4}$ of an hour as being 15 minutes, gr $\frac{1}{4}$ = 15 mg. Likewise, if you think of $\frac{1}{2}$ hour as being 30 minutes, gr $\frac{1}{2}$ = 30 mg, and if you think of $\frac{3}{4}$ of an hour as being 45 minutes, gr $\frac{3}{4}$ = 45 mg.

R&P or DA may be used for conversions as desired.

EXAMPLE 6.7

codeine 15 mg = gr _______

R&P

$$\frac{\text{gr i}}{60\text{ mg}} = \frac{x}{15\text{ mg}}$$

$60x = \text{gr } 15$ Divide both sides by 60.

$x = \frac{1}{4} = \text{gr } \frac{1}{4}$

DA

$$\text{gr} = \frac{\text{gr i}}{60\text{ mg}} \times \frac{15\text{ mg}}{1} = \frac{\text{gr } 15}{60} = \text{gr } \frac{1}{4}$$

EXAMPLE 6.8

NTGSL gr $^1/_{100}$ = ___ mg

R&P

$$\frac{\text{gr i}}{60\text{ mg}} = \frac{\text{gr }\frac{1}{100}}{x}$$

$$x = 60\text{ mg} \bullet \frac{1}{100} = \frac{60}{100}\text{ mg} = 0.6\text{ mg}$$

DA

$$\text{mg} = \frac{60\text{ mg}}{\text{gri}} \times \frac{\text{gr }\frac{1}{100}}{1} = 60\text{ mg} \times \frac{1}{100} = \frac{60}{100}\text{ mg} = \frac{6}{10}\text{ mg} = 0.6\text{ mg}$$

Practice Problems D

Calculate the following practice problems. ***If no medication is specified****, use gr i = 60 mg. Show all of your calculations.*

1. acetaminophen gr v = __________ mg
2. 45 mL = fl℥ __________
3. 15 mg = gr __________
4. 60 mL = flʒ __________
5. 1.5 mL = ♏ ________ (use 1 mL = ♏ xvi)
6. gr viis̄s̄ = __________ g
7. 750 mL = fl℥ __________
8. NTG SL gr $\frac{1}{150}$ = __________ mg
9. codeine gr s̄s̄= __________ mg
10. 15 mL = fl℥ __________
11. NTG SL 0.3 mg = gr __________
12. gr $\frac{3}{4}$ = __________ mcg
13. 4 mL = ♏ __________ (use 1 mL = ♏ xv)

14. A physician writes a medication order for phenobarbital gr $\overline{\text{iss}}$. The available medication is phenobarbital 30 mg tablets.

How many tablets should be administered? ______________

15. A prescription is written for phenobarbital gr $\frac{1}{4}$. The medication stock bottle reads phenobarbital 30 mg per unscored tablet.

What strength in mg should be used for the dose? ______________

Is this the correct medication stock bottle for the prescription? ______________

TECH NOTE

Nitroglycerin sublingual (NTG SL) tablets are available in three strengths, which are ordered in either milligrams or grains. It is a good idea to learn the strength conversions to verify that your conversion calculations are correct.

NTG SL gr $1/200$ 0.3 mg $\left(60 \text{ mg} \times \frac{1}{200}\right)$

NTG SL gr $1/150$ 0.4 mg $\left(60 \text{ mg} \times \frac{1}{150}\right)$

NTG SL gr $1/100$ 0.6 mg $\left(60 \text{ mg} \times \frac{1}{100}\right)$

REVIEW

Conversions between measurement systems are approximations, and some will vary depending on the conversion factor used. The metric system is the most accurate method of measurement and therefore is used exclusively when compounding prescriptions and preparing intravenous medications.

Conversions within and between measurement systems may be accomplished using either R&P or DA. Once you learn the basic equivalencies listed in Table 6.3, you should be able to accomplish almost any conversion needed in the pharmacy setting.

TABLE 6.3 Common Measurements and Conversions

HOUSEHOLD LIQUID MEASUREMENTS (VOLUME)		
1 drop	Gtt	
1 teaspoon	Tsp	60 drops (varies with viscosity and dropper size)
1 tablespoon	Tbsp	3 teaspoons
1 ounce	Oz	2 Tbsp
1 cup	C	8 oz
I pint	Pt	2 c
1 quart	Qt	2 pt
1 gallon	Gal	4 qt
HOUSEHOLD DRY WEIGHT MEASUREMENT		
1 pound	lb or #	16 oz
METRIC WEIGHT MEASUREMENTS		
1 kg = 1,000 g		
1 g = 1,000 mg		
1 mg = 1,000 mcg		
METRIC VOLUME MEASUREMENTS		
1 L = 1,000 mL		
HOUSEHOLD TO METRIC CONVERSIONS		
Volume		
1 tsp = 5 mL		
1 Tbsp = 15 mL		
1 fl oz = 30 mL		
1 pt = 480 mL		
1 gal = 3,840 mL		
Dry Weight		
1# = 454 g		
2.2# = 1 kg		
1 oz = 30 g		
APOTHECARY SYSTEM VOLUME		
1 minim	♏	♏ 60
1 fluid dram	fl ʒ	♏ 60
1 fluid ounce	fl ℥	fl ʒ viii (8)
APOTHECARY SYSTEM WEIGHT		
1 grain	Gr	
1 dram	ʒ	gr 60
1 ounce	℥	ʒ viii (8)
APPROXIMATE CONVERSIONS		
gr i = 60–65 mg		
60 mg with codeine, phenobarbital,[a] and NTG SL		
65 mg with ASA, APAP, and iron		
fl ʒ i = 1 tsp = 5 mL		
fl ℥ i = 2 Tbsp = 30 mL		
MISCELLANEOUS		
Drops: 20 gtt = 1 mL (mostly used for day's supply calculations for insurance companies)		

[a]Some phenobarbital doses are based on gr i = 64.8 mg.

Posttest

Use the correct numeral form (Roman or Arabic) for each system. Be sure the answers are measurable doses. Use either R&P or DA. Round all answers to the nearest tenth. If no medication is specified, use gr i = 60 mg.

1. 3 tsp = fl℥ ____________
2. 6 tsp = ____________ mL
3. codeine gr ¾ = ____________ mg
4. flʒ v = ____________ mL
5. 88# = ____________ kg
6. 0.6 mg = ____________ gr
7. 1,250 mL = ____________ pt
8. 2.5 mL = ____________ gtt
9. 4 qt = ____________ L
10. 45 mg = gr ____________
11. fl℥ 24 = ____________ c
12. 16 Tbsp = fl℥ ____________
13. 17″ = ____________ cm
14. 46# = ____________ kg
15. 0.1 mg = gr ____________
16. 2,500 g = ____________#
17. 12 mL = ____________ gtt
18. 45 mL = flʒ ____________
19. 45 mL = ____________ tsp
20. gr $\frac{1}{200}$ = ____________ mg
21. 5 Tbsp = fl℥ ____________
22. 10 kg = ____________#
23. 328 cm = ____________″
24. 35 mL = ____________ tsp
25. gr 45 = ____________ g (use 1 g = gr xv)
26. aspirin gr x = ____________ mg
27. 2,500 mL = ____________ pt
28. 3 tsp = ____________ mL

Posttest, cont.

29. 50 gtt = ____________ mL

30. 110# = ____________ kg

31. 2 pt = ____________ mL

32. 240 mL = ____________ qt

33. 100 gtt = ____________ mL

34. codeine gr $\overline{\text{iss}}$ = ____________ mg

35. gr 1/60 = ____________ mg

36. 168# = ____________ kg

37. 1 c = ____________ mL

38. 120 mL = ____________ pt

39. 220 # = ____________ kg

40. 4 Tbsp = ____________ mL

41. 5′8″ = ____________ cm

42. 325 mg of aspirin = gr ____________

43. 10 oz = ____________ mL

44. 2 tsp = ____________ mL

45. 2 Tbsp = ____________ mL

46. 12 kg = ____________ #

47. 37.5 mL = ____________ Tbsp

48. An adult places an NTG SL tablet gr 1/150 under his tongue for chest pain. How many milligrams is this?

49. If a patient is prescribed 30 mL of medication, how many tablespoons would this be?

50. A patient is to take 30 mL of an antacid. How many teaspoons should the patient take?

51. A child weighs 68#. How many kilograms does the child weigh?

Continued

Posttest, cont.

52. A female is 5′5″ tall. What is her height in centimeters?

53. Three-fourths of a pint of medication is on the shelf. How many milliliters are left in the container?

54. A prescription requires 90 mL of Zantac (ranitidine) for GERD (gastroesophageal reflux disease). How many ounces are needed to fill this prescription?

55. A medication order in a hospital reads Tylenol (acetaminophen) gr xv ASAP for headache. How many milligrams is this?

56. A prescription calls for 6 oz of cough medicine. How many mL is this?

57. A premature baby weighs 5 ½#. How many *grams* is this?

58. A physician orders acetylsalicylic acid 325 mg. Available are gr v tablets.

PA IN

Should this medication be used for the order? ______________ Why or why not?

59. A child is to receive Benadryl elixir 7.5 mL. The parent needs to give this with a teaspoon.

How many teaspoons should the parent give per dose?

60. A physician orders atropine sulfate 0.4 mg as a preoperative order.

How many grains will the patient receive?

IN SECTION III

SECTION III

Calculations With Prescriptions and Medication Orders

CHAPTER 7

Interpretation of Prescriptions, Medication Orders and Stock Labels

OBJECTIVES

1. Discuss what a prescription indicates, and describe the components of a prescription.
2. Describe what a medication order is, and list the parts of a medication order.
3. Interpret stock medication labels.

KEY WORDS

Auxiliary label Label added to prescriptions to provide important supplementary instructions

Dosage strength Weight of medication in a dose

Generic name Official nonproprietary name approved for a drug by the U.S. Food and Drug Administration (FDA)

Indication Reason to prescribe a medication

Inscription Part of prescription indicating medication name, dosage form, strength, and quantity

Medication order Physician's written or verbal direction for administration of medication in an inpatient health care setting

National Drug Code (NDC) Unique number on a drug product label that identifies the manufacturer, product, and size of container

Pharmacokinetics Movement of drugs through the body; absorption, distribution, metabolism, and excretion

Pharmacotherapeutics Uses and effects of drugs in treatment of conditions and diseases in the body

Prescription Written order by a licensed health care professional for dispensing medications

Scheduled medications **Classification of medications with potential for abuse and misuse:** CII, CIII, CIV, and CV

Signa (Sig) Part of prescription; directions for the patient—how, how much, when, how long

Subscription Part of a prescription that contains instructions for the pharmacist on how to compound if necessary

Superscription Part of a prescription designated with the symbol ℞, meaning, "Take this drug"

Toxicology Study of adverse toxic reactions or toxic levels of chemicals and drugs

Trade/Brand name Proprietary name given to a medication by the manufacturer

Pretest

If you are already comfortable with the subject matter, complete the Pretest to test your knowledge. If not, work your way through the chapter and return to it for extra practice. For the prescriptions, write the directions in lay terms as they should be written on a prescription label for the patient. Inpatient medication orders just need to be interpreted.

1. Prescription: penicillin 250 mg po qid × 10 days
   In stock: penicillin 250 mg tablets
   Label directions: ______________________________
   ____

2. Prescription: nitroglycerin 0.4 mg SL q5min × 3 doses prn; if no relief, call 9-1-1
   In stock: NTG 0.4 mg SL tablets
   Label directions: ______________________________
   ____

3. Prescription: hydrochlorothiazide 25 mg i tab po qam prn swelling
   In stock: HCTZ 25 mg tablets
   Label directions: ______________________________
   ____

ENDO

4. Prescription: Synthroid 0.025 mg po daily @ 8 am
   In stock: Synthroid 25 mcg tablets
   Label directions: ______________________________
   ____

5. Prescription: Premarin 1.25 mg tab po daily × 21 days
   In stock: Premarin 1.25 mg tablets
   Label directions: ______________________________
   ____

6. Prescription: Zithromax 250 mg tab ii po stat, then tab i po daily on days 2 to 5
   In stock: Zithromax 250 mg tablets:
   Label directions: ______________________________
   ____

Pretest, cont.

7. Prescription: Lanoxin 0.25 mg tab po qam if P 60 or ↑

   In stock: Lanoxin 250 mcg tablets

   Label directions: ______________________________

   ____

8. Lawrence Merry, M.D.
   4th Street and Jones Ave.
   Holly, GA 00111
   phone# - 001-555-2176

   Patient Name______________ Date ______
   Address______________ Age ______

   ] Pen-V 250 mg
   #40
   Sig: i tab po q6h

   ______________ Refill ______
   DEA#______________

   Label directions: ______________________________

   ____

9. Lawrence Merry, M.D.
   4th Street and Jones Ave.
   Holly, GA 00111
   phone# - 001-555-2176

   Patient Name______________ Date ______
   Address______________ Age ______

   ] Thorazine 100 mg
   #100
   Sig: tab i po tid

   ______________ Refill ______
   DEA#______________

   Label directions: ______________________________

   ____

Continued

Pretest, cont.

10.

Lawrence Merry, M.D.
4th Street and Jones Ave.
Holly, GA 00111
phone# - 001-555-2176

Patient Name________________________ Date ________
Address____________________________ Age ________

] tetracycline 250 mg
#120
Sig: ii cap po qid x 2wk; i cap po bid x 2wk; then i cap po daily

______________________ Refill ______
DEA#__________________

Label directions: ____

____

11.

Lawrence Merry, M.D.
4th Street and Jones Ave.
Holly, GA 00111
phone# - 001-555-2176

Patient Name________________________ Date ________
Address____________________________ Age ________

] furosemide 40 mg
#30
Sig: i tab po daily @ 10am

______________________ Refill ______
DEA#__________________

Label directions: ____

____

Pretest, cont.

12.

Lawrence Merry, M.D.
4th Street and Jones Ave.
Holly, GA 00111
phone# - 001-555-2176

Patient Name________________________ Date ________
Address___________________________ Age ________

]
lovastatin 10 mg
#30
Sig: i tab po daily c̄ evening meal or at bedtime c̄ snack for hyperlipidemia

________________________ Refill ______
DEA#____________________

Label directions: ____

____

13.

Lawrence Merry, M.D.
4th Street and Jones Ave.
Holly, GA 00111
phone# - 001-555-2176

Patient Name________________________ Date ________
Address___________________________ Age ________

]
Humulin 70/30
10 mL vial
Sig: 22 units subcutaneously qam

________________________ Refill ______
DEA#____________________

Label directions: ____

____

Continued

Pretest, cont.

ENDO 14.

Lawrence Merry, M.D.
4th Street and Jones Ave.
Holly, GA 00111
phone# - 001-555-2176

Patient Name ______________ Date ________
Address ______________ Age ________

]
Reg Insulin
10 mL vial
Sig: 16 units subcutaneously qam and 20 units subcutaneously 30 min ac evening meal

______________ Refill ______
DEA# ______________

Label directions:

____

____

15.

Lawrence Merry, M.D.
4th Street and Jones Ave.
Holly, GA 00111
phone# - 001-555-2176

Patient Name ______________ Date ________
Address ______________ Age ________

]
diazepam 10 mg
#30
Sig: ss – i tab po q4-6h prn anxiety or muscle spasms

______________ Refill ______
DEA# ______________

Label directions:

____

____

Pretest, cont.

16.[a]

Lawrence Merry, M.D.
4th Street and Jones Ave.
Holly, GA 00111
phone# - 001-555-2176

Patient Name__________ Date ______
Address__________ Age ______

] Robitussin DM syrup ℥viii
Sig: ʒii po q4-6h prn cough

__________ Refill ______
DEA#__________

Prescription interpretation: ____________________

Label directions: ____________________

PAIN 17. Medication order: meperidine 50 mg and promethazine 25 mg IM q4–6h prn pain
Interpretation: ____________________

18. Medication order: metoprolol 50 mg po bid
Interpretation: ____________________

19. Medication order: temazepam 7.5 mg i-ii po at bedtime prn sleep
Interpretation: ____________________

[a]Apothecary symbols for drams and ounces are on the ISMP *List of Error-Prone Abbreviations, Symbols, and Dose Designations.*

Continued

Pretest, cont.

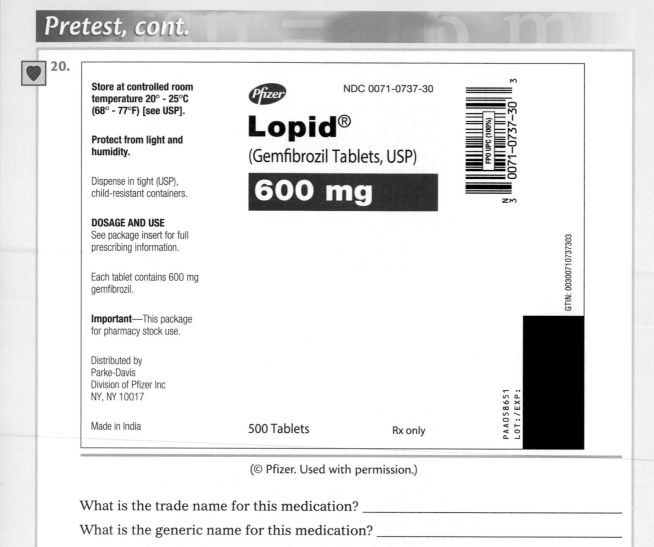

20.

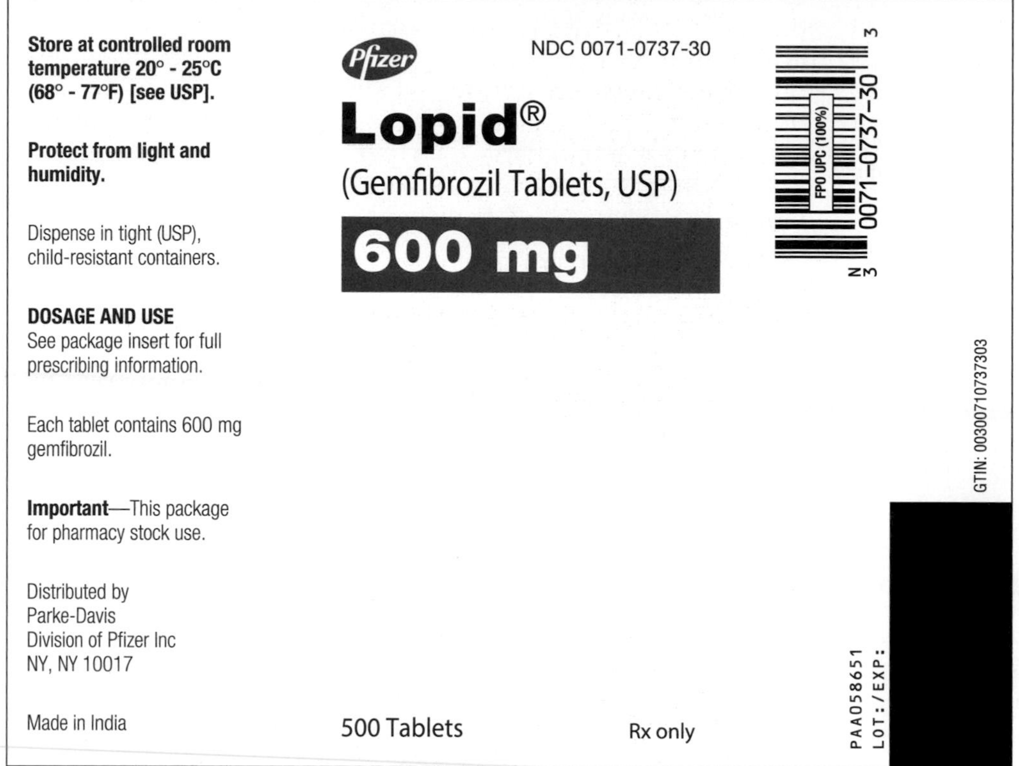
Store at controlled room temperature 20° - 25°C (68° - 77°F) [see USP].
Protect from light and humidity.
Dispense in tight (USP), child-resistant containers.
DOSAGE AND USE
See package insert for full prescribing information.
Each tablet contains 600 mg gemfibrozil.
Important—This package for pharmacy stock use.
Distributed by
Parke-Davis
Division of Pfizer Inc
NY, NY 10017
Made in India
Pfizer
NDC 0071-0737-30
Lopid®
(Gemfibrozil Tablets, USP)
600 mg
500 Tablets
Rx only
FPO UPC (100%)
3 0071-0737-30 3
GTIN: 00300710737303
PAA058651
LOT:/EXP:

(© Pfizer. Used with permission.)

What is the trade name for this medication? ____________________

What is the generic name for this medication? ____________________

What is the NDC number for this medication container? ____________________

What is the total number of tablets in the container? ____________________

INTRODUCTION

Prescriptions are medications ordered by prescribers in outpatient settings, and **medication orders** are medications ordered by prescribers in inpatient settings. Whatever the setting, it is important for the pharmacy technician to be able to read and interpret these orders accurately. This is why it is important to learn the abbreviations from Chapter 1. Every order must be put in writing as soon as possible, and the *pharmacist* must transcribe any verbal orders. Also, a pharmacist is required to handle any clarification of orders with the prescriber. The ability to interpret a medication order or prescription is an essential skill for professionals who work with medications.

The pharmacist is ultimately responsible for dispensing the medication as ordered. A pharmacy technician has the training to perform most functions in the pharmacy. Because the field of medicine is always changing, staying current with new medications and new **indications** for older medications is essential. Patient safety is the most important aspect of dispensing medications.

Knowledge of pharmacy includes **pharmacokinetics**, the movement of the drugs through the body, and **pharmacotherapeutics**, the therapeutic uses and effects of drugs, whether beneficial or harmful. The field of **toxicology** includes the study of the adverse effects of chemical substances on the human body. It is important to learn normal ranges for medication doses so that you can check your calculations to see if your answers make sense. It is easier to check your answers for accuracy when you have an idea of what doses should be. The differences between therapeutic (desired) and toxic (harmful) levels of medications must be considered, as well as possible drug-drug interactions, drug-food interactions, and drug-disease state interactions.

WHAT DOES A PRESCRIPTION INDICATE?

A prescription is a means for a physician or other health professional to provide the information needed by the pharmacist to dispense the desired medication for a patient in an outpatient setting. It is an order written for a specific person by a medical professional licensed to prescribe for a specific condition. The rules about who may prescribe vary from state to state, so the statutes of the state of practice determine the legalities of prescription writing. As a legal document, the prescription indicates the medication desired and the directions for its use. The components of a prescription are included in Fig. 7.1.

TECH NOTE

Legally, the physician's Drug Enforcement Agency (DEA) number must be on a prescription if it is written for a controlled substance!

TECH NOTE

As you work through prescriptions, an understood meaning is that if a tablet or capsule is ordered, the route of administration is by mouth (po) unless otherwise indicated.

When typing prescription labels for the public, make sure that the instructions are clear and easy to understand. Begin oral prescriptions with "Take" and always state the number of tablets, capsules, or milliliters as opposed to the strength. For example, if the prescription is for 500 mg and the medication comes in 250-mg tablets, type "Take 2 tablets," not "Take 500 mg." Other direction words used include "Instill" for eye or ear medications, "Insert" for suppositories, "Apply" for topical preparations and patches, and "Inhale" for nasal and oral inhalers. A few medications, including insulin preparations, are prescribed for subcutaneous use, in which case you could use, "Inject subcutaneously" or "Inject under the skin." Special training should be provided before a patient self-administers subcutaneous medication.

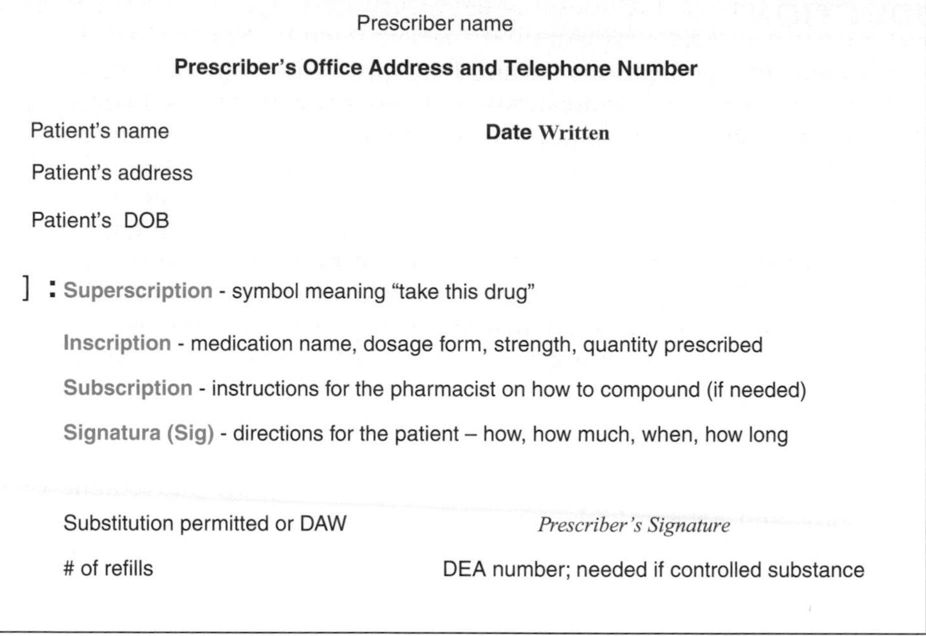

Prescriber name

Prescriber's Office Address and Telephone Number

Patient's name **Date Written**

Patient's address

Patient's DOB

] : Superscription - symbol meaning "take this drug"

Inscription - medication name, dosage form, strength, quantity prescribed

Subscription - instructions for the pharmacist on how to compound (if needed)

Signatura (Sig) - directions for the patient – how, how much, when, how long

Substitution permitted or DAW *Prescriber's Signature*

# of refills DEA number; needed if controlled substance

FIGURE 7.1 **Elements of a Prescription.**

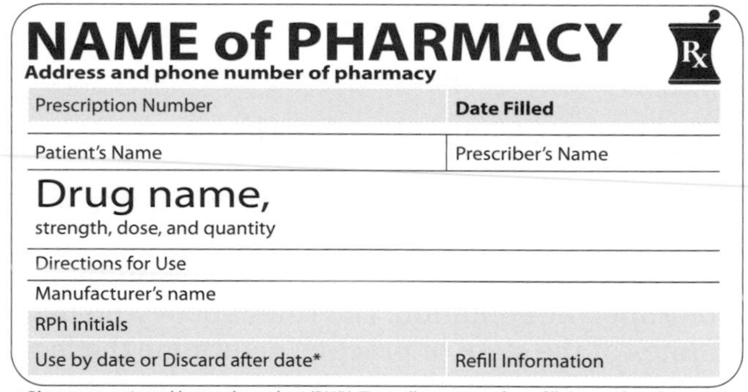

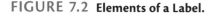

NAME of PHARMACY

Address and phone number of pharmacy

Prescription Number	**Date Filled**
Patient's Name	Prescriber's Name

Drug name,
strength, dose, and quantity

Directions for Use

Manufacturer's name

RPh initials

Use by date or Discard after date*	Refill Information

* Pharmacy assigned beyond use date (BUD); Typically one year from fill date unless the medication is compounded or reconstituted in the pharmacy, has an earlier expiration date, or is an injectable medication

FIGURE 7.2 **Elements of a Label.**

The Institute for Safe Medication Practices (ISMP) recommends the use of numeric rather than alphabetic characters on prescription labels. Therefore, in this text, use numbers such as 1, 2, and 3 on prescription labels as opposed to one, two, and three. In its quest to reduce medication errors, the ISMP also recommends the use of numbers over ambiguous terms such as twice daily (https://www.ismp.org). This should be written, "Take 2 times a day."

TECH NOTE

If a prescription is written for a brand name and substituted with a generic, you must put "generic for (Brand name)," with the specific brand name entered, on the label.

As seen in Figs. 7.1 and 7.2, a prescription must include the *prescriber's* address and phone number and the date it was *written,* whereas a prescription label includes the *pharmacy's* name, address, and phone number and the date it was *filled.* These concepts are bolded in Figs. 7.1 and 7.2 to emphasize this important difference.

A prescription label also includes any necessary **auxiliary labels** which which emphasize important extra instructions. Auxiliary labels include: Shake Well, Take with Food, May Cause Drowsiness, and Avoid Alcohol.

The prescription interpretation is how one would read the prescription without the use of abbreviations. The label directions are written for the patient in language that is easily understood.

EXAMPLE 7.1

Lawrence Merry, M.D.
4th Street and Jones Ave.
Holly, GA 00111
phone# - 001-555-2176

Patient Name________ Date ______
Address________ Age ______

] Zoloft 50 mg
#30
Sig: i tab po qam

________ Refill ______
DEA#________

Prescription interpretation: *Zoloft 50 mg, 30 tablets, one tablet by mouth every morning.*

Label directions: *Take 1 tablet by mouth every morning.*

EXAMPLE 7.2

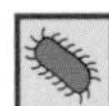

Lawrence Merry, M.D.
4th Street and Jones Ave.
Holly, GA 00111
phone# - 001-555-2176

Patient Name________ Date ______
Address________ Age ______

] Mycostatin Oral Suspension
60 mL
Sig: Agit then swish and swallow 5 mL
q4-6h

________ Refill ______
DEA#________

Prescription interpretation:

Mycostatin Oral Suspension, 60 mL, agitate, then swish and swallow 5 mL every 4 to 6 hours.

Label directions:

Shake well, then swish and swallow 5 mL every 4 to 6 hours.

This prescription should be dispensed with a measuring device appropriate for 5 mL.

Practice Problems A

Interpret the following prescriptions and then write the instructions as they should appear on a prescription label.

1.

Lawrence Merry, M.D.
4th Street and Jones Ave.
Holly, GA 00111
phone# - 001-555-2176

Patient Name________________ Date ______
Address________________ Age ______

] atorvastatin 10 mg
#30
Sig: i tab po nightly at bedtime

________________ Refill ______
DEA#________________

Prescription interpretation: ________________________________

____

Label directions: ______________________________________

2.

Lawrence Merry, M.D.
4th Street and Jones Ave.
Holly, GA 00111
phone# - 001-555-2176

Patient Name________________ Date ______
Address________________ Age ______

] Premarin 0.625 mg
#30
Sig: i tab po daily at approximately
same hour

________________ Refill ______
DEA#________________

Prescription interpretation: ________________________________

____

Label directions: ______________________________________

3.

Lawrence Merry, M.D.
4th Street and Jones Ave.
Holly, GA 00111
phone# - 001-555-2176

Patient Name________________ Date ________
Address________________ Age ________

] Zoloft 50 mg
#30
Sig: i tab po daily $\bar{c}$ morning meal

________________ Refill ______
DEA#________________

Prescription interpretation: ____

____

Label directions: ____

4.

Lawrence Merry, M.D.
4th Street and Jones Ave.
Holly, GA 00111
phone# - 001-555-2176

Patient Name________________ Date ________
Address________________ Age ________

] Prednisone 10 mg
#40
Sig: i tab po qid x 4 d ; i tab po tid x 4 d ; i tab po bid x 4 d ; i tab po daily x 4

________________ Refill ______
DEA#________________

Prescription interpretation: ____

____

____

Label directions: ____

____

____

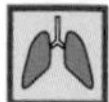

5.

Lawrence Merry, M.D.
4th Street and Jones Ave.
Holly, GA 00111
phone# - 001-555-2176

Patient Name__________ Date ______
Address__________ Age ______

] Allegra 180 mg
#30
Sig: i tab po daily

__________ Refill ______
DEA#__________

Prescription interpretation: ____________________

____

Label directions: ____________________

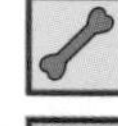

6.

Lawrence Merry, M.D.
4th Street and Jones Ave.
Holly, GA 00111
phone# - 001-555-2176

Patient Name__________ Date ______
Address__________ Age ______

] ibuprofen 800 mg
#100
Sig: i tab po q8h

__________ Refill ______
DEA#__________

Prescription interpretation: ____________________

____

Label directions: ____________________

7.

Lawrence Merry, M.D.
4th Street and Jones Ave.
Holly, GA 00111
phone# - 001-555-2176

Patient Name________ Date ______
Address________ Age ______

] Norvasc 5 mg
#30
Sig: i tab po qam for ↑ B/p

________ Refill ______
DEA#________

Prescription interpretation: ________________

Label directions: ________________

8.

Lawrence Merry, M.D.
4th Street and Jones Ave.
Holly, GA 00111
phone# - 001-555-2176

Patient Name________ Date ______
Address________ Age ______

] furosemide 40 mg
#30
Sig: i tab po daily @ 10am

________ Refill ______
DEA#________

Prescription interpretation: ________________

Label directions: ________________

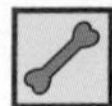

9.

Lawrence Merry, M.D.
4th Street and Jones Ave.
Holly, GA 00111
phone# - 001-555-2176

Patient Name________________________ Date ________
Address____________________________ Age ________

] Fosamax 70 mg
#4
Sig: i po on same d qwk

________________________ Refill ______
DEA#____________________

Prescription interpretation: ____

____

Label directions: ____

10.

Lawrence Merry, M.D.
4th Street and Jones Ave.
Holly, GA 00111
phone# - 001-555-2176

Patient Name________________________ Date ________
Address____________________________ Age ________

] diazepam 5 mg
#100
Sig: i po tid prn anxiety

________________________ Refill ______
DEA# AM123321

Prescription interpretation: ____

____

Label directions: ____

11.

Lawrence Merry, M.D.
4th Street and Jones Ave.
Holly, GA 00111
phone# - 001-555-2176

Patient Name____________________ Date ________
Address____________________ Age ________

] Neurontin 600 mg
#50
Sig: i po daily x 5 d ; i po bid x 5 d ;
then i po tid

____________________ Refill ______
DEA#____________________

Prescription interpretation: ____

____

Label directions: ____

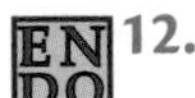

12.

Lawrence Merry, M.D.
4th Street and Jones Ave.
Holly, GA 00111
phone# - 001-555-2176

Patient Name____________________ Date ________
Address____________________ Age ________

] Glucotrol XL 10 mg
#30
Sig: i tab po $\bar{c}$ am meal

____________________ Refill ______
DEA#____________________

Prescription interpretation: ____

____

Label directions: ____

Write the instructions as they should appear on the patient's label.

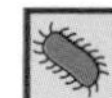

13. Rx: doxycycline 100 mg

Sig: i tab po bid × 7 days

Stock available: doxycycline 100 mg tablets (antibiotic)

____

14. Rx: Lanoxin (digoxin) 0.25 mg

#30

Sig: i tab daily in am if P ↑60 bpm

Stock: Lanoxin 250 mcg tablets (for congestive heart failure)

____

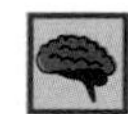

15. Rx: Keppra (levetiracetam) 500 mg

#60

Sig: i tab po bid

Stock: Keppra 500 mg tablets (anticonvulsant)

____

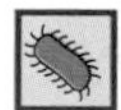

16. Rx: amoxicillin suspension 250 mg/5 mL

150 mL

Sig: 1 tsp tid until gone

Stock: amoxicillin 250 mg/5 mL for oral suspension 150 mL bottle (antibiotic)

____

17. Rx: Prozac (fluoxetine) 20 mg

#90

Sig: i cap po qam

Stock: fluoxetine 20 mg capsules (antidepressant)

____

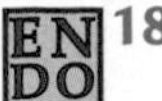

18. Rx: Synthroid (levothyroxine) 25 mcg

#90

Sig: i tab qam ā eating c̄ full glass of water

Stock: Synthroid 25 mcg tablets (thyroid replacement)

19. Rx: Zocor (simvastatin) 5 mg

#30

Sig: i tab po qpm c̄ low fat snack

Stock: Zocor 5 mg tablets (antihypercholesterolemic)

20. Rx: Zyban (bupropion) 150 mg

#60

Sig: i tab qam and i tab 8 hours later × 7 weeks

Stock: Zyban 150 mg tablets (smoking cessation aid)

What Is a Medication Order?

A medication order is a method of providing the same information found on an outpatient prescription, but it is used in an inpatient environment (Fig. 7.3). Whereas a prescription is written for either the number of doses or length of time of therapy, a medication order tells a health care professional what drug or drugs should be administered, how to administer them, the strength of the medication, and the frequency with which they should be given to an inpatient. The medication order contains the date, patient name, medication name, dose, route of administration, time and frequency of administration, and the signature of the prescribing professional. Although only recommended in emergency situations, medication orders may be verbally communicated. For legal purposes, each order should be transcribed into writing by the health care professional receiving the order, and then countersigned by the licensed health care professional ordering the medication.

PHYSICIAN'S ORDERS

Patient, James A.

DATE	ORDERS			TRANS BY
	Diagnosis:	Weight:	Height:	
	Sensitivities/Drug Allergies:			
1/12/17	0900 Lasix 80 mg. p.o. b.i.d.			
	Digoxin 0.125 mg. p.o. q.d.			
	Slow-K 10 mEq. p.o. b.i.d.			
	A. Physician, M.D.			

MEDICAL RECORDS COPY	PHYSICIAN'S ORDERS							T-5
B-CLIN. NOTES	E-LAB	G-X-RAY	K-DIAGNOSTIC	M-SURGERY	Q-THERAPY	T-ORDERS	W-NURSING	Y-MISC.

A

Transcription of Med Sheet by: ______

Reviewed by: ______ Page ____ of ____

Initials	Signature
NJ	N. Jones R.N.
AN	A. Nurse R.N.

Allergies: ☑ NKDA

Injection Sites:
A = RUE
B = LUE E = Abdomen
C = RLE F = R Glut
D = LLE G = L Glut

Special Notes:

See Legend on Back

Patient, James A.

☐ Inpatient ☐ Outpatient

DATE	DRUG			08 09 10 11	12 13 14 15	16 17 18 19	20 21 22 23	24 01 02 03	04 05 06 07	1/12/17		1/13/17		1/14/17	1/15/17	1/16/17
1 1/12	Lasix									09 AN	21 NJ	09 AN	21 NJ			
	80 mg dose	p.o. route	b.i.d. interval	09			21									
2 1/12	Digoxin									09 AN		09 AN				
	0.125 mg dose	p.o. route	q.d. interval	09												
3 1/12	Slow-K									09 AN	21 NJ	09 AN	21 NJ			
	10 mEq dose	p.o. route	b.i.d. interval	09			21									
4																
	dose	route	interval													
5																
	dose	route	interval													

MEDICATION PROFILE								
B-CLIN. NOTES	E-LAB	G-X-RAY	K-DIAGNOSTIC	M-SURGERY	Q-THERAPY	T-ORDERS	W-NURSING	Y-MISC.

B

FIGURE 7.3 **Examples of Physician's Orders:** (A) a patient's medication administration record (B) with appropriate drug interpretations. (Forms courtesy Clarian Health, Indianapolis, IN.)

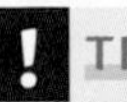

TECH ALERT

Even though, in most inpatient pharmacies, a pharmacist enters medication orders into the computer, the pharmacy technician still has a responsibility to check as he or she is filling orders and report any concerns to the pharmacist.

When interpreting medication orders, simply restate the order without the use of abbreviations (other than dose strengths such as mg, g, mL, etc.). Include the name of the drug ordered and strength because these are orders that will only be seen by other health care professionals, not patients.

EXAMPLE 7.3

PAIN Discontinue naproxen 375 mg; start naproxen 500 mg po bid

Discontinue naproxen 375 mg; start naproxen 500 mg by mouth twice daily

Practice Problems B

Interpret the following medication orders.

1. Discontinue Zocor; add Lipitor 10 mg tab i po at bedtime

____

____

2. amoxicillin suspension 250 mg po tid until discontinued

____

3. cephalexin 500 mg po q8h × 3 days

____

4. ENDO metformin-XR 500 mg po qd c̄ pm meal

____

5. Discontinue Septra; start Cipro 500 mg po bid × 2 days

____

____

6. albuterol sulfate 2 puffs q4h SOB

____

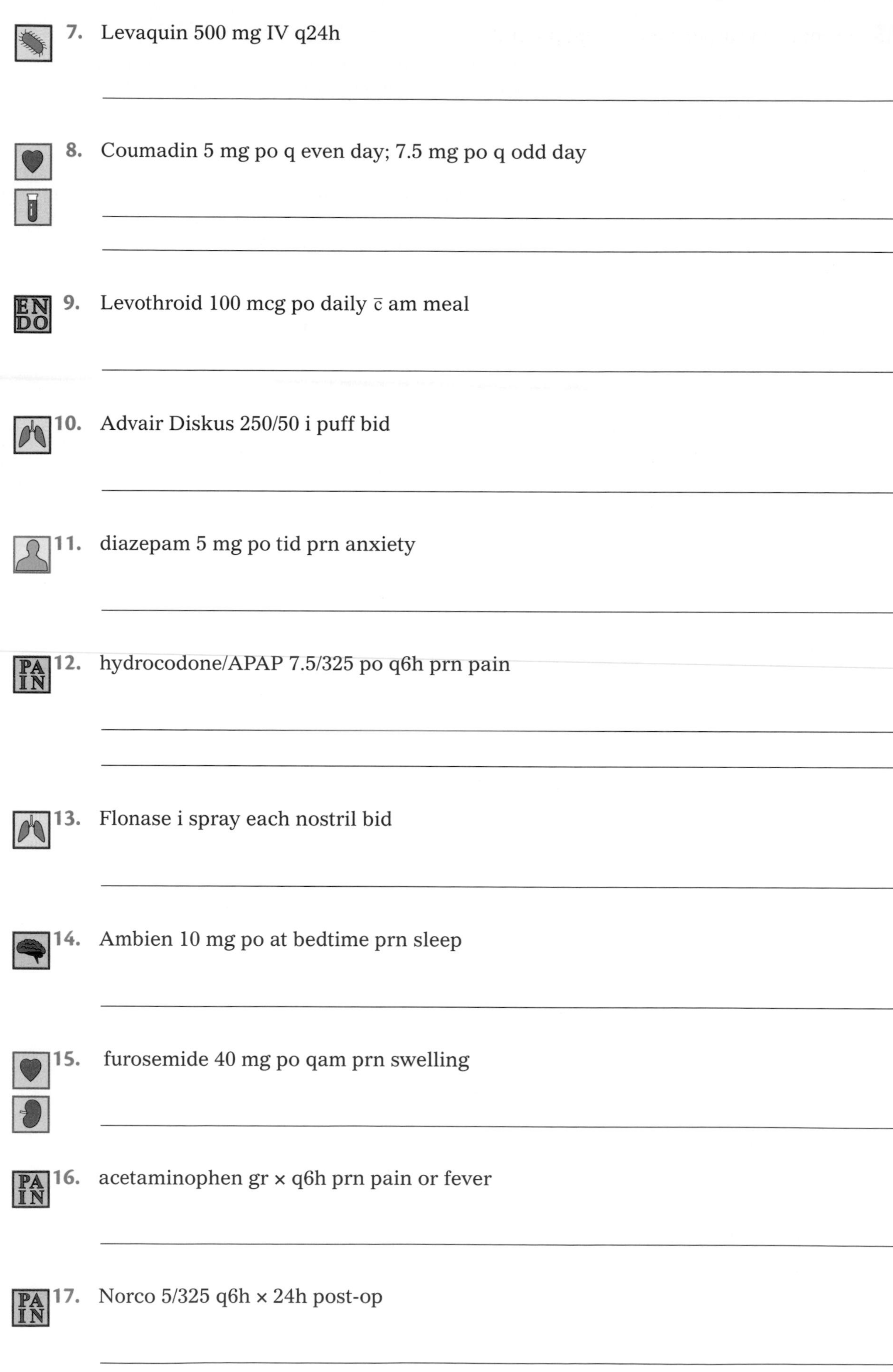

7. Levaquin 500 mg IV q24h

8. Coumadin 5 mg po q even day; 7.5 mg po q odd day

9. Levothroid 100 mcg po daily c̄ am meal

10. Advair Diskus 250/50 i puff bid

11. diazepam 5 mg po tid prn anxiety

12. hydrocodone/APAP 7.5/325 po q6h prn pain

13. Flonase i spray each nostril bid

14. Ambien 10 mg po at bedtime prn sleep

15. furosemide 40 mg po qam prn swelling

16. acetaminophen gr x q6h prn pain or fever

17. Norco 5/325 q6h × 24h post-op

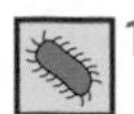
18. cephalexin suspension 500 mg po q12h

____

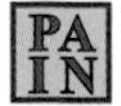
19. midazolam 0.1 mg/kg IV push over at least 5 minutes

____

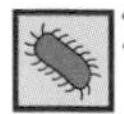
20. Discontinue amoxicillin; start Bactrim DS po bid

____

INTERPRETING STOCK MEDICATION LABELS

Labels on stock medication bottles identify the drug within the container. They also indicate the important information needed (**in bold**) to dispense the drug as follows:

- Generic name—the official name that is assigned to a medication after approval by the FDA; found in the *U.S. Pharmacopeia–National Formulary* (USP-NF)
- Trade/Brand name—the name assigned by the manufacturer
- National Drug Code (NDC) number—a 10-digit, 3-segment number that identifies the manufacturer (labeler), the product, and the size of the container in which the medication is packaged; a universal product identifier in the United States
- **Strength**—the amount of active ingredient found in the medication, such as micrograms (mcg), milligrams (mg), grams (g), grains (gr), units, or milliequivalents (mEq), per dose
- **Total quantity of medication**—amount in the container as packed by the manufacturer
- **Dosage form**—tablet, capsule, solution, suspension, suppository, etc.
- **Name of the manufacturer**
- **Special instructions** for mixing or compounding if indicated by the manufacturer
- **Storage requirements** for the medication
- **Lot and batch numbers or control number** of the medication that can be used for identification if the medication is recalled
- **Expiration date**
- **Controlled substance indicators** as appropriate—indicated by a large "C" with the schedule number in Roman numerals within the "C"

TECH NOTE

The generic name should be expressed with a lowercase letter, such as diazepam. The brand name is expressed with a capital letter, such as Valium. If the medication is a generic form of the drug, a trade name will not be found on the manufacturer's label.

One of the most important aspects of patient safety is the careful interpretation of the medication label. To ensure that the proper medication is provided, the label (drug name, strength, form, expiration date, and NDC number) should be read when taking the medication from the shelf, before preparing the medication for dispensing, and when returning the medication container to the shelf for storage. By reading medication labels carefully, you can reduce errors and avoid confusion, and the therapeutic potential of the drug is maximized. The pharmacy technician must be fully aware of the information on the label, including the expiration date, to ensure that the medicine dispensed is of the highest quality and exactly as ordered.

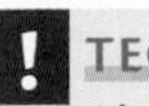

TECH ALERT

Always read medication labels at least three times. Read before removing from the storage place; before counting when preparing the prescription; and before passing it to the pharmacist for the final check.

EXAMPLE 7.4

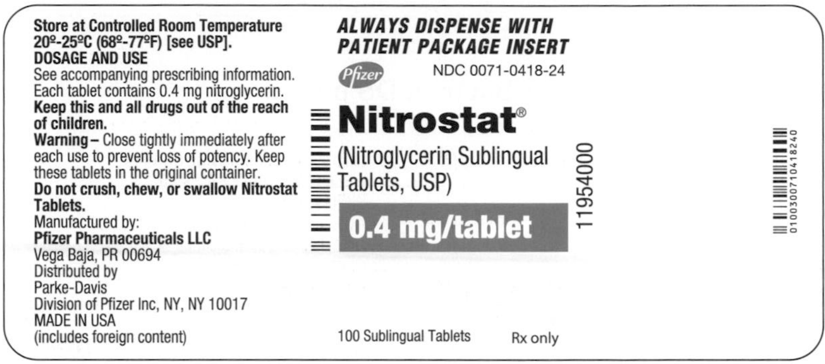

Store at Controlled Room Temperature 20º-25ºC (68º-77ºF) [see USP].
DOSAGE AND USE
See accompanying prescribing information.
Each tablet contains 0.4 mg nitroglycerin.
Keep this and all drugs out of the reach of children.
Warning – Close tightly immediately after each use to prevent loss of potency. Keep these tablets in the original container.
Do not crush, chew, or swallow Nitrostat Tablets.
Manufactured by:
Pfizer Pharmaceuticals LLC
Vega Baja, PR 00694
Distributed by
Parke-Davis
Division of Pfizer Inc, NY, NY 10017
MADE IN USA
(includes foreign content)
ALWAYS DISPENSE WITH PATIENT PACKAGE INSERT
Pfizer
NDC 0071-0418-24
Nitrostat®
(Nitroglycerin Sublingual Tablets, USP)
0.4 mg/tablet
11954000
100 Sublingual Tablets
Rx only

(© Pfizer. Used with permission.)

What is the NDC number for this medication? *0071-0418-24*

0071—manufacturer (labeler), 0418—product identification, 24—package size

How many tablets are in a full container? *100*

What is the strength of this medication? *0.4 mg/tablet*

Who manufactures this medication? *Pfizer Pharmaceuticals LLC*

Where is it manufactured? *Vega Baja, Puerto Rico*

What is the trade name of this medication? *Nitrostat*

What is the generic name of this medication? *nitroglycerin*

What are the warnings that must accompany a prescription for Nitrostat?

Close tightly immediately after use to prevent loss of potency. Keep these tablets in the original container. Do not crush, chew, or swallow.

Practice Problems C

Using the following labels, answer the questions that follow.

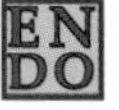

1.

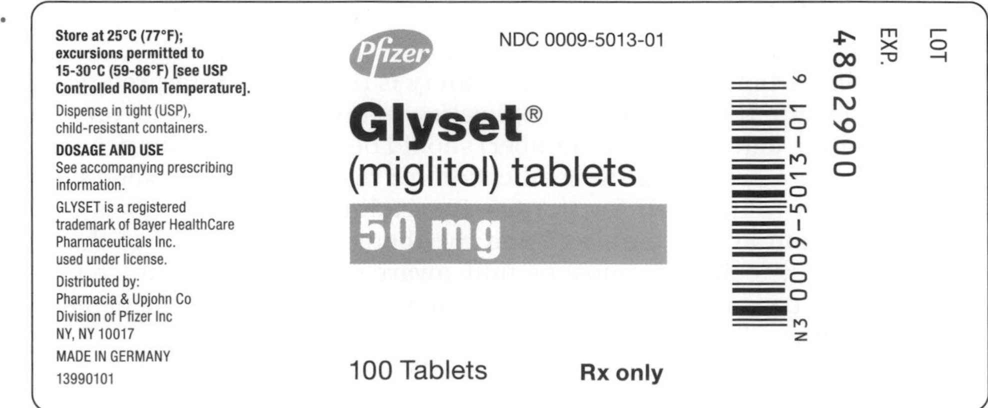

Store at 25°C (77°F); excursions permitted to 15-30°C (59-86°F) [see USP Controlled Room Temperature].
Dispense in tight (USP), child-resistant containers.
DOSAGE AND USE
See accompanying prescribing information.
GLYSET is a registered trademark of Bayer HealthCare Pharmaceuticals Inc. used under license.
Distributed by:
Pharmacia & Upjohn Co
Division of Pfizer Inc
NY, NY 10017
MADE IN GERMANY
13990101
Pfizer
NDC 0009-5013-01
Glyset®
(miglitol) tablets
50 mg
100 Tablets
Rx only
N3 0009-5013-01 6
LOT
EXP.
4802900

(© Pfizer. Used with permission.)

Who is the manufacturer of this medication? ______________________

What is the NDC number on this container? ______________________

What is the trade name for this medication? ______________________

What is the generic name for this medication? ______________________

What is the strength of this medication? ______________________

How many tablets are in an unopened container? ______________________

2.

ALWAYS DISPENSE WITH MEDICATION GUIDE

NDC 0071-2214-20

Pfizer

Dilantin-125®

(Phenytoin Oral Suspension, USP)

125 mg per 5 mL

IMPORTANT–SHAKE WELL BEFORE EACH USE

NOT FOR PARENTERAL USE

8 fl oz (237 mL) Rx only

THIS PRODUCT MUST BE SHAKEN WELL ESPECIALLY PRIOR TO INITIAL USE.

Each 5 mL contains 125 mg phenytoin, with a maximum alcohol content not greater than 0.6 percent.

DOSAGE AND USE

Adults, 1 teaspoonful (5 mL) three times daily; pediatric patients, see package insert.

Advice to Pharmacist and Patient–Patient must be advised to use an accurate measuring device when using this product.

See package insert for complete prescribing information.

Store at Controlled Room Temperature 20°-25°C (68°-77°F) [see USP].

Protect from freezing and light.

Keep this and all drugs out of the reach of children.

Distributed by
Parke-Davis
Division of Pfizer Inc
NY, NY 10017

N 3 0071-2214-20 8

PAA063621

LOT/EXP

Imprint Area
NO VARNISH

Who manufactures the medication? ______________________

What is the dosage form of this medication? ______________________

What are the specific directions (capitalized information) accompanying this medication? ______________________

____

What is the dosage strength? ______________________

What is the total volume in metric measurements? ______________________

What is the trade name? ______________________

What is the generic name? ______________________

3.

NDC 6304-7633-56

100 Tablets
(10 blisterpacks of 10 tablets each)

UNIT DOSE PACK

Digoxin Tablets

Each scored tablet contains
250 mcg (0.25 mg)

See package insert for
Dosage and Administration.

Store at 25°C (77°F);
excursions permitted to
15 to30°C(59 to 86°F)
[see Usp Controlled Room
Temperature] in a dry place.

What is the type of packaging for this medication? ______________________

How many tablets are found in the total package? ______________________

What is the strength of the medication in mcg?____________ in mg? __________

What are the storage requirements of the medication? ______________________

____

What is the dosage form of the medication? ______________________

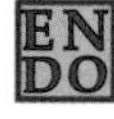

4.

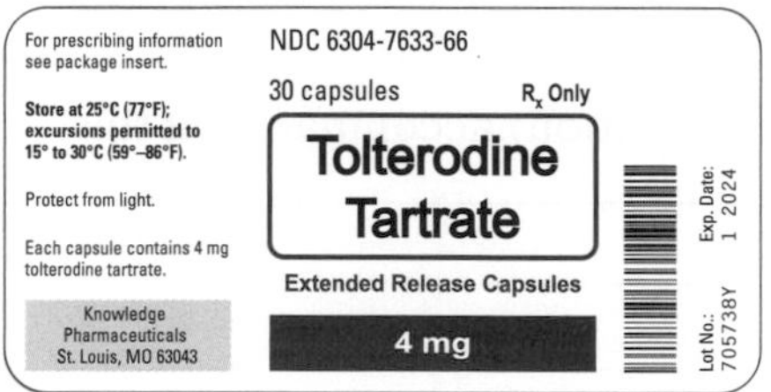
For prescribing information see package insert.
Store at 25°C (77°F); excursions permitted to 15° to 30°C (59°–86°F).
Protect from light.
Each capsule contains 4 mg tolterodine tartrate.
Knowledge Pharmaceuticals St. Louis, MO 63043
NDC 6304-7633-66
30 capsules
Rx Only
Tolterodine Tartrate
Extended Release Capsules
4 mg
Exp. Date: 1 2024
Lot No.: 705738Y

What is the dosage form of this medication? ______________________

Who manufactures this medication? ______________________

What type capsules are found in this container? ______________________

How many capsules are in the container? ______________________

REVIEW

It is absolutely necessary to interpret medication orders and prescriptions correctly. There must be checks and balances among the prescriber, the pharmacist, and the person responsible for obtaining the medications for dispensing, such as the pharmacy technician, as well as the person administering the medication. Any break in this checking process could result in the patient getting the wrong medication or strength, which could have dire consequences.

TECH NOTE

As a pharmacy technician, you are responsible for understanding orders and prescriptions. Ask for verification if you have any concerns. Never make assumptions! As part of the medical team, you must assist in continuous quality control for patient safety.

Posttest

Interpret the following prescriptions or medication orders as directed and write the directions as they should appear on a prescription label. If the prescription calls for the liquid form of a medication, use the metric system and assume that a dispensing utensil is provided.

1.

Lawrence Merry, M.D.
4th Street and Jones Ave.
Holly, GA 00111
phone# - 001-555-2176

Patient Name______________________ Date ________
Address______________________ Age ________

] Xanax 500 mcg
#30
Sig: i tab po at bedtime

______________________ Refill ______
DEA#______________________

Label directions: ______________________

____

Continued

Posttest, cont.

2.

Lawrence Merry, M.D.
4th Street and Jones Ave.
Holly, GA 00111
phone# - 001-555-2176

Patient Name________________________ Date ________
Address____________________________ Age ________

] K-Clor 20 mEq ℥xvi
Sig: ʒ $\overline{\dot{s}\dot{s}}$ po qam $\bar{p}$ breakfast

________________________ Refill ______
DEA#____________________

Prescription interpretation: ____

Label directions: ____

3.

Lawrence Merry, M.D.
4th Street and Jones Ave.
Holly, GA 00111
phone# - 001-555-2176

Patient Name________________________ Date ________
Address____________________________ Age ________

] Dilantin 100 mg caps
#120
Sig: cap iv po stat then cap $\bar{\dot{i}}$ po qid

________________________ Refill ______
DEA#____________________

Prescription interpretation: ____

____

Label directions: ____

____

Posttest, cont.

4.

Lawrence Merry, M.D.
4th Street and Jones Ave.
Holly, GA 00111
phone# - 001-555-2176

Patient Name__________ Date ______
Address__________ Age ______

] amlodipine 5 mg
#30
Sig: tab i po daily @ 10 am

__________ Refill ______
DEA#__________

Label directions: ____________________

5.

Lawrence Merry, M.D.
4th Street and Jones Ave.
Holly, GA 00111
phone# - 001-555-2176

Patient Name__________ Date ______
Address__________ Age ______

] Vasotec 10 mg
#30
Sig: tab ss po x 1 wk then i tab po daily.
Check B/p and record daily.

__________ Refill ______
DEA#__________

Prescription interpretation: ____________________

Label directions: ____________________

Continued

Posttest, cont.

6.

Lawrence Merry, M.D.
4th Street and Jones Ave.
Holly, GA 00111
phone# - 001-555-2176

Patient Name__________ Date _____
Address__________ Age _____

] Antivert 12.5 mg
#60
Sig: tab i po q4-6h prn

__________ Refill _____
DEA#__________

Label directions: ____________________

7.

Lawrence Merry, M.D.
4th Street and Jones Ave.
Holly, GA 00111
phone# - 001-555-2176

Patient Name__________ Date _____
Address__________ Age _____

] Ocuflox Ophthalmic Solution
5 mL
Sig: i gtt each eye qid x 5 d

__________ Refill _____
DEA#__________

Prescription interpretation: ____________________

____

Label directions: ____________________

____

Posttest, cont.

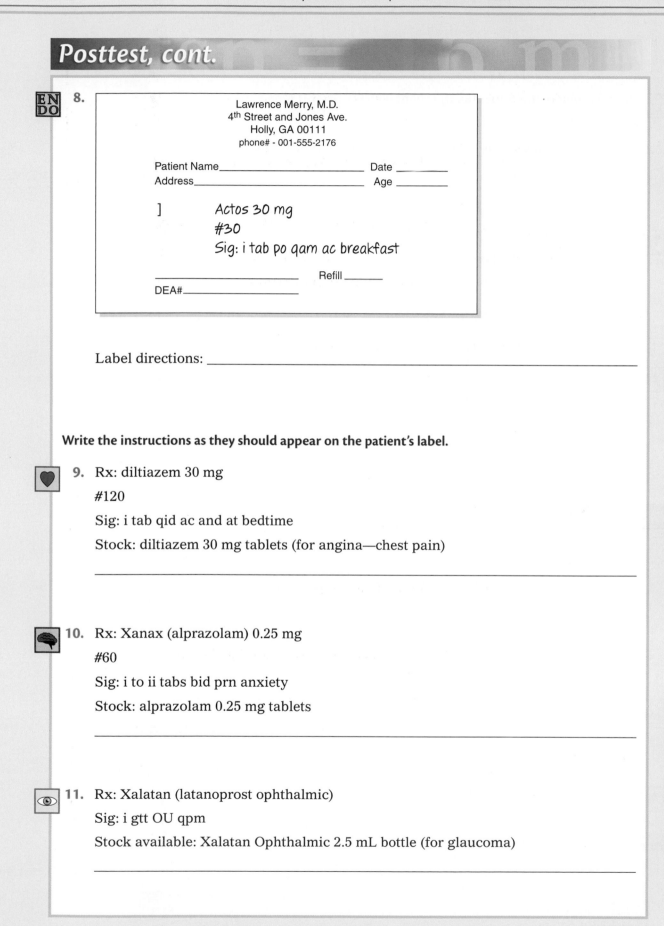

8.

Lawrence Merry, M.D.
4th Street and Jones Ave.
Holly, GA 00111
phone# - 001-555-2176

Patient Name______________________ Date ________
Address__________________________ Age ________

] Actos 30 mg
#30
Sig: i tab po qam ac breakfast

______________________ Refill ______
DEA#________________

Label directions: ____

Write the instructions as they should appear on the patient's label.

9. Rx: diltiazem 30 mg
#120
Sig: i tab qid ac and at bedtime
Stock: diltiazem 30 mg tablets (for angina—chest pain)

____

10. Rx: Xanax (alprazolam) 0.25 mg
#60
Sig: i to ii tabs bid prn anxiety
Stock: alprazolam 0.25 mg tablets

____

11. Rx: Xalatan (latanoprost ophthalmic)
Sig: i gtt OU qpm
Stock available: Xalatan Ophthalmic 2.5 mL bottle (for glaucoma)

____

Continued

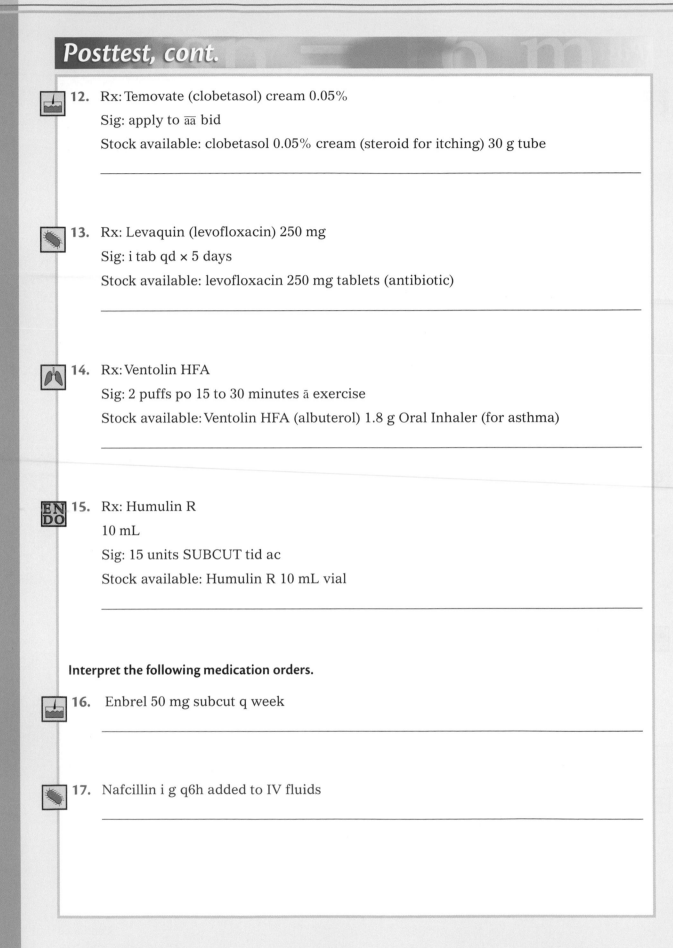

Posttest, cont.

12. Rx: Temovate (clobetasol) cream 0.05%

Sig: apply to $\overline{aa}$ bid

Stock available: clobetasol 0.05% cream (steroid for itching) 30 g tube

____

13. Rx: Levaquin (levofloxacin) 250 mg

Sig: i tab qd × 5 days

Stock available: levofloxacin 250 mg tablets (antibiotic)

____

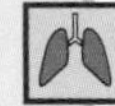

14. Rx: Ventolin HFA

Sig: 2 puffs po 15 to 30 minutes $\bar{a}$ exercise

Stock available: Ventolin HFA (albuterol) 1.8 g Oral Inhaler (for asthma)

____

15. Rx: Humulin R

10 mL

Sig: 15 units SUBCUT tid ac

Stock available: Humulin R 10 mL vial

____

Interpret the following medication orders.

16. Enbrel 50 mg subcut q week

____

17. Nafcillin i g q6h added to IV fluids

____

Posttest, cont.

ENDO 18. Humulin 70/30 25 units subcut qam ac breakfast and ac supper

____

____

19. cimetidine 300 mg IM stat

____

20. ampicillin 250 mg po qid c̄ meals and hs c̄ snack

____

____

21. warfarin 5 mg po on even days and 2.5 mg po on odd days

____

____

22. digoxin 250 mcg po qam c̄ pulse ↑60

____

____

23. Sudafed 60 mg po q4–6h prn nasal congestion

____

____

24. Maalox 20 mL po 1 hour pc prn gastric distress

____

25. Lunesta 1 mg po at bedtime prn sleep

____

Continued

Posttest, cont.

26. labetalol 5 to 10 mg IV q4h prn BP >150/90

27. cefazolin 500 mg IM q8h

28. furosemide 80 mg po qam

29. Singulair 10 mg qpm

30. Reglan 10 mg po qid 30 minutes ac and at bedtime

31. digoxin 0.25 mg po qam

32. Epogen 20 units/kg SUBCUT on Mon, Wed, Sat

33. Narcan 0.2 mg IV stat; may rep until desired response up to 0.8 mg total (opioid antagonist)

Posttest, cont.

34. cefazolin 1 g IV 1 hour pre-op and q8h post-op × 24 hours

____

____

Interpret these labels by answering the following questions.

35.

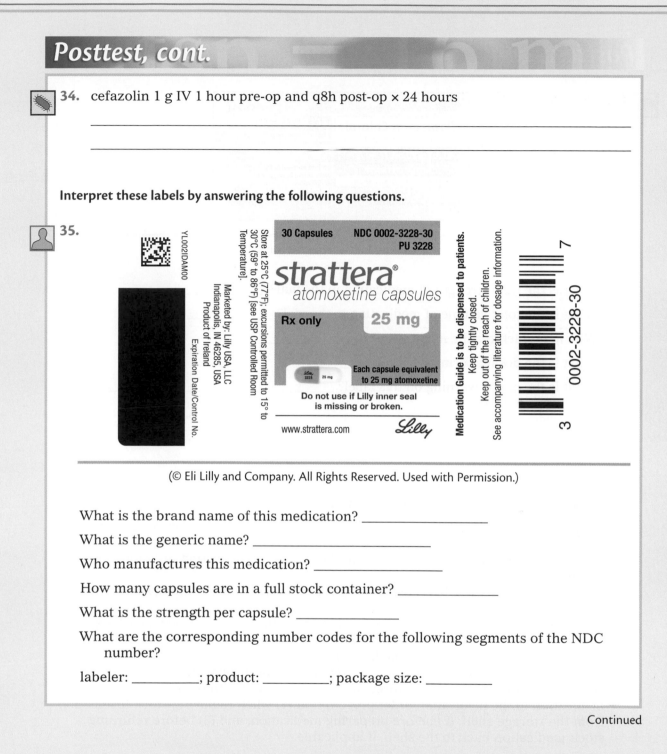

30 Capsules NDC 0002-3228-30
PU 3228
strattera®
atomoxetine capsules
Rx only 25 mg
Each capsule equivalent to 25 mg atomoxetine
Do not use if Lilly inner seal is missing or broken.
www.strattera.com Lilly

Store at 25°C (77°F); excursions permitted to 15° to 30°C (59° to 86°F) [see USP Controlled Room Temperature].
Marketed by: Lilly USA, LLC
Indianapolis, IN 46285, USA
Product of Ireland
Expiration Date/Control No.
YL002IDAM00

Medication Guide is to be dispensed to patients.
Keep tightly closed.
Keep out of the reach of children.
See accompanying literature for dosage information.
3 0002-3228-30 7

What is the brand name of this medication? ______________

What is the generic name? ____________________

Who manufactures this medication? ______________

How many capsules are in a full stock container? ___________

What is the strength per capsule? ___________

What are the corresponding number codes for the following segments of the NDC number?

labeler: _______; product: _______; package size: _______

Continued

Posttest, cont.

36.

20 mL Single-dose For Intravenous use. Rx only NDC 0409-6653-18

Potassium Chloride
for Injection **Concentrate**, USP
40 mEq/20 mL (2 mEq/mL)
CONCENTRATE
MUST BE DILUTED BEFORE USE.

KCl Each mL contains potassium chloride, 2 mEq (149 mg). May contain HCl for pH adjustment. Sterile, nonpyrogenic. 4 mOsmol/mL (calc). Usual dosage: See insert. **Discard unused portion. Contains no more than 100 mcg/L of aluminum.**

Hospira, Inc., Lake Forest, IL 60045 USA RL-4578 Hospira

What is the total strength of medication in the vial? ____________

What is the total volume of medication in the vial? ____________

Who manufactures the medication? ________________

What is the dosage form? ________________

What is the major warning on this label? ____

REVIEW OF RULES

Interpreting Medication Labels and Orders

- Always read the entire label/prescription/medication order before making decisions concerning the medication to be dispensed.
- Solid medications are usually ordered in the weight of medication per tablet or capsule.
- Liquid medications will be found as weight per volume of medication, such as mg/mL.
- The generic name for the medication should be written in lowercase letters, whereas the trade or proprietary name will begin with a capital letter and may be followed by ®.
- If there is a question about the medication ordered, always ask the pharmacist to verify before beginning the process of preparing it for dispensing.
- Always read medication labels three times to ensure correctness of the dispensed medication to the medication order/prescription (1) when removing stock medication from the storage shelf; (2) before preparing medication; and (3) before returning stock medication back to the shelf, if applicable.

Calculation of Oral Solid Doses

OBJECTIVES

1. Calculate solid oral medication doses using both ratio and proportion and dimensional analysis
2. Convert equivalent measurements of oral solid doses between different units or measurement systems.
3. Maintain patient safety.

KEY WORDS

Buccal Between gum and cheek

Dosage Size, frequency, and number of doses of medication prescribed *over a period of time*

Dosage form Physical structure of a dose; for example capsule, tablet, solution

Dose Amount of a medication to be administered *at one time*

Enteric-coated tablet Dosage form that allows medication to pass through stomach unchanged; to prevent stomach irritation or prevent degradation of the active ingredient by stomach acid

Oral medications Medications taken by mouth (po)

Stock strength Strength or weight of medication available for doses

Sublingual medications Medications placed under the tongue to dissolve (SL)

Pretest

If you are already comfortable with the subject matter, perform the following calculations to test your knowledge. If not, work your way through the chapter and return to them for extra practice. Determine how many capsules or tablets must be given per dose of the stock available. Brand names have been paired with their appropriate generic substitutions. Any labels included represent the stock strength available. Show your calculations.

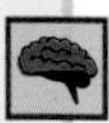

1. Dose ordered: phenobarbital 30 mg
   Stock strength: phenobarbital 60 mg tablets ______________

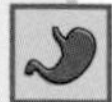

2. Dose ordered: AcipHex 60 mg
   Stock strength: AcipHex (rabeprazole) 20 mg tablets ______________

3. Dose ordered: Lanoxin 0.25 mg
   Stock strength: digoxin 250 mcg tablets ______________

Continued

Pretest, cont.

4. Dose ordered: Mobic 7.5 to 15 mg
   Stock strength: meloxicam 7.5 mg tablets ____________

5. Dose ordered: theophylline 0.4 g
   Stock strength: theophylline 200 mg capsules ____________

6. Dose ordered: potassium chloride 10 mEq
   Stock strength: potassium chloride 20 mEq scored tablets ____________

7. Dose ordered: aspirin gr x
   Stock strength: aspirin gr v tablets ____________

8. Dose ordered: Pepcid 40 mg
   Stock strength: famotidine 20 mg tablets ____________

9. Dose ordered: amoxicillin 1 g
   Stock strength: amoxicillin 500 mg capsules ____________

10. Dose ordered: Haldol 2 mg
    Stock strength: haloperidol 1 mg tablets ____________

11. Dose ordered: Synthroid 350 mcg
    Stock strength: levothyroxine 0.175 mg tablets ____________

12. Dose ordered: ferrous sulfate 324 mg
    Stock available: ferrous sulfate 5 grain tablets ____________

Pretest, cont.

13. Dose ordered: Glyset 50 mg

    Number of tablets needed: _____________

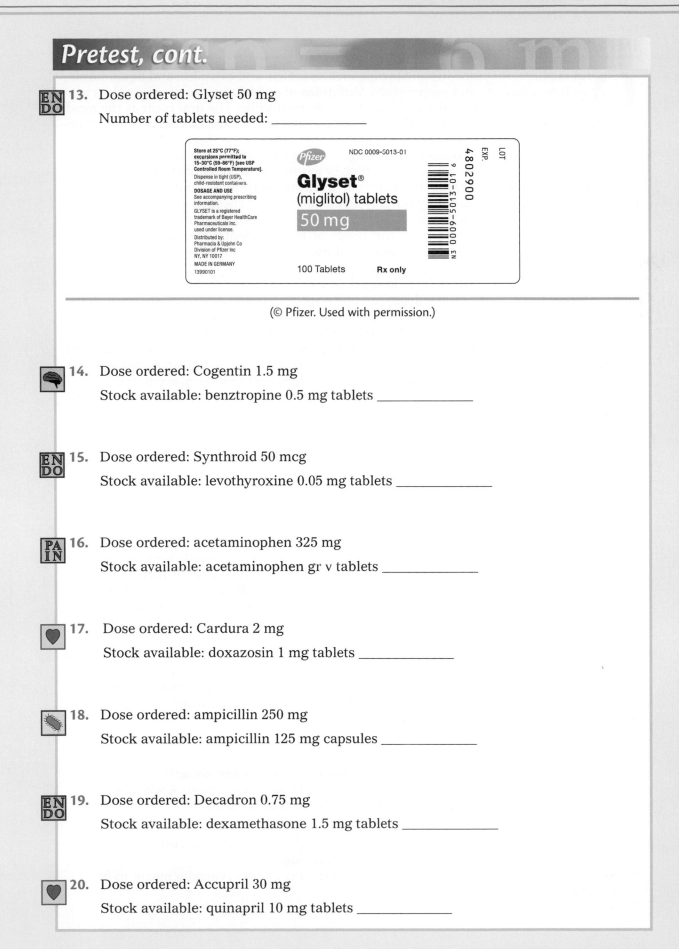

Store at 25°C (77°F); excursions permitted to 15-30°C (59-86°F) [see USP Controlled Room Temperature].
Dispense in tight (USP), child-resistant containers.
DOSAGE AND USE
See accompanying prescribing information.
GLYSET is a registered trademark of Bayer HealthCare Pharmaceuticals Inc. used under license.
Distributed by: Pharmacia & Upjohn Co Division of Pfizer Inc NY, NY 10017
MADE IN GERMANY
13990101

Pfizer
NDC 0009-5013-01
Glyset®
(miglitol) tablets
50 mg
100 Tablets
Rx only

N3 0009-5013-01 6
4802900
EXP.
LOT

14. Dose ordered: Cogentin 1.5 mg

    Stock available: benztropine 0.5 mg tablets _____________

15. Dose ordered: Synthroid 50 mcg

    Stock available: levothyroxine 0.05 mg tablets _____________

16. Dose ordered: acetaminophen 325 mg

    Stock available: acetaminophen gr v tablets _____________

17. Dose ordered: Cardura 2 mg

    Stock available: doxazosin 1 mg tablets _____________

18. Dose ordered: ampicillin 250 mg

    Stock available: ampicillin 125 mg capsules _____________

19. Dose ordered: Decadron 0.75 mg

    Stock available: dexamethasone 1.5 mg tablets _____________

20. Dose ordered: Accupril 30 mg

    Stock available: quinapril 10 mg tablets _____________

INTRODUCTION

Oral medications come in solid forms, such as tablets and capsules, and liquid forms, such as solutions and suspensions. Variations of solid forms, such as powders and granules, may be dissolved in liquid for administration. The oral route is the most frequently used due to convenience for the patient, safety, and reduced cost of administration and manufacturing.

Oral medications are absorbed in the gastrointestinal tract, primarily in the small intestine. A prescription or medication order is written to accommodate individual differences due to age, weight, and concurrent medical conditions, among others. These differences must be considered by the physician and further checked and verified by the pharmacy professional as a means of checks and balances. Drug manufacturers provide drugs in different strengths to meet the needs of most patients. The pharmacy technician must be aware of the various strengths of medications and choose the correct drug strength to dispense.

Calculation of exact doses and dosages is a critical factor in both dispensing and administering medications. Many drugs are prescribed in the exact amount found in stock, whereas others must be calculated. When the dose ordered is available in the ordered strength and form, no calculations are needed and fewer errors occur.

Some tablets are scored to allow breaking them in half or even thirds. Medications that are not scored are generally not to be divided into smaller doses. Some tablets are enteric-coated to delay release until they pass through the stomach to either prevent irritation of the stomach or avoid the inactivation of the medication by stomach acid. Enteric-coated medications should *never* be divided, crushed, or chewed. This rule also applies to most extended-release (over time) formulations and delayed-release formulations. Capsules should not be crushed, chewed, or divided, although a few can be opened and sprinkled on food for ease of administration. Be certain of these restrictions when calculating solid doses.

CALCULATING SOLID ORAL MEDICATION DOSES

The pharmacy technician must be sure to calculate the correct amount of medicine to be given to the patient both for an individual dose and the entire course of therapy. A **dose** is the amount of medicine to be given at *one specific time*, whereas **dosage** indicates the size, frequency, and number of doses of medication prescribed *over a period of time*. Also, be sure that the medication name is correct because many medications have sound-alike or look-alike names. If there is ever a doubt about the medicine to be used or if the answer calculated is not what you expect, obtain clarification from the pharmacist, a practice that is always safe, important, and acceptable. The pharmacist is the person ultimately responsible for dispensing the medication and would prefer to answer questions before medication preparation rather than make a medication error by dispensing incorrect doses, dosages, or medications.

TECH NOTE

Remember that dose refers to the amount of medication given at *a single time*; dosage refers to the amount of medication needed to fill the physician's entire order *over a period of time*. A helpful hint to remember this is the word dosage includes age, which refers to a period of time.

Rules that should be considered when calculating medication doses follow:

- *Most* capsules are not meant to be opened or divided.
- Scored tablets may be divided, but unscored tablets are not typically meant to be divided.

- **Enteric-coated, buccal,** and **sublingual** tablets, as well as most extended- and delayed-release capsules, are not intended for crushing, dividing, or chewing.
- Buccal and sublingual tablets should not be swallowed whole but should be dissolved within the oral cavity in the designated location.
- If a part of a tablet (usually ½) is the answer to a dose problem, be sure dividing the tablet will not alter the pharmaceutical action, the calculations are correct, and the correct medication and strength have been chosen.

! TECH ALERT

Always double-check your calculations! If your answer seems incorrect, recalculate. If the answer still does not seem correct, ALWAYS ask for help from a pharmacist. Never fill an order or prescription if you have a question regarding the accuracy of your calculations.

Single-step calculations are easily performed with the ratio and proportion (R&P) method, using cross-multiplication and division. Any of these calculations can also be performed with dimensional analysis (DA). Choose which method is best for you.

Calculating Medication Doses Using Ratio and Proportion

First, write the relationships as fractional units. Note that the **known** dose and the **dosage form** are on the left side of the proportion. Remember that the units of the numerators must be the same and the units of the denominators must be the same, since these are equivalent fractions.

If you have 250 mg capsules available and you need a 500 mg dose:

$$\frac{250 \text{ mg}}{1 \text{ cap}} = \frac{500 \text{ mg}}{x} \quad \text{1 times 500 divided by 250 equals 2 capsules.}$$

This is read as follows: If there are 250 mg in 1 capsule, there are 500 mg in x capsules.

! TECH ALERT

ONLY cross-multiply and divide with the **R&P** method!

EXAMPLE 8.1

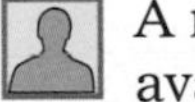

A medication order is written for fluoxetine (Prozac) 80 mg and the stock medication available is Prozac 40 mg capsules. What is the dose to be given to the patient?

$$\frac{40 \text{ mg}}{1 \text{ cap}} = \frac{80 \text{ mg}}{x} \quad \text{Cross-multiply.}$$

The units "mg" cancel.

$$40x = 80 \text{ caps} \quad \text{Divide both sides by 40.}$$

$$x = 2 \text{ caps}$$

EXAMPLE 8.2

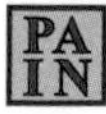 A medication order is written for gr 3⁄4 codeine.

Stock strength available is codeine gr 1⁄4 tablet. What is the dose to be given to the patient?

$$\frac{\text{gr } 1/4}{1 \text{ tab}} = \frac{\text{gr } 3/4}{x} \quad \text{Cross-multiply:}$$

The units "gr" cancel.

$$\frac{1}{4}x = \frac{3}{4} \text{ tabs} \quad \text{Multiply both sides by 4.} \quad x = 3 \text{ tabs}$$

Calculating Medications Using Dimensional Analysis

Although DA is most useful when performing calculations with more than one step, to keep track of units, it can be used for single-step calculations. To use DA, fractional units must allow for the cancellation of measurements from one fraction to the next. When orders are written in different measurement systems or units, DA is used to incorporate a conversion factor.

TECH NOTE

Remember to always start with whatever unit you want for your answer, follow it with an equal sign, and place the known quantity with that unit in the numerator of the first fraction to the right of the equal sign. Continue with this process until you cancel all but your desired unit.

If you have 250 mg capsules available and you need a 500 mg dose, start with the unit needed for the answer, capsules, and follow with an equal sign. Then use the known quantity with that unit as the numerator first. Follow with the fraction that will cancel the unit of the previous denominator, and solve.

$$\text{caps} = \frac{1 \text{ cap}}{250 \text{ mg}} \bullet \frac{500 \text{ mg}}{1} = 2 \text{ caps}$$

 **TECH ALERT**

DA is multiplication of fractions. NEVER cross-multiply unless using R&P!
As we have seen previously, this one-step problem was solved more simply with R&P.
The following examples show Examples 8.1 and 8.2 performed with DA.

EXAMPLE 8.3

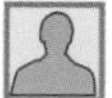 A medication order is written for Prozac (fluoxetine) 80 mg, and the stock medication available is Prozac 40 mg capsules. What is the dose to be given to the patient?

$$\text{caps} = \frac{1 \text{ cap}}{40 \text{ mg}} \bullet \frac{80 \text{ mg}}{1}$$ Milligrams are canceled because this is a fraction multiplication:

$$\text{caps} = \frac{80 \text{ caps}}{40} = 2 \text{ caps}$$

EXAMPLE 8.4

PA
IN

A medication order is written for gr 3/4 codeine to be given, and stock strength available is codeine gr 1/4/tablet. What is the dose to be given to the patient?

$$\text{tabs} = \frac{1 \text{ tab}}{\text{gr } 1/4} \bullet \frac{\text{gr } 3/4}{1}$$ gr cancel because this is a fraction multiplication

$$\text{tabs} = \frac{3}{4} \text{ tabs} \Big/ \frac{1}{4}$$ Invert the second fraction and multiply.

$$\text{tabs} = \frac{3}{4} \text{ tabs} \bullet \frac{4}{1} = 3 \text{ tabs}$$

Either method can be used for Practice Problems A, but DA should be used for Practice Problems B, which are multistep problems.

Practice Problems A

Calculate the number of tablets or capsules required per dose in the following orders. Show your calculations.

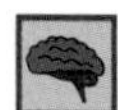

1. Order: Dilantin (phenytoin) 200 mg po

   Number of capsules needed: ____________

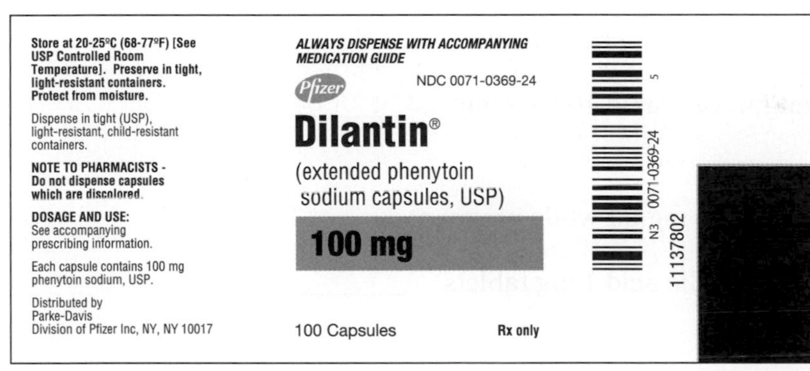
Store at 20-25°C (68-77°F) [See USP Controlled Room Temperature]. Preserve in tight, light-resistant containers. Protect from moisture.
Dispense in tight (USP), light-resistant, child-resistant containers.
NOTE TO PHARMACISTS - Do not dispense capsules which are discolored.
DOSAGE AND USE: See accompanying prescribing information.
Each capsule contains 100 mg phenytoin sodium, USP.
Distributed by Parke-Davis Division of Pfizer Inc, NY, NY 10017
ALWAYS DISPENSE WITH ACCOMPANYING MEDICATION GUIDE
Pfizer
NDC 0071-0369-24
Dilantin®
(extended phenytoin sodium capsules, USP)
100 mg
100 Capsules
Rx only
N3 0071-0369-24 5
11137802

(© Pfizer. Used with permission.)

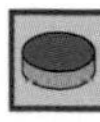

2. Order: ferrous sulfate gr x po qam

   Stock strength: ferrous sulfate gr v tablets ____________

3. Order: digoxin cap 0.1 mg po qam c̄ P ↑60 until changed by MD

   Stock strength: Lanoxicaps 0.05 mg (50 mcg) capsules ____________

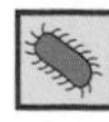

4. Order: Biaxin 500 mg po bid c̄ food

   Stock strength: clarithromycin 250 mg tablets ____________

5. Order: Pravachol 20 mg po daily

   Stock strength: pravastatin 10 mg tablets _____________

6. Order: Ativan 0.5 mg po q6–8h prn anxiety

   Stock strength: lorazepam 1 mg tablets _____________

7. Order: Retrovir 200 mg po qpm

   Stock strength: Retrovir (zidovudine) 100 mg capsules _____________

8. Order: ASA gr × po q4–6h prn aching; do not exceed 8 tab q24h

   Stock strength: aspirin gr v tablets _____________

9. Order: Decadron 0.75 mg daily @ same time

   Stock strength: dexamethasone 0.25 mg tablets _____________

10. Order: isoniazid 250 mg tid c̄ meals

    Stock strength: isoniazid 100 mg tablets _____________

11. Order: folic acid 4 mg qd while pregnant

    Stock strength: folic acid 1 mg tablets _____________

12. Order: ASA 650 mg po q4–6h prn aching; do not exceed 8 tab q24h

    Stock strength: aspirin 325 mg tablets _____________

13. Order: Paxil (paroxetine) 40 mg qam

    Stock strength: Paxil 20 mg tablets _____________

14. Order: Accupril (quinapril) 7.5 mg

    Stock strength: Accupril 5 mg tablets _____________

15. Order: Lyrica (pregabalin) 150 mg bid

Stock strength: Lyrica 75 mg capsules ____________

PA IN 16. Order: Imitrex 75 mg po at onset of migraine, may repeat after 2 hours prn

Stock strength: sumatriptan 25 mg tablets ____________

EN DO 17. Order: Premarin 1.25 mg po qd for 3 weeks, then 1 week off

Stock strength: conjugated estrogens 0.625 mg tablets ____________

PA IN 18. Order: colchicine 1.2 mg po at first sign of gout attack

Stock strength: colchicine 0.6 mg tablets ____________

19. Order: Valium 2.5 mg po tid prn anxiety

Stock strength: diazepam 5 mg tablets ____________

20. Order: LaMICtal 25 mg qd × 2 weeks, then 50 mg qd × 2 weeks, then 100 mg qd × 1 week, then 200 mg qd

Stock strength: lamoTRIgine 25 mg tablets

How many tablets are needed per dose for the first 2 weeks? ____________

How many tablets are needed per dose for the second 2 weeks? ____________

How many tablets are needed per dose for the fifth week? ____________

How many tablets are needed per dose after 5 weeks? ____________

Combination products need to be considered carefully, such as Lotrel 2.5/10. Each tablet contains 2.5 mg of amlodipine and 10 mg of benazepril. If a different dose of Lotrel is ordered, it must be ordered in equal multiples of each component. An order of *Lotrel 5/20 daily in am* is for 2 times the amount of amlodipine (2 × 2.5 = 5) and 2 times the amount of benazepril (2 × 10 = 20); therefore the dose can be provided with 2 tablets of Lotrel 2.5/10. If it were not ordered in equal multiples, the order could not be filled with this medication.

CALCULATIONS INVOLVING DIFFERENT UNITS OF MEASUREMENT

If the units of measurement differ, a conversion factor is required. This becomes a multistep problem, which is better performed with DA in order to keep track of units. DA allows you to make the entire conversion in one equation.

EXAMPLE 8.5

A physician orders metformin 1 g qam. Available stock is 500 mg tablets. How many tablets are needed for one dose?

This requires the use of a conversion factor between g and mg.

$$\frac{\text{tabs}}{\text{dose}} = \frac{1 \text{ tab}}{500 \text{ mg}} \bullet \frac{1{,}000 \text{ mg}}{1 \text{ g}} \bullet \frac{1 \text{ g}}{\text{dose}} = 2 \text{ tabs/dose}$$

Frequently this type of problem is set up without using per dose each time, as that is understood from the question:

$$\text{tabs} = \frac{1 \text{ tab}}{500 \text{ mg}} \bullet \frac{1{,}000 \text{ mg}}{1 \text{ g}} \bullet \frac{1 \text{ g}}{1} = 2 \text{ tabs}$$

TECH NOTE

DA is best when conversions between or within measurement systems are necessary.

EXAMPLE 8.6

A physician orders phenobarbital gr ½ tid. Available stock is phenobarbital 15 mg tablets. How many tablets are needed for one dose?

This requires the use of a conversion factor between gr and mg.

$$\frac{\text{tabs}}{\text{dose}} = \frac{1 \text{ tab}}{15 \text{ mg}} \bullet \frac{60 \text{ mg}}{\text{gr i}} \bullet \frac{\text{gr } 1/2}{\text{dose}} = 2 \text{ tabs/dose}$$

TECH NOTE

When converting, the answer may be approximate rather than exact. Depending on the medication, answers *may* be rounded to the nearest whole number of capsules or tablets. An answer such as 1.9 tablets would be rounded to 2. If tablets are scored, they can be rounded to the nearest half tablet.

Practice Problems B

Calculate the number of tablets, capsules, or packets to be given per dose with each of the following orders using DA. Show calculations.

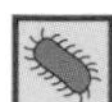

1. Order: ciprofloxacin 1.5 g po qam

   Stock available: ciprofloxacin 750 mg tablets ____________

2. Order: Lopid 1.2 g qam c̄ am meal ____________

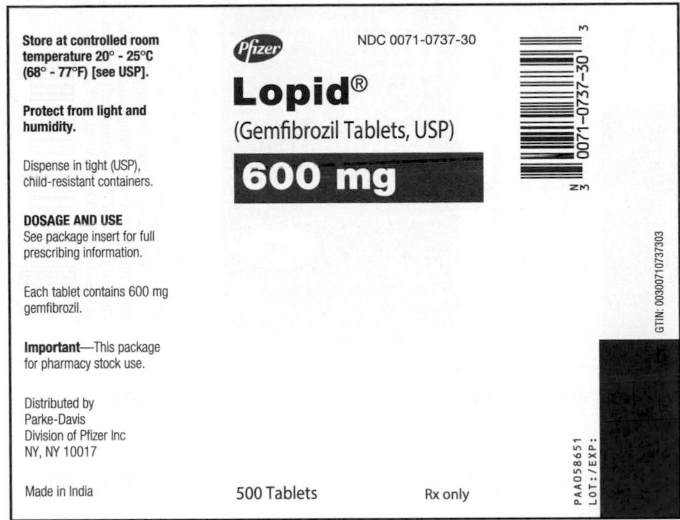

Store at controlled room temperature 20° - 25°C (68° - 77°F) [see USP].
Protect from light and humidity.
Dispense in tight (USP), child-resistant containers.
DOSAGE AND USE
See package insert for full prescribing information.
Each tablet contains 600 mg gemfibrozil.
Important—This package for pharmacy stock use.
Distributed by Parke-Davis Division of Pfizer Inc NY, NY 10017
Made in India
Pfizer
NDC 0071-0737-30
Lopid®
(Gemfibrozil Tablets, USP)
600 mg
500 Tablets
Rx only
N 3 0071-0737-30 3
GTIN: 00300710737303
PAA058651
LOT:/EXP:

(© Pfizer. Used with permission.)

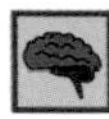

3. Order: Dilantin 0.3 g bid c̄ breakfast and evening meal ____________

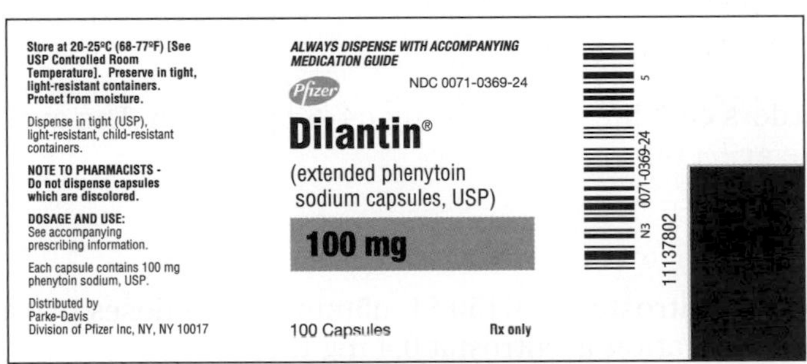

(© Pfizer. Used with permission.)

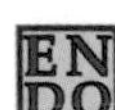

4. Order: Glucophage 1 g po bid c̄ meals

Stock available: metformin 500 mg tablets ____________

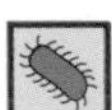

5. Order: cephalexin 0.75 g po bid

Stock available: cephalexin 250 mg capsules ____________

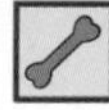 6. Order: Evista 0.12 g po daily ____________

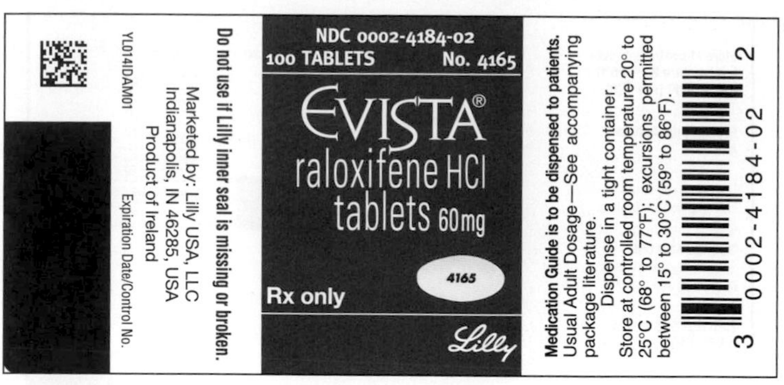

NDC 0002-4184-02
100 TABLETS No. 4165
EVISTA®
raloxifene HCl
tablets 60mg
4165
Rx only
Lilly
Do not use if Lilly inner seal is missing or broken.
Marketed by: Lilly USA, LLC
Indianapolis, IN 46285, USA
Product of Ireland
YL0141DAM01
Expiration Date/Control No.
Medication Guide is to be dispensed to patients.
Usual Adult Dosage—See accompanying package literature.
Dispense in a tight container.
Store at controlled room temperature 20° to 25°C (68° to 77°F); excursions permitted between 15° to 30°C (59° to 86°F).
3 0002-4184-02 2

(© Eli Lilly and Company. All Rights Reserved. Used with Permission.)

7. A physician orders ferrous sulfate gr v po bid. The available stock medication is ferrous sulfate 325 mg tabs. ____________

8. A physician orders phenobarbital gr $\overline{ss}$ po qpm. The available stock medication is phenobarbital 60 mg tabs. (use gr i = 60 mg) ____________

9. A physician orders codeine sulfate 60 mg q4–6h prn pain. The available stock is codeine sulfate gr 1/4 tab. ____________

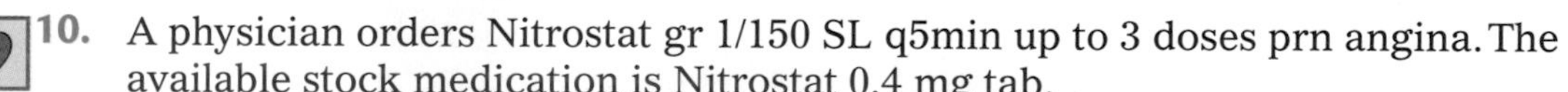

10. A physician orders Nitrostat gr 1/150 SL q5min up to 3 doses prn angina. The available stock medication is Nitrostat 0.4 mg tab. ____________

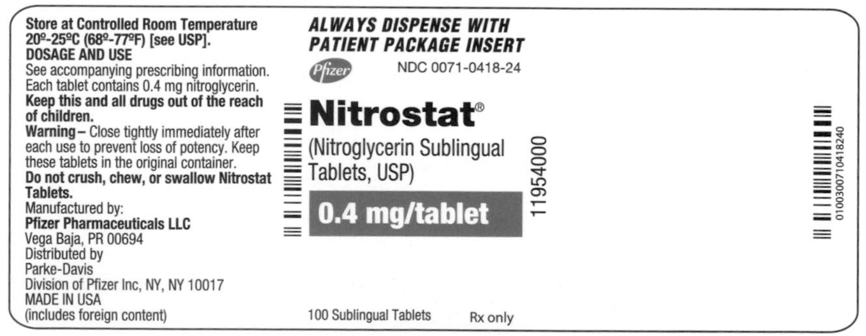

Store at Controlled Room Temperature 20°-25°C (68°-77°F) [see USP].
DOSAGE AND USE
See accompanying prescribing information.
Each tablet contains 0.4 mg nitroglycerin.
Keep this and all drugs out of the reach of children.
Warning– Close tightly immediately after each use to prevent loss of potency. Keep these tablets in the original container.
Do not crush, chew, or swallow Nitrostat Tablets.
Manufactured by:
Pfizer Pharmaceuticals LLC
Vega Baja, PR 00694
Distributed by
Parke-Davis
Division of Pfizer Inc, NY, NY 10017
MADE IN USA
(includes foreign content)
ALWAYS DISPENSE WITH PATIENT PACKAGE INSERT
Pfizer
NDC 0071-0418-24
Nitrostat®
(Nitroglycerin Sublingual Tablets, USP)
0.4 mg/tablet
11954000
100 Sublingual Tablets
Rx only

(© Pfizer. Used with permission.)

11. Order: Robaxin (methocarbamol) 1.5 g

Stock available: methocarbamol 500 mg tablets ____________

12. Prescription: Relafen (nabumetone) 1 g qd with or without food for arthritis pain

    Stock available: Relafen 500 mg tablets ____________

13. Order: codeine phosphate gr $\overline{ss}$ po stat and q4–6h prn pain

    Stock available: codeine phosphate 30 mg tablets ____________

14. Order: Tylenol gr x q4–6h prn fever

    Stock available: acetaminophen 325 mg tablets ____________

15. Order: phenobarbital gr i$\overline{ss}$ po bid

    Stock available: phenobarbital 32.4 mg tablets (use gr i = 64.8 mg) ____________

16. Order: Cogentin 1 mg po qd

    Stock available: benztropine 500 mcg tablets ____________

17. A physician orders Plaquenil 500 mg qd for 4 weeks, then 300 mg qd, for rheumatoid arthritis maintenance therapy. Hydroxychloroquine is available in 0.2 g tablets.

    How many tablets are needed per dose for the first 4 weeks? ____________

    How many tablets are needed per dose for maintenance therapy? ____________

18. A physician orders ibuprofen 0.6 g q8h for rheumatoid arthritis. The patient has ibuprofen 200 mg tablets at home.

    How many tablets are needed per dose? ____________

19. A physician orders levothyroxine 0.2 mg qd on an empty stomach with a glass of water. The stock available is 50 mcg tablets.

    How many tablets are needed per dose? ____________

20. Order: Lamisil granules 0.25 g qd × 6 wk, sprinkle on 1 spoonful of nonacidic food like pudding or mashed potatoes and swallow. Do Not Chew.

    Stock available: terbinafine 125 mg/packet ____________

PATIENT SAFETY WHEN CALCULATING DOSES AND DOSAGES

Accurate calculations are essential for patient safety. Medication orders or prescriptions are the physician's determination of what medication and dosage should be safe for the patient. The physician, pharmacist, pharmacy technician, nurse, and other health care team members work together to ensure this safety. The patient is dependent on health care professionals to provide medications that are as risk-free as possible.

To be certain that the medication and dose are correct, follow the safety rules:

- Always recheck calculations after the dose has been determined. Learn and practice calculations until you are confident using them.
- If you have any calculation questions, check with the pharmacist. Remember that he or she is ultimately responsible.
- As you work from either a medication order or a prescription, verify that what you have on hand is the medication ordered and that it is in the dosage form required.
- Check labels three times before presenting the prescription to the pharmacist for verification—before taking the medication from the shelf, before preparing the medication, and before passing it to the pharmacist.
- Compare the label on the medication with the order from the physician. Be sure these are the same, being careful of look-alike and sound-alike medications. Do not allow yourself to be distracted; keep your full attention on the task at hand.
- Know your medication and the average dose that is required for a patient of the age, gender, and weight of the person for whom the prescription or medication order is written. If in doubt, read the package insert or other reference materials related to the specific medication before preparing it so that you are aware of the usual dose.
- Finally, remember that the pharmacist would rather have you ask a question than have the incorrect medication dispensed to the patient.

REVIEW

When calculating solid oral medication doses, the amount of medication should be calculated to that of the physician's order. If the medication order and the available medication are in different measurement systems, use a conversion factor and DA.

Single-step medication doses can be calculated using R&P or DA. As a pharmacy technician, find the method that is most comfortable for you. Multistep problems involving one or more conversion factors have been taught using DA.

Posttest

Determine the number of capsules or tablets to be given *per dose*. Show all calculations.

1. Order: Tagamet 0.8 g bid

   Stock available: cimetidine 400 mg tablets ______________

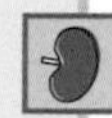

2. Order: HydroDIURIL 100 mg qam pc meal

   Stock strength available: hydrochlorothiazide 50 mg tablets ______________

Posttest, cont.

3. Order: Cipro 0.5 g tid c̄ meals × 7 days
   Stock strength available: ciprofloxacin 250 mg capsules ______________

4. Order: cefaclor 0.75 g daily *in 3 divided doses*
   Stock strength: cefaclor 250 mg capsules ______________

5. Order: Urecholine 20 mg po bid c̄ meals × 10 days
   Stock available: bethanechol 10 mg tablets ______________

6. Order: Benadryl 50 mg po tid prn itching
   Stock strength: diphenhydramine 50 mg capsules ______________

7. Order: Cipro 0.75 g po bid × 10 days
   Stock available: ciprofloxacin 750 mg tablets ______________

8. Order: ampicillin 1 g po stat, then 500 mg po qid × 12 days
   Stock strength available: ampicillin 500 mg capsules
   Number of capsules to be given stat: ______________
   Number of capsules to be given qid: ______________

9. Order: Restoril 0.015 g po at bedtime prn sleep
   Stock strength available: temazepam 15 mg capsules ______________

10. Order: Lopressor 100 mg po bid today, then 50 mg po bid
    Stock strength: metoprolol 50 mg tablets
    What is the *total dosage* to be given today (mg)? ______________
    How many tablets are needed *per dose* today? ______________
    What is the *total daily dosage* to be given starting tomorrow (mg)? ______________
    How many tablets are needed *per dose* starting tomorrow? ______________

Continued

Posttest, cont.

11. Order: tetracycline 500 mg qid × 5 days; then 500 mg bid × 5 days; then 500 mg daily × 5 days for acne

    Stock available: tetracycline 500 mg capsules

    How many capsules are needed *per dose*? ____________

    What is the total number of capsules that will be given over the first 5 days?

    What is the total number of capsules that will be given over days 6 through 10?

    What is the total number of capsules that will be given over the last 5 days?

    What is the total number of capsules necessary to fill the prescription?

    What is the total dosage per day in the first 5 days (g)?

    What is the total dosage per day for days 6 to 10 (g)?

    What is the total dosage per day for the last 5 days (mg)?

12. Order: Strattera 0.05 g po daily c̄ breakfast

    How many capsules are needed for one dose? ____________

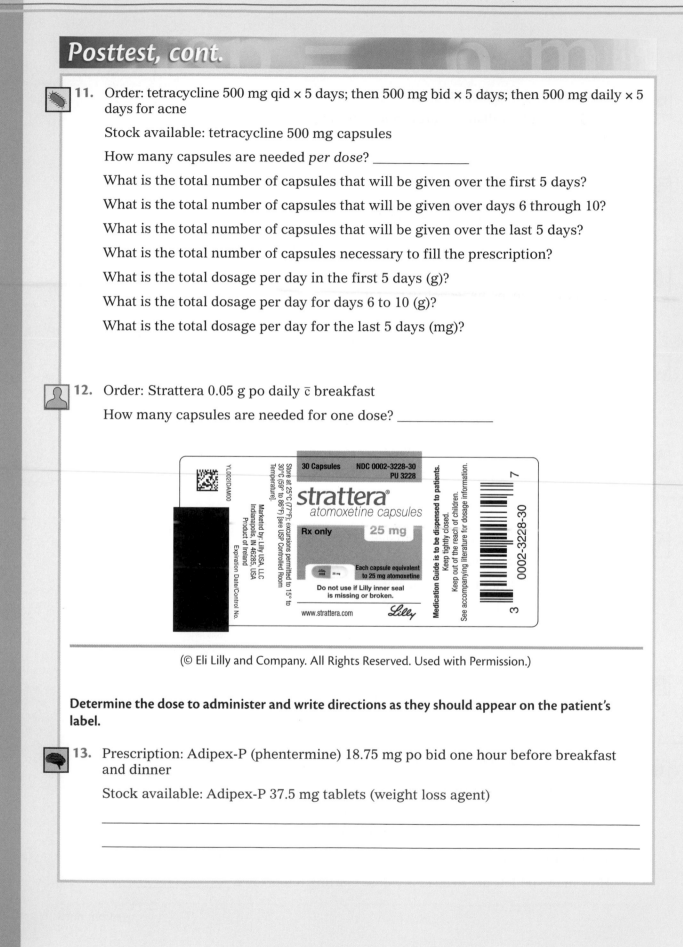

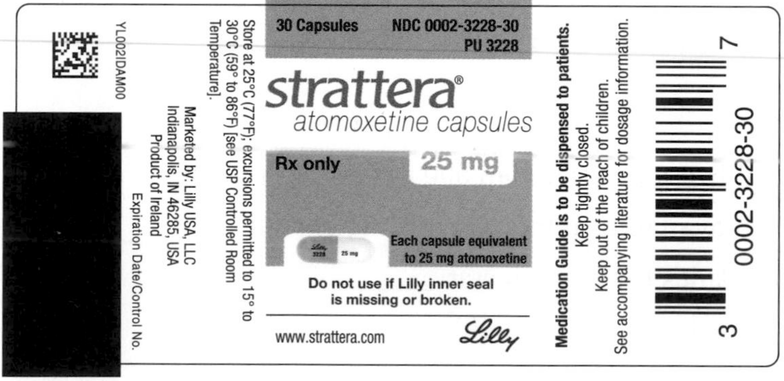

Determine the dose to administer and write directions as they should appear on the patient's label.

13. Prescription: Adipex-P (phentermine) 18.75 mg po bid one hour before breakfast and dinner

    Stock available: Adipex-P 37.5 mg tablets (weight loss agent)

    ____

    ____

Posttest, cont.

14. Prescription: Zyloprim 200 mg q8h for gout

    Stock available: allopurinol 100 mg tablets

    ____

15. Prescription: Elavil 40 mg at bedtime

    Stock available: amitriptyline 10 mg tablets (antidepressant)

    ____

16. Prescription: Zithromax (azithromycin) 500 mg po now, then 250 mg po qd × 4 days

    Stock available: azithromycin 250 mg tablets (antibiotic)

    ____

    ____

17. Prescription: Elavil 10 mg po tid and 20 mg at bedtime

    Stock available: amitriptyline 10 mg tablets (antidepressant)

    ____

18. Prescription: Seroquel (quetiapine) 50 mg po at bedtime on first day, 100 mg po at bedtime on second day, 200 mg po at bedtime on third day, and then 300 mg po at bedtime

    Stock available: quetiapine 50 mg tablets (antipsychotic)

    ____

    ____

    ____

Continued

Posttest, cont.

19. Prescription: Klonopin (clonazepam) 0.25 mg po bid

Stock available: clonazepam 0.5 mg tablets (antianxiety/anticonvulsant)

____

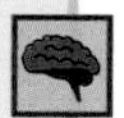

20. Prescription: Namenda (memantine) 5 mg po qd for 1 week, then 5 mg bid for 1 week, then 10 mg bid

Stock available: Namenda 10 mg tablets (Alzheimer agent)

____

REVIEW OF RULES

Calculating Solid Oral Medications

- Calculations for oral solid medications may be accomplished by using R&P or DA.
- Use DA if the problem requires a conversion factor.
- Solid medications usually have a quantity of a single solid form such as per tablet, per capsule, or per package of powder.
- Scored tablets may be broken at scores or on indented marks.
- To solve using R&P, place the known measurements on the left side of the equation and the unknowns on the right. Remember to place the values in each ratio so that the units are in the same position to make the proportion equal. Cross-multiply and divide.
- To solve using DA, always start with the unit of the numerator of your desired answer as the numerator of the first fraction and add the remaining known information as fractions in the order that will cancel unwanted units by multiplication of the fractions.

Calculation of Oral Liquid Doses

OBJECTIVES

1. Interpret orders and calculate the volume of oral liquid medication necessary to administer ordered doses using either ratio and proportion or dimensional analysis.
2. Discuss the process of reconstitution of powders into oral liquid medications.

KEY WORDS

Beyond use date (BUD) Date assigned by the pharmacy to a reconstituted or repackaged medication beyond which the preparation is no longer considered usable

Diluent Agent that dilutes a substance; in pharmacy, the liquid added to a powder to change the powder to a liquid or the liquid used to dilute another liquid; also known as **solvent**

Elixir Sweetened, flavored medication dissolved in a mixture of alcohol and water

Expiration date Date assigned by the manufacturer of a medication beyond which it is not considered usable (no longer valid once a medication is repackaged or reconstituted)

Graduates Containers, calibrated in the metric system, that are used to measure liquid

Meniscus Curved line that develops on the upper surface of a liquid when poured into a container; always read at the bottom of the curve at eye level

Powder volume Space occupied by the powdered active ingredient relative to the total volume of medication after reconstitution; also known as **displacement value;** a measurement of the amount of active substance that displaces (takes the place of) some of the liquid diluent

Reconstitution Process of adding fluid, such as distilled water, to a powdered or crystalline form of medication to make a specific liquid dosage strength

Solution Dosage form in which the medication is completely dissolved in the liquid

Solute Substance that is being dissolved; in this chapter, the powdered medication

Solvent Substance doing the dissolving; aka **diluent**

Suspension Dosage form in which small particles of medication are dispersed throughout the liquid; most require shaking before dispensing and administering

Syrup Aqueous solution sweetened with sugar or a sugar substitute to disguise taste

Tincture A nonvolatile solution of alcohol or alcohol and water, containing plant or chemical substances; examples: Iodine Tincture USP and Vanilla Tincture USP

Pretest

If you are already comfortable with the subject matter, perform the following calculations to test your knowledge. If not, work your way through the chapter and return to them for extra practice. Show your work. Answer in mL unless otherwise specified. Round answers to the nearest tenth.

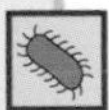

1. A physician orders Ceclor 250 mg po tid for a child with otitis media.

   Stock strength: cefaclor 125 mg/5 mL

   What volume of medication is needed for one dose?

   What is one dose in household measurements?

Continued

Pretest, cont.

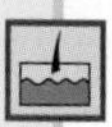

2. Rx: hydroxyzine hydrochloride syrup 10 mg/5 mL
   Sig: 15 mg po qid prn itching
   What volume of medication is needed per dose?

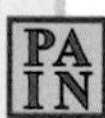

3. A physician orders a child Tylenol gr v q4h prn fever.
   The drug available is acetaminophen suspension 160 mg/5 mL.
   What volume of medication is needed per dose? (Round to nearest whole number.)

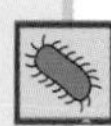

4. A physician orders Amoxil 62.5 mg po tid for an infant.
   The drug available is amoxicillin suspension 125 mg/5 mL.
   What volume of medication is needed per dose?

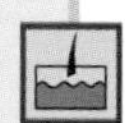

5. A physician orders Benadryl 25 mg tid prn for severe itching.
   The strength available is diphenhydramine 12.5 mg/5 mL.
   What volume of medication is needed per dose?

   What volume is needed in household measurements?

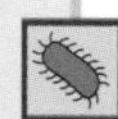

6. Ordered medication: amoxicillin 375 mg po tid × 7 days
   Stock available: amoxicillin oral suspension 250 mg/5 mL
   What volume of medication is needed per dose?

   What is the equivalent household measurement in teaspoons?

Pretest, cont.

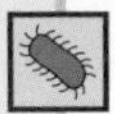

7. Ordered medication: erythromycin 0.3 g po tid × 5 days

   Stock available: erythromycin ethylsuccinate oral suspension 200 mg/5 mL

   What volume of medication is needed per dose?

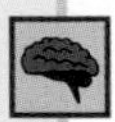

8. Rx: phenobarbital elixir 20 mg/5 mL

   Sig: 30 mg po at bedtime

   What volume of medication is needed per dose?

9. Rx: Prozac (fluoxetine) 20 mg/5 mL

   Sig: 10 mg po qam

   What volume of medication is needed per dose?

   What is this volume in household measurements?

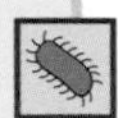

10. A bottle of ampicillin suspension is marked 125 mg/5 mL. The 200-mL bottle instructs that 158 mL of water be added for an oral suspension. The physician wants the child to receive ampicillin 250 mg qid.

    What volume of water should be added to the powder?

    What is the powder volume?

    What is the volume per dose that the child should receive?

    What is this dose in household measurements?

INTRODUCTION

Oral liquid formulations include **solutions**, **tinctures**, **elixirs**, **suspensions**, and **syrups.** Oral medications given in liquid form are absorbed more quickly than solids that have to dissolve before absorption. Most oral medications are absorbed in the small intestine, although some are absorbed beginning in the mouth or stomach. For some patients, solid medications such as tablets and capsules are difficult to swallow so the physician will order oral liquid formulations. This is most common with children and elderly patients. Liquid preparations are labeled as weight per unit of volume such as milligrams per milliliter. Most liquid medications are dosed in household or metric units, with metric being preferred. As with solid medications, conversions may be accomplished by either ratio and proportion (R&P) or dimensional analysis (DA). Some medications for oral administration are supplied in a powder form for reconstitution to a liquid form before dispensing.

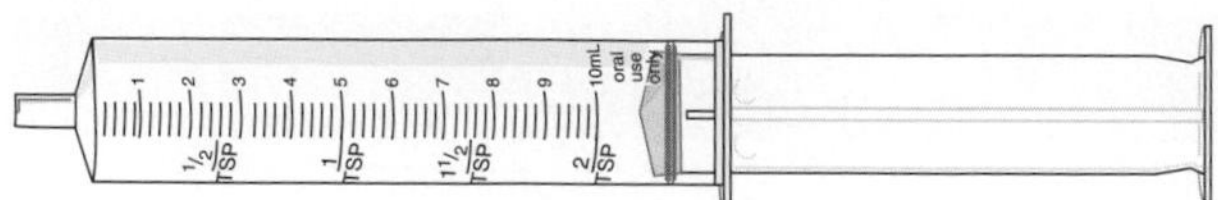

FIGURE 9.1 **Typical Oral Syringe.** (Fulcher EM, Soto CD, Fulcher RM: *Pharmacology: principles and applications*, ed 3, St. Louis, Saunders, 2012.)

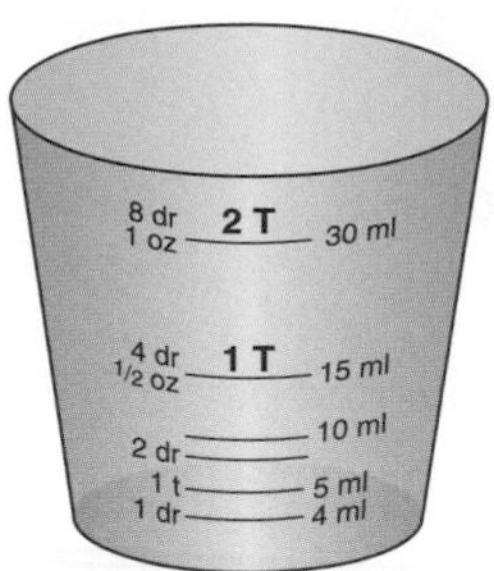

FIGURE 9.2 **Typical Medication Cup.** (Kee J, Hayes E, McCuistion LE: *Pharmacology: a nursing process approach*, ed 7, St. Louis, Saunders, 2012.)

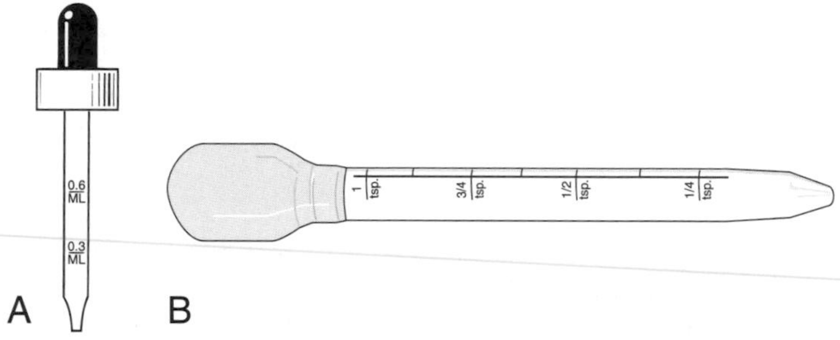

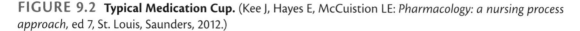

FIGURE 9.3 **Typical Medicine Droppers.** (A, From Brown M, Mulholland JM: *Drug calculations: process and problems for clinical practice*, ed 8, St. Louis, Mosby, 2008. B, From Fulcher EM, Soto CD, Fulcher RM: *Pharmacology: principles and applications*, ed 3, St. Louis, Saunders, 2012.)

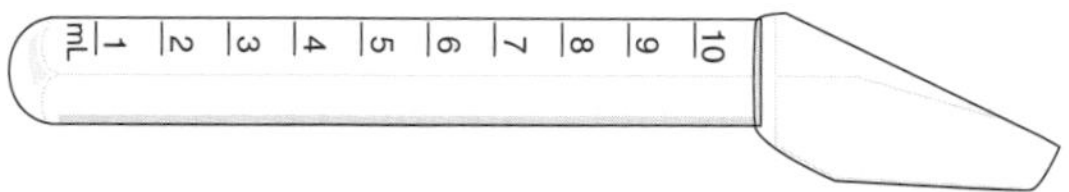

FIGURE 9.4 **Typical Dosespoon Found With Oral Liquid Pediatric Medications.** (Fulcher EM, Soto CD, Fulcher RM: *Pharmacology: principles and applications*, ed 3, St. Louis, Saunders, 2012.)

ADMINISTRATION OF ORAL LIQUID MEDICATIONS

Liquid medications may be administered with oral syringes that are available in 1-mL, 3-mL, 5-mL, 6-mL, and 10-mL sizes (Fig. 9.1), medication cups (Fig. 9.2), droppers that are available in different measurements frequently tailored by the manufacturer for a specific drug (Fig. 9.3), dosespoons (Fig. 9.4), pacifiers that hold a measured amount of medication (Fig. 9.5), or household devices such as teaspoons and tablespoons (not recommended). The choice of administration device depends on the volume of medication to be administered and the availability of supplies. Teaspoons and tablespoons are sometimes used for doses in the home setting when calibrated devices are not available. The use of kitchen utensils is discouraged because of inaccuracy.

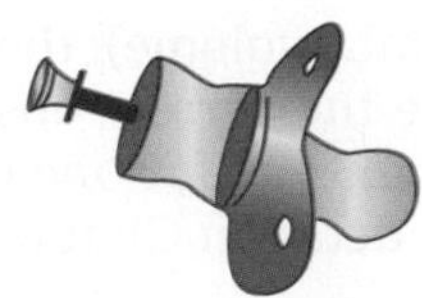

FIGURE 9.5 Pacifier Used to Administer Oral Liquid Medication to Infant. (Modified from Kee J, Hayes E, McCuistion LE: *Pharmacology: a nursing process approach*, ed 7, St. Louis, Saunders, 2012.)

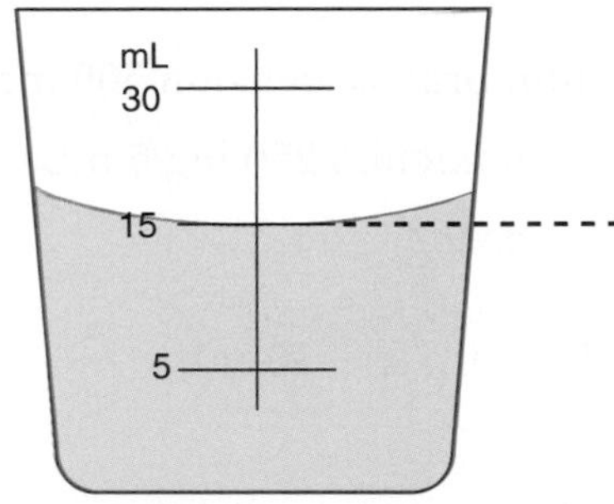

FIGURE 9.6 Reading the Meniscus or Curved Line to 15 mL. (Clayton BD, Stock, YN, Cooper S: *Basic pharmacology for nurses*, ed 15, St. Louis, Mosby, 2010.)

TECH NOTE

When a medication dropper is provided by the manufacturer, it should be used for administration of that particular medication.

When measuring oral liquid medications using a medicine cup, read the line of the medication to the **meniscus** at eye level. The meniscus is the curved line that develops when a liquid is poured into a container (Fig. 9.6) and should be measured at the lowest point. For medications that must be more accurately measured, an oral syringe should be used. With the 1-mL and 3-mL oral syringes, the dose is measured using 0.1-mL increments. With the 5-mL, 6-mL, and 10-mL oral syringes, the calibrations are in 0.2-mL increments.

! TECH ALERT

Household utensils are sources of potential errors and are not the ideal means of measuring doses. The abbreviations for teaspoon (tsp) and tablespoon (Tbsp) can be easily confused, leading to errors in administration. Also, when people use their own flatware to measure, there is too much variation. Patient safety is better ensured if calibrated medication administration utensils are used. However, household utensils are still used in some instances, so understanding these conversions is needed to assist people with proper dosing.

CALCULATION OF ORAL LIQUID MEDICATION

Liquid drug preparations are labeled with the weight of the drug per unit of volume. Most are expressed in the metric units mg/mL. Occasionally you will still see per teaspoon or per tablespoon on a manufacturer's label. Even more rare is the use of the apothecary system. Most labels using grains will include the metric measurement as well.

TECH NOTE

Volume is the unknown value when calculating oral liquid medication doses and dosages.

Remember, the *dose* is the amount of medication to be administered at a specific time, whereas the *dosage* is the total amount of medication that will be dispensed and administered over a particular length of time. A physician may order amoxicillin 500 mg tid for 7 days for a patient who requests a liquid dosage form. If the medication on hand is amoxicillin 250 mg (weight) per 5 mL (volume), the known amounts can be placed into a R&P or a DA equation to determine the correct dose of medication. The total dosage to dispense is found by multiplying the amount for one dose by the number of doses per day by 7 days, which will be discussed in detail in Chapter 11.

Calculating Oral Liquid Medications Using Ratio and Proportion

EXAMPLE 9.1

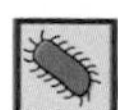

A physician orders amoxicillin oral suspension 500 mg tid for 7 days.

The medication available is amoxicillin 250 mg/5 mL.

How many mL are needed for one dose?

$$\frac{250\text{ mg}}{5\text{ mL}} = \frac{500\text{ mg}}{x} \quad 250x = 2{,}500\text{ mL} \quad x = 10\text{ mL}$$

EXAMPLE 9.2

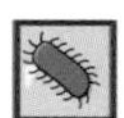

A physician orders Ceftin oral suspension 200 mg every 12 hours for 10 days.

The medication on hand is cefuroxime 125 mg/5 mL.

What volume should be given per dose?

$$\frac{125\text{ mg}}{5\text{ mL}} = \frac{200\text{ mg}}{x} \quad 125x = 1{,}000\text{ mL} \quad x = 8\text{ mL}$$

This prescription should be dispensed with an administration device such as an oral syringe to accurately measure the 8 mL dose.

Calculating Oral Liquid Medications Using Dimensional Analysis

Examples 9.1 and 9.2 are rewritten in prescription format.

EXAMPLE 9.3

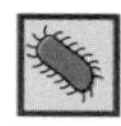

Rx: amoxicillin 250 mg/5 mL

Sig: 500 mg tid × 7 days

How many mL are needed for one dose?

$$\text{mL} = \frac{5\text{ mL}}{250\text{ mg}} \bullet \frac{500\text{ mg}}{1} = 10\text{ mL}$$

Because "mg" is found in both the numerator and denominator, these units cancel.

The amount needed for a 10-day supply is 10 mL/dose × 3 doses/day × 7 days = 210 mL.

EXAMPLE 9.4

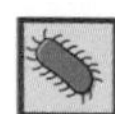

Rx: Ceftin 125 mg/5 mL

Sig: 200 mg po q12h × 10 days

What volume should be given for one dose?

$$\text{mL} = \frac{5\text{ mL}}{125\text{ mg}} \bullet \frac{200\text{ mg}}{1} = 8\text{ mL}$$

To obtain the answer in teaspoons, one more step of fractional components needs to be added to the calculation.

$$\text{tsp} = \frac{1\ \text{tsp}}{5\ \text{mL}} \bullet \frac{5\ \text{mL}}{125\ \text{mg}} \bullet \frac{200\ \text{mg}}{1} = 1\frac{6}{10}\text{tsp or } 1\frac{3}{5}\text{tsp}$$

This is not a measurable amount and would need to be rounded to 1½ tsp. This leads to variation in the actual dose and is not the recommended system to use. 8 mL is much more accurate than rounding to 1½ tsp, which is equivalent to only 7.5 mL.

TECH NOTE

An apothecary dram is approximately 4–5 mL and is considered a teaspoon in the household measurement system. Neither the apothecary nor the household measurement system is extremely accurate.

TECH ALERT

When it is necessary to compute medication doses and equivalencies, the equivalent should be no more than 10% above or below the amount of the prescribed dose. Some doses will require rounding to a measurable quantity; however, the dose, once rounded, should be within the 10% margin. Be aware that some medications require that rounding be within a much lower percentage of variation. This is due to the narrow range between effectiveness and toxicity. If you have questions regarding acceptable rounding techniques, ask your pharmacist for assistance.

Practice Problems A

Calculate the following medication orders, and answer the questions listed. If there is a dispensing device shown, mark the correct dose. Show your work.

Remember to use the method of calculation and conversion that is most comfortable for you.

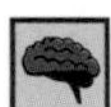

1. Medication order: phenobarbital elixir 60 mg po qid

   Stock strength: phenobarbital elixir 20 mg/5 mL

   What volume of medication is needed per dose?

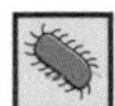

2. Prescribed: Diflucan suspension 60 mg po stat, then 30 mg po qd × 20 days

   Stock strength available: fluconazole oral suspension 10 mg/mL

   What volume of medication is needed for the stat dose?

   What volume of medication is needed per dose thereafter?

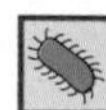

3. Rx: cephalexin susp 125 mg/5 mL

Sig: 62.5 mg po tid c̄ food × 7 days

What volume of medication is needed per dose?

What is the equivalent in the household measurement system?

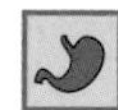

4. Rx: Colace (docusate sodium) syrup 20 mg/5 mL

Sig: 100 mg po at bedtime prn dry, hard stools

What volume of medication is needed per dose?

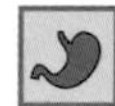

5. Rx: ranitidine syrup 15 mg/mL

Sig: 150 mg po bid q12h

What volume of medication is needed per dose?

6. Rx: fluoxetine 20 mg/5 mL

Sig: 10 mg po bid

What volume of medication is needed per dose?

What is the equivalent volume in the household measurement system?

What types of medication administration devices could be used to administer this dose?

____

7. Prescribed: Lanoxin pediatric 75 mcg bid if P ↑ 60

Stock available: digoxin 0.05 mg/mL solution

What volume of medication is needed per dose?

This medication increases the strength of heart contractions.

Would it be appropriate to measure the dose with household utensils? Why or why not?

____

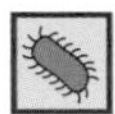

8. Rx: amoxicillin susp 125 mg/5 mL

Sig: 375 mg po tid q8h

What volume of medication is needed per dose?

What is the equivalent in household measurements?

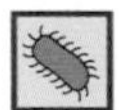

9. Prescribed: cefaclor oral suspension 250 mg tid c̄ food

What volume of cefaclor oral suspension 125 mg/5 mL should be given per dose?

What volume of cefaclor oral suspension 250 mg/5 mL should be given per dose?

What volume of cefaclor oral suspension 375 mg/5 mL should be given per dose?

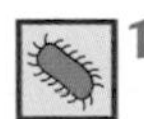

10. Prescribed: amoxicillin oral suspension 0.75 g daily in three divided doses

Stock strength available: amoxicillin 250 mg/5 mL oral suspension

What volume of medication is needed per dose?

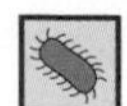 **11.** Prescribed: cephalexin oral suspension 0.375 g tid

What volume of cephalexin oral suspension 125 mg/5 mL would be given per dose?

What volume of cephalexin oral suspension 250 mg/5 mL would be given per dose?

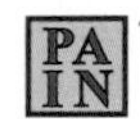 **12.** Prescribed: acetaminophen 19 mg q4h prn fever and aching

Stock strength available: acetaminophen liquid 160 mg/5 mL

What volume of medication is needed per dose? (Round answer to nearest tenth.)

Show the appropriate dose on the following dropper:

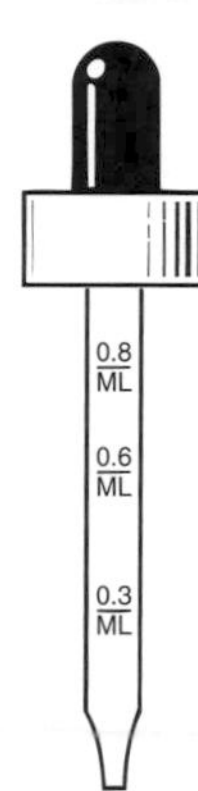

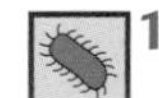 **13.** Rx: penicillin VK susp 125 mg/5 mL

Sig: 62.5 mg po qid c̄ food

What volume of medication is needed per dose?

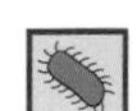 **14.** Order: Vibramycin (doxycycline) susp 25 mg/5 mL

Rx: 100 mg po q12h for the first day, then 50 mg po q12h with fluid for acne

What is the volume of the first 2 doses?

What is the volume of the maintenance doses?

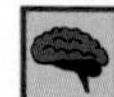

15. Rx: phenobarbital elixir 20 mg/5 mL

Sig: 15 mg po stat

*What is the **measurable** volume for this dose?*

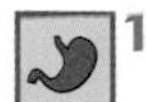

16. Rx: docusate sodium syrup 20 mg/5 mL

Sig: 80 mg po at bedtime

What volume of medication is needed per dose?

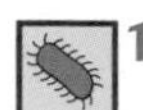

17. Rx: Keflex (cephalexin) susp 125 mg/5 mL

Sig: 32 mg q6h × 7 days

*What is the **measurable** volume for this dose?*

18. Rx: Risperdal (risperidone) 1 mg/mL

Sig: 3 mg po qd

What volume of medication is needed per dose?

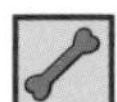

19. Rx: alendronate 70 mg/75 mL

Sig: 35 mg po q week

What volume is needed per dose?

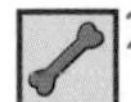

20. Rx: alendronate 70 mg/75 mL

Sig: 10 mg po qd

*What is the **measurable** volume for this dose?*

TECH ALERT

If the answer to a dose calculation does not agree with an anticipated answer based on the amount of medication prescribed and the medication on hand, ALWAYS recalculate and ask for assistance as necessary. A dose that seems too large or too small should always be questioned.

RECONSTITUTION OF POWDERS INTO ORAL LIQUID MEDICATIONS

Medications that are unstable in liquid form for extended periods of time are manufactured in a powdered form that needs to be reconstituted before administration. **Reconstitution** is the process of dissolving the powdered medication, the **solute,** with the appropriate liquid **diluent,** the **solvent.** Follow the reconstitution instructions on medication labels *exactly* to prepare them to the correct strength. Before use, the dry medication must be completely dissolved or suspended into liquid form.

The most important step in reconstituting a powder is to read the label or package insert carefully because it provides the directions for reconstitution. The label states the total quantity of the drug in the container, the volume and type of diluent to use for reconstitution, and the final strength of the medication after reconstitution. The label also includes information on stability and storage needs after reconstitution. These directions must be read carefully and followed exactly each time a medication is reconstituted.

TECH NOTE

Tap the bottle of medication to be reconstituted to loosen any medication that may be attached to the side of the container before adding any diluent.

Many oral liquid antibiotics are supplied in powdered form. Most are manufactured in bottles that are larger than the final medication volume to allow space for shaking before administration. Because the usual vehicle for reconstitution of oral medications is distilled water, **graduates** are used to measure the quantity of liquid to be added (Fig. 9.7). The diluent should be added in increments according to the label, shaking after each addition. In some pharmacies, a computerized dispenser for distilled water is available.

The label on every medication to be reconstituted provides the necessary information for the volume of diluent to be mixed with the powder to provide the desired dosage per unit of volume. When medication is supplied as a dry powder, the space occupied by the powder is known as **powder volume.** The powder actually displaces, or takes the place of, some of the liquid needed to achieve the correct total volume. For example, a powdered medication for oral suspension may require only 78 mL of diluent to be added to produce a total of 100 mL of suspension (Fig. 9.8). The powder takes the place of the other 22 mL. The total liquid volume of the medication will be that of the amount of powder medication displacement plus the amount of added liquid.

Product manufacturers have already calculated the powder volume, or **displacement value**, for medications, and the appropriate amount of diluent to add is listed on every bottle of medication. With medications supplied as reconstitutable powders, the manufacturer's container usually provides the volume needed for a normal course of therapy. For example, most oral antibiotic suspensions will provide enough medication for the necessary 7- to 10-day supply required. Sometimes a drug normally intended for pediatric use will be prescribed for an adult, and more than one bottle of the selected liquid medication may be needed to fill an entire prescription for the desired length of time. This will be covered in Chapter 11.

Before reconstitution, these medications are labeled with an **expiration date** from the manufacturer. Once the pharmacy reconstitutes the medication, the expiration date is no longer valid since these medications begin to degrade. The pharmacy must then assign a **beyond use date**, or **BUD**, according to the directions on the manufacturer's label regarding stability. The BUD should be clearly visible on the prescription label.

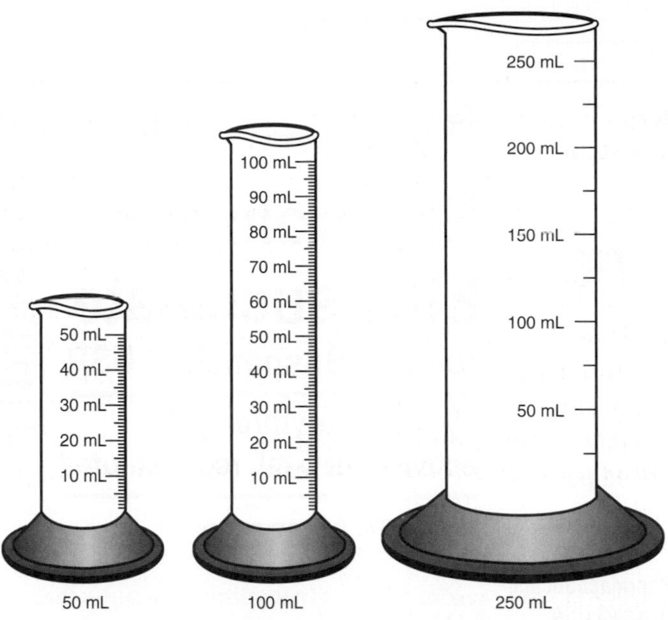

FIGURE 9.7 **Examples of Graduated Cylinders.**

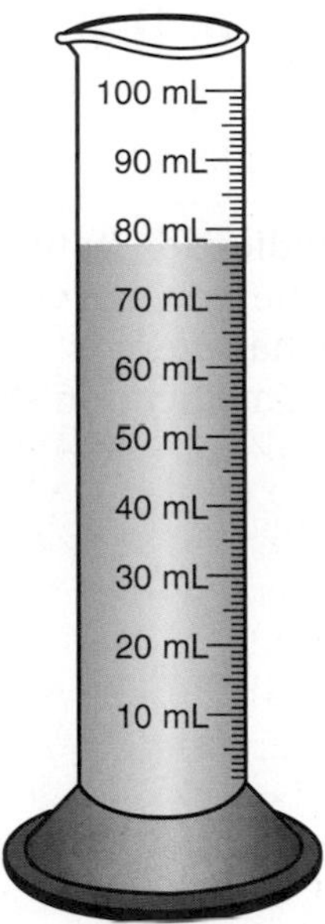

FIGURE 9.8 **Graduated Cylinder Shows 78 mL of Diluent.**

EXAMPLE 9.5

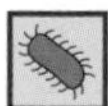

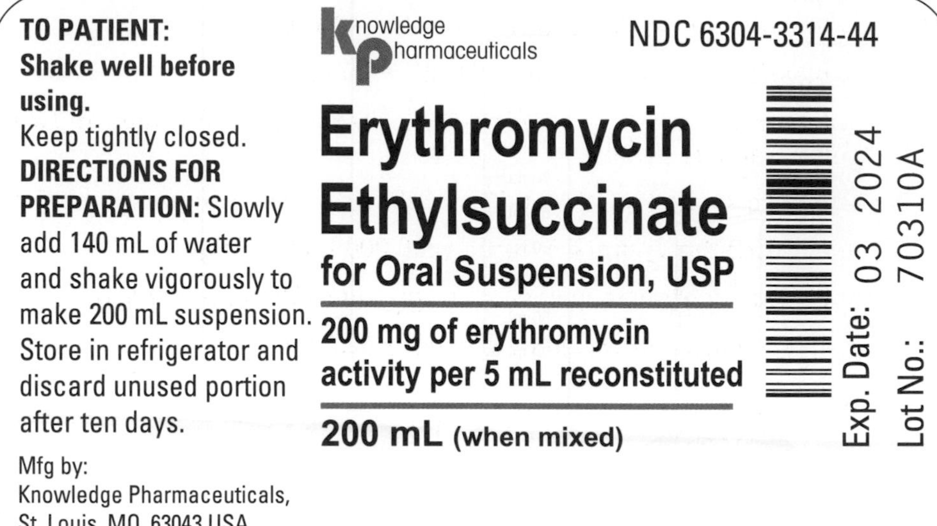

According to the "DIRECTIONS FOR PREPARATION," the bottle of erythromycin will contain a total volume of 200 mL after reconstitution with 140 mL of distilled water. It must then be kept refrigerated and any unused portion discarded after 10 days. The expiration date of 03/2024 must be replaced with a BUD of 10 days from the time of reconstitution. The strength will be 200 mg/5 mL.

The powder volume calculation is: 200 mL − 140 mL = 60 mL

Remember that the final volume of medication in the container will always be greater than the amount of diluent added due to the powder volume. Thus the total volume prepared should always be checked to ensure that there is an adequate amount for dispensing the prescription; if not, be sure the correct medication strength has been chosen and reconstituted as ordered.

EXAMPLE 9.6

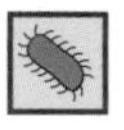

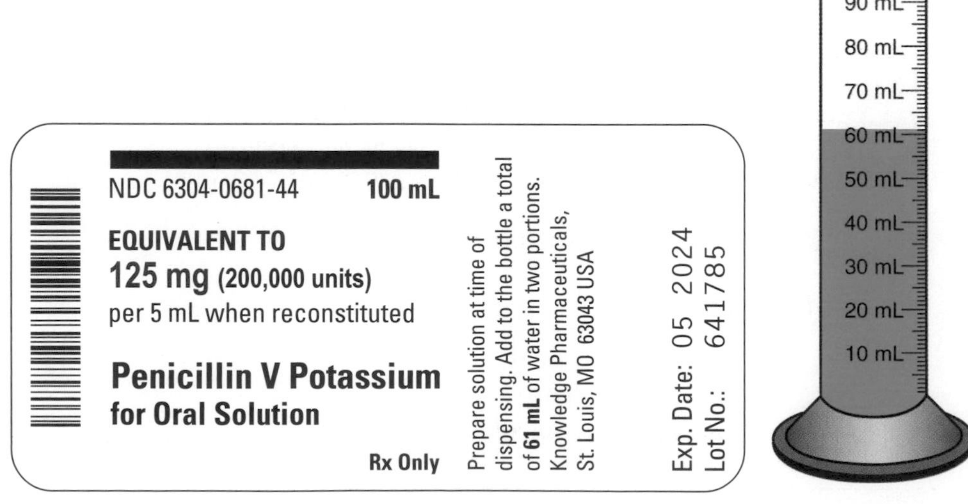

What is the total volume of medication after reconstitution? 100 mL

What diluent is indicated to be added to powder for reconstitution? Water

What volume of diluent is added to the powder? 61 mL

What is the powder volume? 100 mL – 61 mL = 39 mL

What special instructions are given for adding the diluent? Add water in *two* portions; shake well after each addition

What is the metric strength of the solution after reconstitution? 125 mg/5 mL

What is the medication strength in units? 200,000 units/5 mL

What volume of medication is necessary to provide 125 mg of medication? 5 mL

What volume of medication would be given for 62.5 mg?

$$\frac{125 \text{ mg}}{5 \text{ mL}} = \frac{62.5 \text{ mg}}{x} \quad 125x = 5 \bullet 62.5 \text{ mL} \quad 125x = 312.5 \text{ mL}$$

$$x = 2.5 \text{ mL}$$

Practice Problems B

Answer the following questions. Show your work.

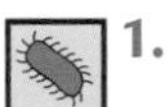

1.

FOR ORAL USE ONLY
Shake well before each use. Discard unused portion after 14 days.

MIXING DIRECTIONS
Tap bottle lightly to loosen powder. Add 24 mL of distilled water to the bottle. Shake well.

NDC 6304-0002-44

35 mL when reconstituted

FLUCONAZOLE
for Oral Suspension, USP
10 mg/mL
*each teaspoonful (5 mL) contains 50 mg of fluconazole when reconstituted

This package contains 350 mg of fluconazole in orange flavor

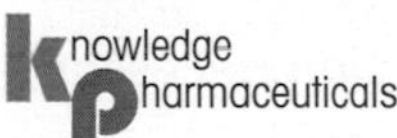

Exp. Date: 03 2024
Lot No.: 70310A

What is the total volume of medication after reconstitution? ____________

What diluent is indicated to be added to powder for reconstitution? ____________

What volume of diluent is added to the powder? ____________

What is the powder volume?

What special instructions are given for adding the diluent? ____________

____

What is the metric strength of the suspension per milliliter after reconstitution? ________

What volume of medication provides 50 mg of medication?

What volume of medication provides 30 mg of medication?

2.

AMOXICILLIN
125 mg/ 5mL

Directions for mixing:
Tap bottle until all powder flows freely. Add approx. 2/3 of total water for re–constitution (total of 67 mL) Add remaining water and shake well Must be refrigerated. Discard after 10 days. .

Keep tightly closed.
Shake well before using.

125mg/5mL
NDC 6304-3314-44
AMOXICILLIN/ CLAVULANATE POTASSIUM
FOR ORAL SUSPENSION
When reconstituted, each 5 mL contains:
AMOXICILLIN, 125 MG, as the trihydrate
CLAVULANIC ACID, 31.25 MG, as clavulanate potassium
75 mL (when reconstituted)
Knowledge Pharmaceuticals

Mfg By:
Knowledge Pharmaceuticals
St. Louis, MO 63043

LOT 170508-A
EXP 05 2024

100 mL
90 mL
80 mL
70 mL
60 mL
50 mL
40 mL
30 mL
20 mL
10 mL

What two drugs are in this medication? ______________________________

What is the total volume of medication after reconstitution? ____________

What volume of diluent should be added? ____________

On the graduate, show the volume of diluent to be added.

What is the powder volume?

On the label, what is the first direction necessary for reconstitution? ____________

What special directions are necessary when adding the diluent? ______________

____

What volume of medication provides a dose of 250 mg of amoxicillin?

What is the volume of this dose in household measurements?

What instructions must be given to the patient when dispensing? ______________

____

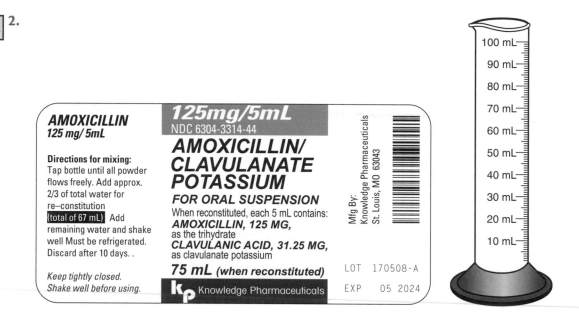

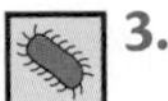

3.

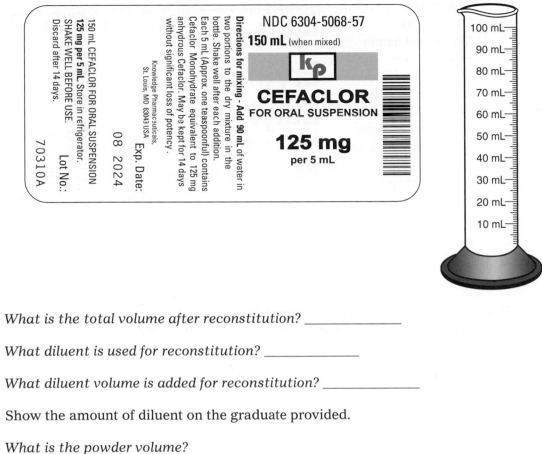

NDC 6304-5068-57
150 mL (when mixed)
kp
CEFACLOR
FOR ORAL SUSPENSION
125 mg
per 5 mL

Directions for mixing - Add 90 mL of water in two portions to the dry mixture in the bottle. Shake well after each addition. Each 5 mL (Approx. one teaspoonful) contains Cefaclor Monohydrate equivalent to 125 mg anhydrous Cefaclor. May be kept for 14 days without significant loss of potency.

Knowledge Pharmaceuticals,
St. Louis, MO 63043 USA

Exp. Date:
08 2024

150 mL CEFACLOR FOR ORAL SUSPENSION
125 mg per 5 mL. Store in refrigerator.
SHAKE WELL BEFORE USE.
Discard after 14 days.

Lot No.:
70310A

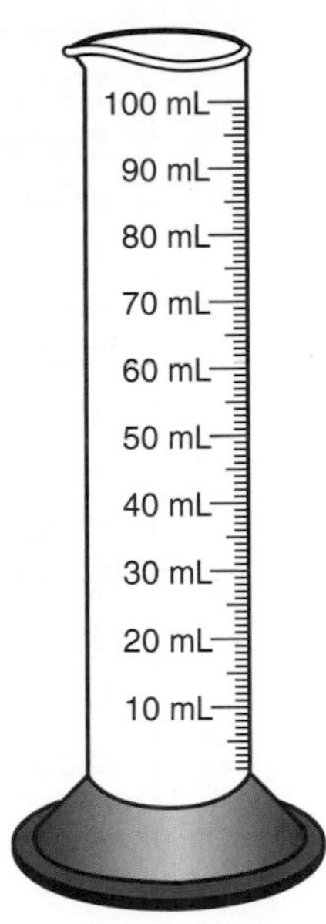

What is the total volume after reconstitution? ______________

What diluent is used for reconstitution? ______________

What diluent volume is added for reconstitution? ______________

Show the amount of diluent on the graduate provided.

What is the powder volume?

What special directions are necessary for reconstitution? __________________________

____

What is the medication strength after reconstitution? ______________

What directions must be given to the patient? __________________________

How long can the medication be kept without loss of potency? ____________________

How many milliliters are needed for a 375 mg dose?

4.

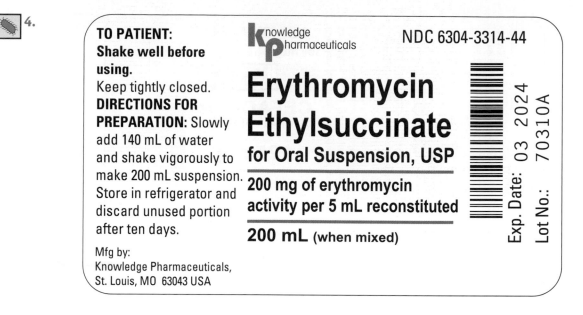

TO PATIENT:
Shake well before using.
Keep tightly closed.
DIRECTIONS FOR PREPARATION: Slowly add 140 mL of water and shake vigorously to make 200 mL suspension. Store in refrigerator and discard unused portion after ten days.

Mfg by:
Knowledge Pharmaceuticals,
St. Louis, MO 63043 USA

knowledge pharmaceuticals

NDC 6304-3314-44

Erythromycin Ethylsuccinate
for Oral Suspension, USP

200 mg of erythromycin activity per 5 mL reconstituted

200 mL (when mixed)

Exp. Date: 03 2024
Lot No.: 70310A

What is the diluent volume that should be added to the medication when reconstituting to the strength designated on the container? ____________

What is the powder volume in the bottle?

What is the strength of the medication after reconstitution? ____________

How long is the medication stable after reconstitution when stored in the refrigerator? ____________

What information needs to be supplied to the patient when this medication is dispensed? ____________

What volume of medication is necessary for a dose of 400 mg?

What is the dose in household measurements?

REVIEW

The same methods for calculation—R&P and DA—are used for oral solid and liquid dosing calculations. Liquid medications are dispensed using the measurements for liquids in the three systems—metric, household, and, rarely, apothecary. Conversions for the correct volume of medication depend on the measurement system to be used for administration. The household system is often used for home delivery of oral medications when a more accurate utensil for administration is not provided. The metric system is always used in inpatient settings.

Reconstitution is necessary when a medication is unstable in a liquid form. Most oral antibiotic liquid medications come in powders that require reconstitution with a diluent. Distilled water or purified water USP are the usual diluents used. Follow the reconstitution directions printed on the medication label exactly to attain the correct strength.

Liquid oral medications may be administered from a medicine cup, dosespoon, oral syringe, medicine dropper, or medication pacifier depending on the volume of medication and the age and ability of the patient. Always provide an appropriate dosage delivery device when dispensing oral medications. As with all medications, the proper calculation and appropriate containers for administration are important for patient safety, which should always be the utmost concern.

Posttest

Interpret the orders and calculate the ordered doses. Show your work. Round to the nearest tenth after completing calculations. Make sure the answer is a measurable volume.

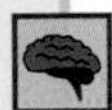

1. Rx: Benadryl (diphenhydramine) elixir 12.5 mg/5 mL
   Sig: 50 mg po at bedtime
   What is the volume per dose?

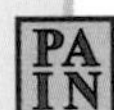

2. Order: acetaminophen suspension 400 mg
   Stock available: Children's acetaminophen liquid suspension 160 mg/5 mL
   What is the volume for the dose?

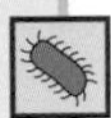

3. Rx: cephalexin 250 mg/5 mL susp
   Sig: cephalexin 375 mg po tid × 7 days
   What volume of medication should be taken per dose?

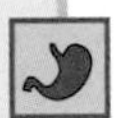

4. Rx: Pepcid (famotidine) susp 40 mg/5 mL
   Sig: 30 mg po bid
   What is the measurable volume per dose?

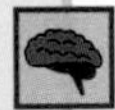

5. Rx: methylphenidate solution 10 mg/5 mL
   Sig: 5 mg bid before breakfast and lunch for ADHD
   What volume of medication should be taken per dose?

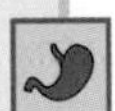

6. Rx: Colace (docusate sodium) syrup 20 mg/5 mL
   Sig: 60 mg po at bedtime
   What is the volume per dose?

Continued

Posttest, cont.

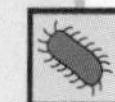

7. Order: Dynapen (dicloxacillin) 125 mg

   Strength available: dicloxacillin suspension 62.5 mg/5 mL

   What is the volume for the dose?

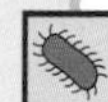

8. Order: Diflucan (fluconazole) 25 mg

   Strength available: fluconazole suspension 10 mg/mL

   What is the volume for the dose?

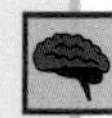

9. Rx: Dilantin-125 Suspension

   Sig: 100 mg q8h

ALWAYS DISPENSE WITH MEDICATION GUIDE

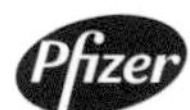

NDC 0071-2214-20

Dilantin-125®

(Phenytoin
Oral Suspension, USP)

125 mg per 5 mL

IMPORTANT–SHAKE WELL BEFORE EACH USE

NOT FOR PARENTERAL USE

8 fl oz (237 mL) **Rx only**

THIS PRODUCT MUST BE SHAKEN WELL ESPECIALLY PRIOR TO INITIAL USE.

Each 5 mL contains 125 mg phenytoin, with a maximum alcohol content not greater than 0.6 percent.

DOSAGE AND USE
Adults, 1 teaspoonful (5 mL) three times daily; pediatric patients, see package insert.

Advice to Pharmacist and Patient–Patient must be advised to use an accurate measuring device when using this product.

See package insert for complete prescribing information.

Store at Controlled Room Temperature 20°-25°C (68°-77°F) [see USP].

Protect from freezing and light.

Keep this and all drugs out of the reach of children.

Distributed by
Parke-Davis
Division of Pfizer Inc
NY, NY 10017

PAA063621

LOT/EXP

Imprint Area
NO VARNISH

What volume of medication is needed per dose?

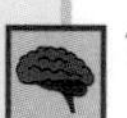

10. Prescribed: phenobarbital elixir gr $\overline{ss}$ q4h for epilepsy

    Stock strength available: phenobarbital elixir 20 mg/5 mL (use gr i = 60 mg)

    Interpret the order: ______________________________

    ____

    What volume of medication is needed per dose?

Posttest, cont.

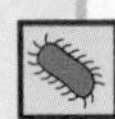

11. Rx: Pen VK (penicillin V potassium) 125 mg/5 mL
Sig: 0.25 g po qid × 10 days

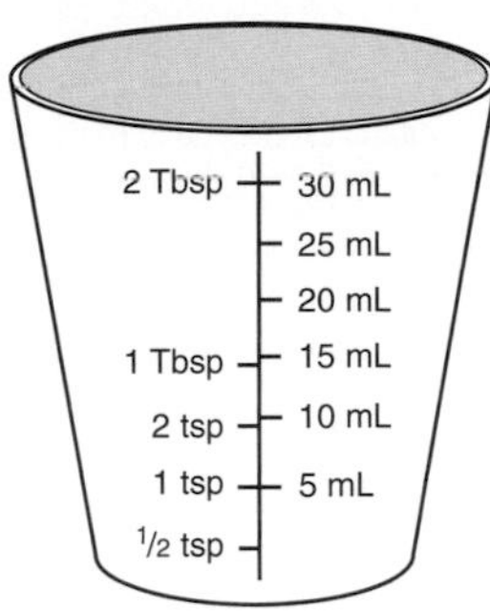

What volume of medication is needed per dose?

What is the equivalent in household measurements?

Indicate the amount of medication in the medication cup.

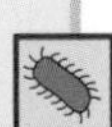

12. Rx: amoxicillin susp 250 mg/5 mL
Sig: 125 mg po q8h × 7d
What volume of medication is needed per dose?

What is the equivalent in household measurements?

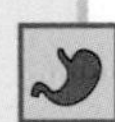

13. Rx: Zantac (ranitidine) syrup 15 mg/mL
Sig: 75 mg bid 30 min ac
What volume of medication is needed per dose?

What is the equivalent in household measurements?

Continued

Posttest, cont.

Indicate the volume of medication on each of the utensils to be used for administration.

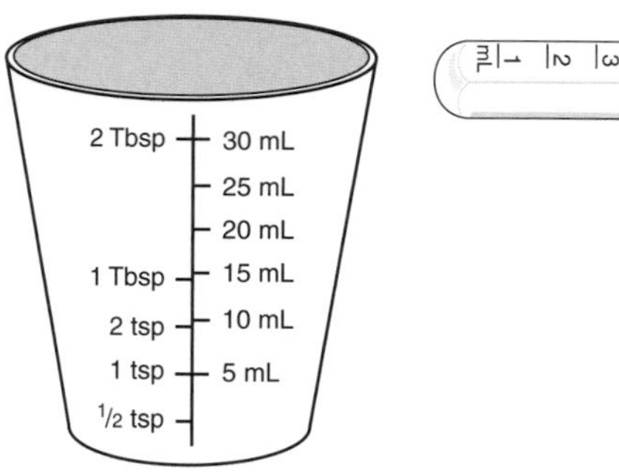

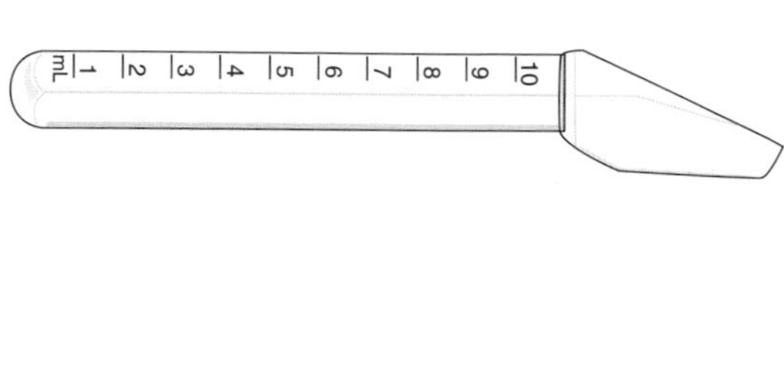

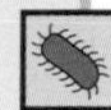

14. Prescribed: Duricef Suspension 750 mg po stat then 0.5 g q12h

Stock strengths available: cefadroxil 250 mg/5 mL and cefadroxil 500 mg/5 mL

Interpret the order: ______________________________

____

Which strength should be used? ______________

What volume of medication should be given for the stat dose in the metric system?

What volume of medication should be given for the stat dose in the household system?

What volume of medication should be given q12h in the metric system?

What volume of medication should be given q12h in household measurements?

How would the answers differ if the other strength had to be used? ______________

____

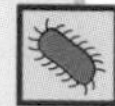

15. A physician orders Mycostatin Oral Suspension 300,000 units to be administered bid. The available medication is nystatin oral suspension 100,000 units/mL.

What total volume of medication should be administered with each dose?

Each dose is to be divided between each side of the mouth.

Posttest, cont.

What volume of medication should be placed in each side? ___________

Write the patient label directions for the following prescriptions.

16. Rx: Prozac (fluoxetine) sol 20 mg/5 mL

Sig: 30 mg po qam

____

17. Rx: Lanoxin (digoxin) Elixir 50 mcg/mL

Sig: 0.125 mg po qam

____

18. Rx: Zantac (ranitidine) syrup 15 mg/mL

Sig: 45 mg po bid 30 minutes ac

____

____

19. Rx: nitrofurantoin susp 25 mg/5 mL

Sig: 100 mg po qid with food × 7 days

____

____

20. Prescription: Septra DS i po q12h × 10 days (patient requires liquid medications)

Stock available: Septra DS tablets: 800 mg sulfamethoxazole and 160 mg trimethoprim
Oral Susp: 200 mg sulfamethoxazole and 40 mg trimethoprim /5 mL

____

Continued

Posttest, cont.

21. Prescription: nystatin 400,000 units po ½ dose in each side of mouth qid, swish as long as possible and swallow

    Stock available: nystatin oral suspension 500,000 units/5 mL

    ____

    ____

    ____

22. Rx: amoxicillin 125 mg/5 mL susp

    Sig: 300 mg po q8h × 7 days

    ____

23. Rx: penicillin V potassium 125 mg/5 mL susp

    Sig: 62.5 mg po qid × 7 days

    ____

24. Rx: griseofulvin susp 125 mg/5 mL

    Sig: 500 mg po q12h with a high fat snack × 6 months for nail fungus

    ____

    ____

Posttest, cont.

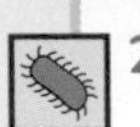

25.

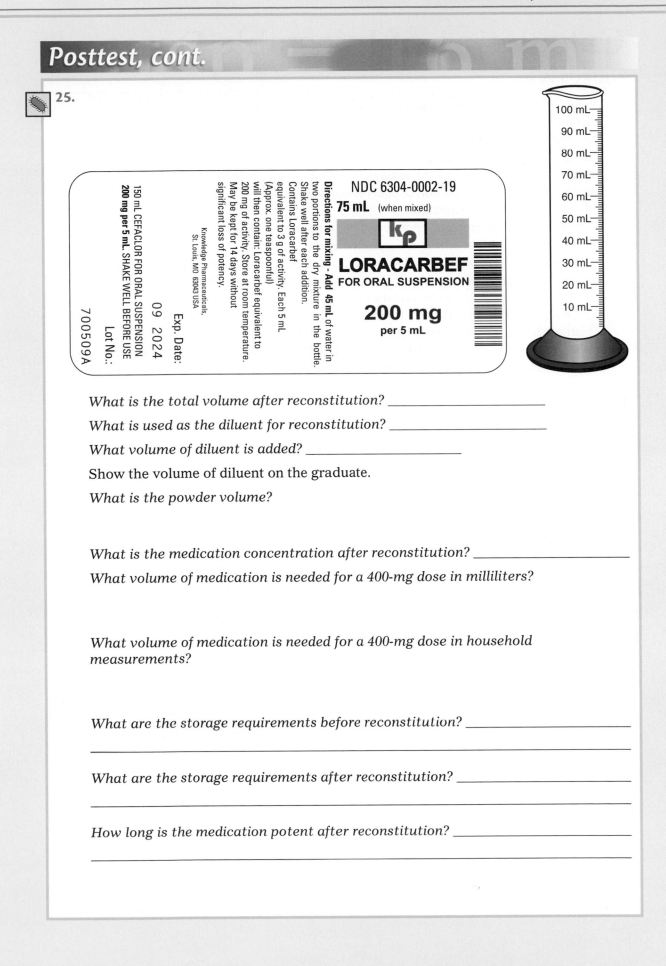

NDC 6304-0002-19
75 mL (when mixed)
kp
LORACARBEF
FOR ORAL SUSPENSION
200 mg
per 5 mL

Directions for mixing - Add 45 mL of water in two portions to the dry mixture in the bottle. Shake well after each addition. Contains Loracarbef equivalent to 3 g of activity. Each 5 mL (Approx. one teaspoonful) will then contain: Loracarbef equivalent to 200 mg of activity. Store at room temperature. May be kept for 14 days without significant loss of potency.

Knowledge Pharmaceuticals,
St. Louis, MO 63043 USA

Exp. Date:
09 2024
Lot No.:
700509A

150 mL CEFACLOR FOR ORAL SUSPENSION
200 mg per 5 mL. SHAKE WELL BEFORE USE

100 mL
90 mL
80 mL
70 mL
60 mL
50 mL
40 mL
30 mL
20 mL
10 mL

What is the total volume after reconstitution? ____________________

What is used as the diluent for reconstitution? ____________________

What volume of diluent is added? ____________________

Show the volume of diluent on the graduate.

What is the powder volume?

What is the medication concentration after reconstitution? ____________________

What volume of medication is needed for a 400-mg dose in milliliters?

What volume of medication is needed for a 400-mg dose in household measurements?

What are the storage requirements before reconstitution? ____________________

____

What are the storage requirements after reconstitution? ____________________

____

How long is the medication potent after reconstitution? ____________________

____

Calculation of Injectable Doses

OBJECTIVES

1. Discuss injectable medications and how they are administered.
2. Measure injectable medications with appropriate syringes.
3. Describe ampules and vials, and discuss their uses.
4. Discuss the rules for calculating injectable medication doses
5. Interpret orders and calculate the volume of injectable medication necessary to administer doses using either ratio and proportion or dimensional analysis.
6. Calculate insulin and heparin doses.
7. Discuss the role of pharmacy technicians in the vaccination process.
8. Describe the following as related to reconstitution:
   - Interpret labels of reconstitutable medications to determine correct type and volume of diluent needed, expiration dates, storage conditions before and after reconstitution, and instructions for assigning beyond use dates.
   - Understand the importance of labeling multidose reconstituted medications with date, time, strength, and initials of person performing the reconstitution.
   - Determine the appropriate dilution concentration when more than one strength is possible, and then determine the correct amount of diluent necessary to achieve this concentration.

KEY WORDS

Ampule Sealed glass container that holds a single dose of medication, usually for injection

Anticoagulant Substance that stops or delays the clotting of blood

High-alert medications Medications that have a high risk of causing significant harm to a patient if dosed or used incorrectly

Injection A dose of medication administered with a needle and syringe

Infusion Slow administration of fluids, other than blood, into a vein

Intradermal Into or within the dermis of the skin (ID)

Intramuscular Into or within the muscle (IM)

Intravenous Into or within a vein (IV)

Parenteral Administration outside the gastrointestinal tract; mostly considered to be by injection or infusion

Patent Open and unobstructed as in IV lines or blood vessels

Subcutaneous Beneath the skin; medications injected into the subcutaneous tissue (subcut)

Therapeutic range A dosage or blood concentration range that normally produces desired results; too much may be toxic and too little may not achieve the desired effect

Vaccination Act of introducing a vaccine into the body to produce immunity

Vaccine Substance causing the immune system to respond better when it is exposed to a disease-causing agent; prepared from the disease-causing agent or a synthetic (manmade) substitute

Vial Glass or plastic container with metal-enclosed rubber seal for injectable medications; may contain single or multiple doses

Pretest

If you are already comfortable with the subject matter, perform the following calculations to test your knowledge. If not, work your way through the chapter and return to them for extra practice. These are medication orders, so assume generic substitution is permitted. Indicate the volume of medication to be administered on any syringes, based on the route of administration, to provide the most accurate dose. Round any dose less than 1 mL to the nearest hundredth and those over 1 mL to the nearest tenth.

1. A physician orders Zofran 2 mg IM 30 minutes before chemotherapy treatment.

   Available stock: ondansetron 2 mg/mL (20-mL multidose vial)

   Interpret the order:

   ____

   How many milliliters should be administered?

2. Order: vitamin B_{12} 500 mcg IM qwk

   Available stock: cyanocobalamin injection 1,000 mcg/mL

   Interpret the order:

   ____

   How many milliliters should be administered to the patient as a weekly dose?

3. Order: Dilaudid 1.3 mg Subcut q6h prn pain

   Available stock: hydromorphone injection 2 mg/mL (1-mL vial)

   Interpret the order: ________________________________

   How many milliliters should be administered per dose?

Continued

Pretest, cont.

4. Order: 25 mg meperidine and 25 mg promethazine IM q4–6h prn pain and nausea
   Available stock: meperidine 50 mg/mL and promethazine 25 mg/mL
   Interpret the order:

   ____

   ____

   How many milliliters of meperidine are needed per dose?

   How many milliliters of promethazine are needed per dose?

   What is the total volume of medication needed if this is administered in one syringe?

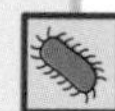

5. A physician orders streptomycin 750 mg IM
   After reconstitution, the strength of the streptomycin is 400 mg/mL.
   Interpret the order:

   ____

   How many milliliters should be administered?

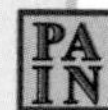

6. Order: codeine phosphate gr $\overline{ss}$ subcut q4h prn
   Stock available: codeine phosphate injection 30 mg (½ gr)/mL (1-mL ampule)
   Interpret the order:

   ____

   How many milliliters should be administered per dose?

Pretest, cont.

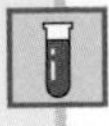

7. Order: heparin sodium 1,500 units subcut stat

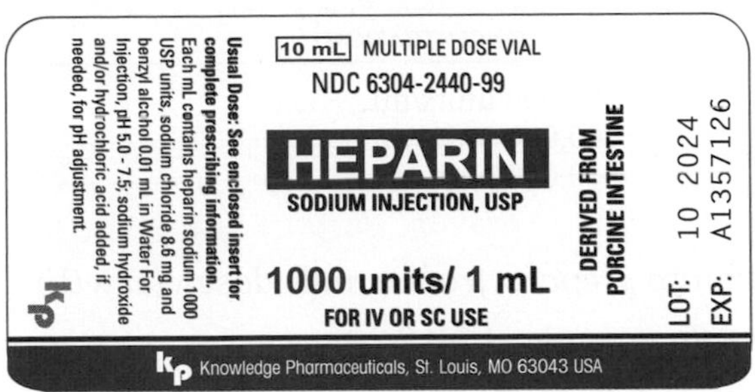

10 mL MULTIPLE DOSE VIAL
NDC 6304-2440-99
HEPARIN
SODIUM INJECTION, USP
1000 units/ 1 mL
FOR IV OR SC USE
DERIVED FROM PORCINE INTESTINE
LOT: 10 2024
EXP: A1357126
Usual Dose: See enclosed insert for complete prescribing information.
Each mL contains heparin sodium 1000 USP units, sodium chloride 8.6 mg and benzyl alcohol 0.01 mL in Water For Injection, pH 5.0 - 7.5; sodium hydroxide and/or hydrochloric acid added, if needed, for pH adjustment.
kp
kp Knowledge Pharmaceuticals, St. Louis, MO 63043 USA

Interpret the medication order:

____

What is the measurable volume of medication that should be given to the patient?

What size syringe should be used? ______________

What is the total volume of medication in the vial? ______________

What is the total number of units of heparin in the vial? ______________

ENDO

8. Rx: Humulin R subcut 14 units tid ac

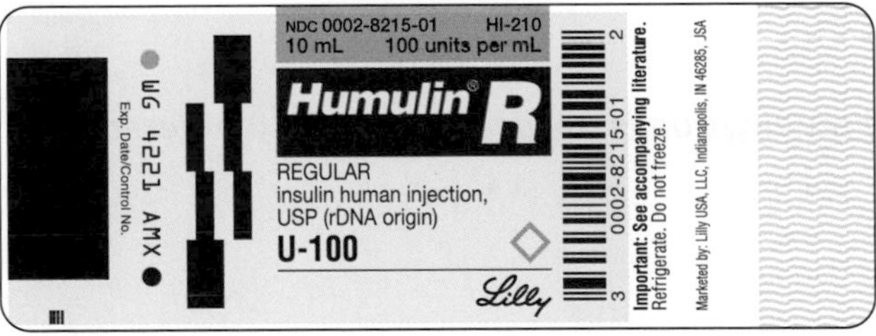

NDC 0002-8215-01 HI-210
10 mL 100 units per mL
Humulin R
REGULAR
insulin human injection,
USP (rDNA origin)
U-100
Lilly
3 0002-8215-01 2
Important: See accompanying literature.
Refrigerate. Do not freeze.
Marketed by: Lilly USA, LLC, Indianapolis, IN 46285, USA
WG 4221 AMX
Exp. Date/Control No.

Write the directions as they should appear on the prescription label:

____

What syringe is most appropriate for this dose? ______________

Continued

Pretest, cont.

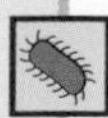

9. A physician orders penicillin G 250,000 units IM q4h × 5 days for a child.

DILUENT	FINAL CONCENTRATION
9.6 mL	100,000 units/mL
4.6 mL	200,000 units/mL
1.6 mL	500,000 units/mL

What is the appropriate concentration to prepare, from a multidose vial with the above choices, to keep the dose volume under 1 mL? ____________

What volume of diluent is needed to meet the requirement for this dose? ________

After reconstitution, what volume of medication is needed per dose?

10. Order: ampicillin 500 mg IM q6h

The available medication is a 1-g vial with the following information on the label:

Ampicillin Concentration: 250 mg/mL

Amount of Diluent: 3.4 mL

What is the total amount (weight) of medication in the vial? ____________

What is the total volume after reconstitution? ____________

What is the powder volume? ____________

What volume of medication is needed for the dose ordered?

INTRODUCTION

Parenteral medications technically include anything administered outside of the gastrointestinal tract but are commonly considered to be those given by **injection** or **infusion**. They are commonly administered directly within the bloodstream (**intravenous**), within the muscle (**intramuscular**), under the skin (**subcutaneous**), or within the skin (**intradermal**). With the exception of slow-release injectable medications, which are ***never*** given intravenously, injectable medications have a quicker onset of action than oral medications. They may be administered if a person is unable to swallow solid medications, if a quick effect is needed, if a person is combative, or if the particular medication would be degraded (broken down) by stomach acid before it has a chance to exert an effect on the body.

> **! TECH ALERT**
>
> All medications administered by injection must be in a sterile liquid form. Once these medications have been injected, the medication cannot be retrieved, so special care is needed to ensure that the medication and its dose are correct before administration.

Most injectable medications are supplied in **ampules** or **vials** (Fig. 10.1) and are prepared as a liquid either in an aqueous (water) or occasionally an oil base by the drug manufacturer. Some medications, especially those used for cardiac emergencies, are supplied as prefilled syringes from the manufacturer. Medications that are not stable in the liquid form come in powders that must be reconstituted before administration. These medications are not stable in liquid form for an extended period of time, so stability must be considered at the time of reconstitution and administration. As with oral liquid medications, most strengths of parenteral medications are identified by weight of medication in a specific volume of liquid. The weight is usually provided in the metric system—milligrams, grams, or micrograms—and the volume in milliliters. Electrolytes are typically measured in mEq/mL. The apothecary system unit of grains per milliliter may also be used, although

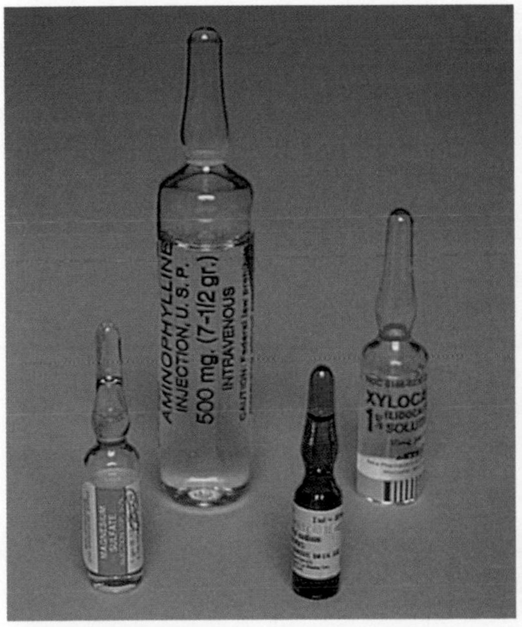

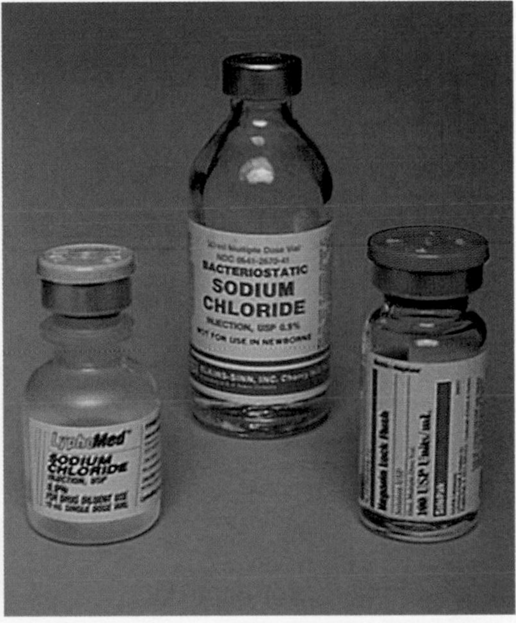

FIGURE 10.1 Typical Ampule and Vial Containers. (Potter P, Perry A: *Fundamentals of nursing*, ed 9, St. Louis, Mosby, 2017.)

this is not common. International Units are used for biologic medications. Some parenteral medication strengths are expressed as a percentage or ratio, but these are often expressed on the manufacturer's label in weight per volume strength as well.

TECH NOTE

Injectable labels express the amount of medication per mL, such as mcg/mL, mg/mL, mg/L, g/mL, g/L, units/mL, mEq/mL, and occasionally gr/mL.

Syringes

Because all injectable medications must be prepared using sterile technique, sterile needles and syringes must be used. Pharmacy staff uses syringes ranging from 1 to 60 mL when preparing injectable medication. Tuberculin (TB) syringes have a 1-mL capacity and are calibrated in 0.01-mL increments (Fig. 10.2). 3-mL syringes are calibrated in 0.1-mL increments (Fig. 10.3). 5-mL and 10-mL syringes are calibrated in 0.2-mL increments (Fig. 10.4). 20-mL syringes are calibrated in 1-mL increments. 60-mL syringes are calibrated in 2-mL increments.

TECH NOTE

Calibrations between markings on a syringe are usually four spaces, as in increments of 0.1 mL on the 3-mL syringe or 0.2 mL on the 5-mL syringe. Always be sure to understand the markings before using the syringe for preparing medications to ensure that the correct amount of medication is being prepared.

Once the dose has been calculated, the correct syringe must be chosen based on the amount of medication to be administered or added to other intravenous (IV) fluids. If the volume of a medication dose is less than 1 mL, it should be measured with a 1-mL TB syringe except in the case of insulin U-100, which is measured in specially calibrated insulin syringes (covered later in this chapter). Doses less than 1 mL that require rounding are rounded to the hundredths place because that is measurable on a TB syringe. A 3-mL syringe is the usual choice for measuring volumes between 1 mL and 3 mL, which would be rounded to the tenths position if necessary. A 5-mL syringe is used for doses between 3 mL and 5 mL, and a 10-mL syringe is used for doses between 5 mL and 10 mL. These doses

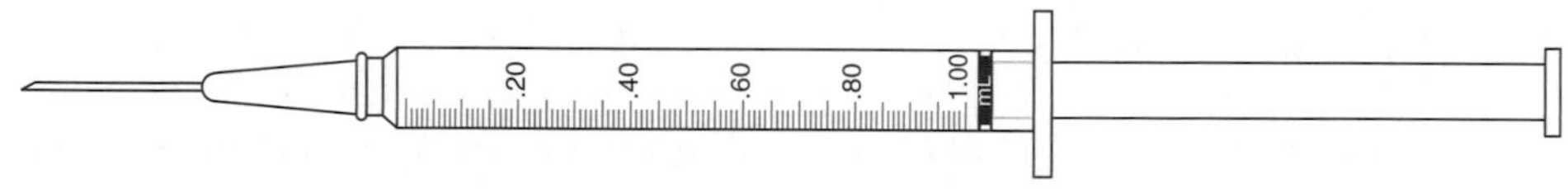

FIGURE 10.2 **Typical Tuberculin Syringe Measured in 0.01 mL.** (Fulcher EM, Soto CD, Fulcher RM: *Pharmacology: principles and applications*, ed 3, St. Louis, Saunders, 2012.)

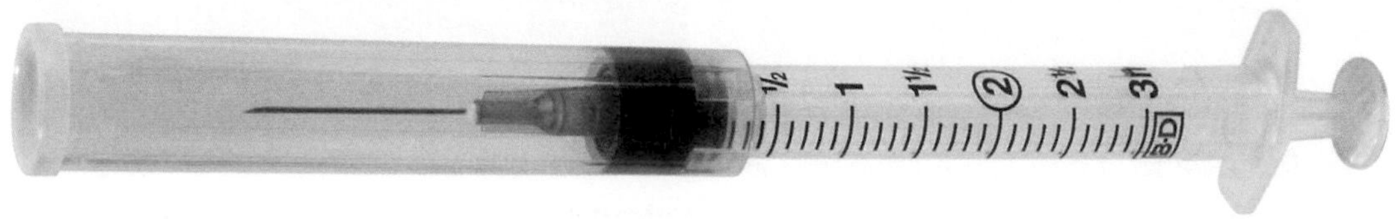

FIGURE 10.3 **BD Safety-LOK 3-mL Syringe.** (Courtesy and copyright Becton, Dickinson and Company.)

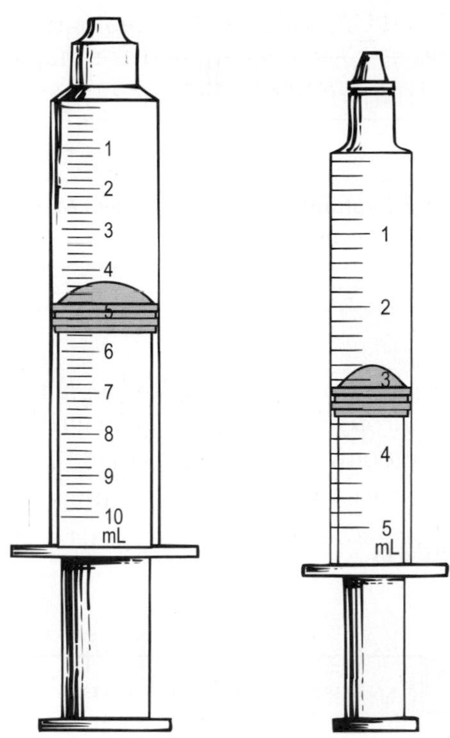

FIGURE 10.4 Measurement of Liquids in Larger Syringes in 0.2-mL Increments. (Brown M, Mulholland JM: *Drug calculations: process and problems for clinical practice*, ed 8, St. Louis, Mosby, 2008.)

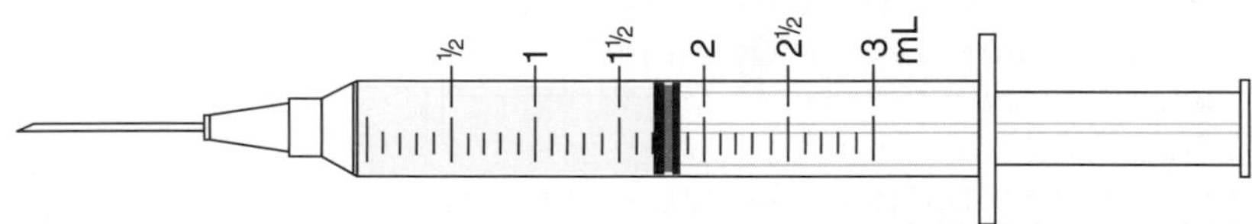

FIGURE 10.5 Syringe Containing a Volume of 1.7 mL. (Fulcher EM, Soto CD, Fulcher RM: *Pharmacology: principles and applications*, ed 3, St. Louis, Saunders, 2012.)

should also be rounded to the tenths position if necessary. A 20-mL syringe is generally used when measuring medication to be added to a larger bag of IV fluid or for an IV push.

Injectable medications may be prepared for direct administration to a patient or for addition to IV bags, which will be covered in Chapter 15. Some medications *must be further diluted* to be safely administered to a patient.

TECH NOTE

Large syringes are seldom used for medication administration (other than for an IV push or use in a syringe pump) but are frequently used in the preparation of IV fluids.

The accuracy of measurement of medications decreases as the syringe size increases. The selection of the correct syringe depends on the volume of medication and the precision needed. The liquid volume in a syringe is measured from the top ring of the plunger, not the raised portion in the middle. In Fig. 10.4, the 10-mL syringe is pulled back to the 4.8-mL mark and the 5-mL syringe to the 3.1-mL position (halfway between the 3.0 mL and 3.2 mL marks). Fig. 10.5 indicates 1.7 mL, and Fig. 10.6 indicates 2.3 mL.

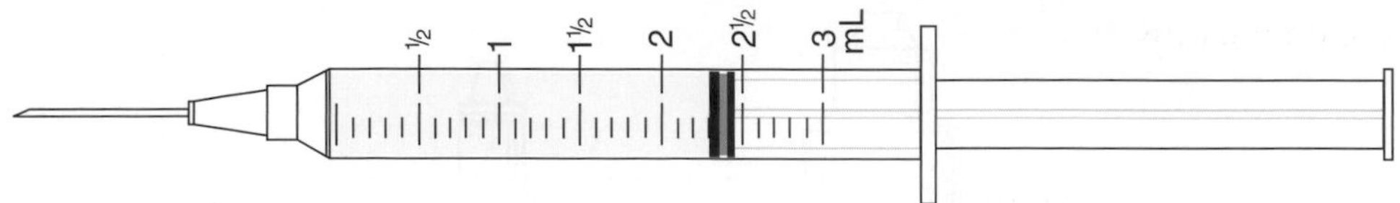

FIGURE 10.6 Syringe Containing a Volume of 2.3 mL. (Fulcher EM, Soto CD, Fulcher RM: *Pharmacology: principles and applications*, ed 3, St. Louis, Saunders, 2012.)

Practice Problems A

Record the volume in the syringes for numbers 1 through 4 and mark the correct volume on the syringes in numbers 6 through 10. Remember to write your answers with decimals, since mL is a metric measurement, even though some of the syringes are labeled with fractions!

1. The amount in the syringe is _____________.

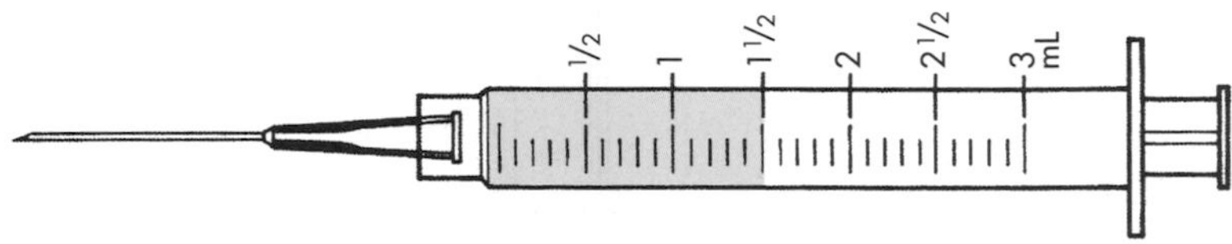

2. The amount in the syringe is _____________.

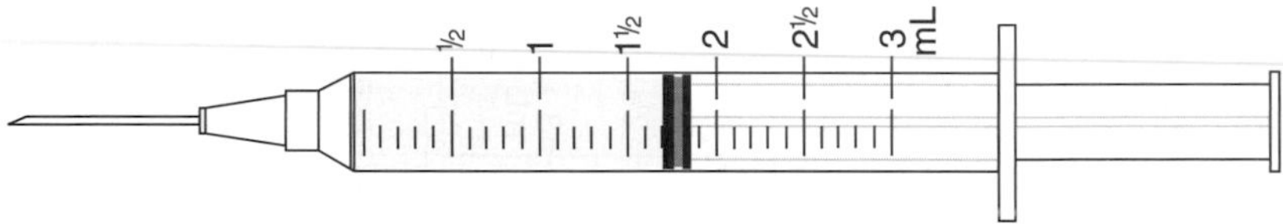

3. The amount in the syringe is _____________.

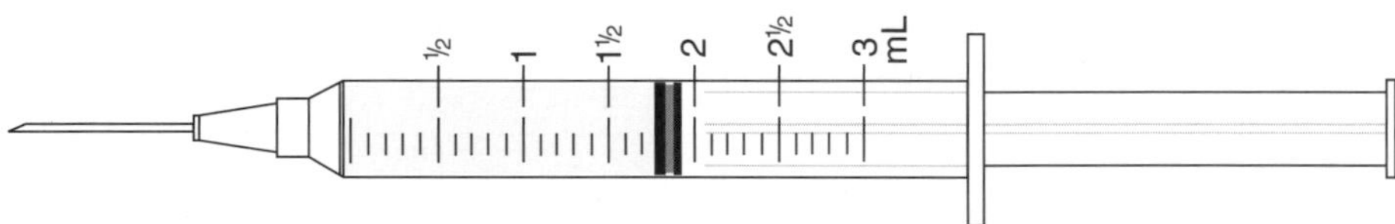

4. The amount in the syringe is _____________.

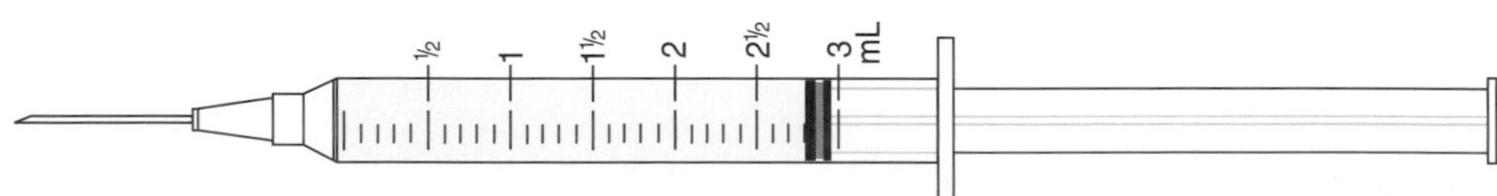

5. Indicate 9.4 mL.

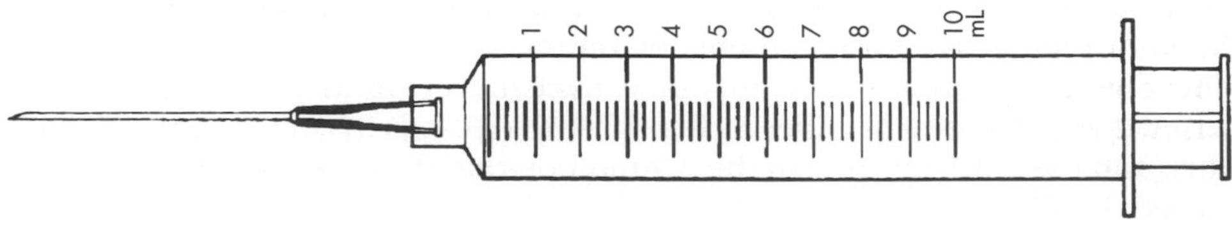

6. Indicate 0.64 mL.

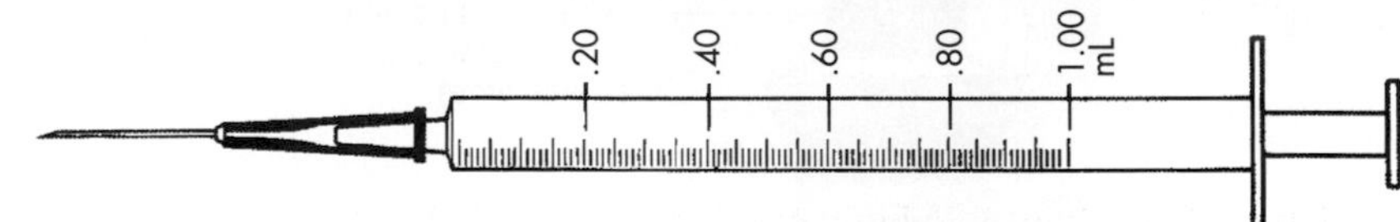

7. Indicate 6.8 mL.

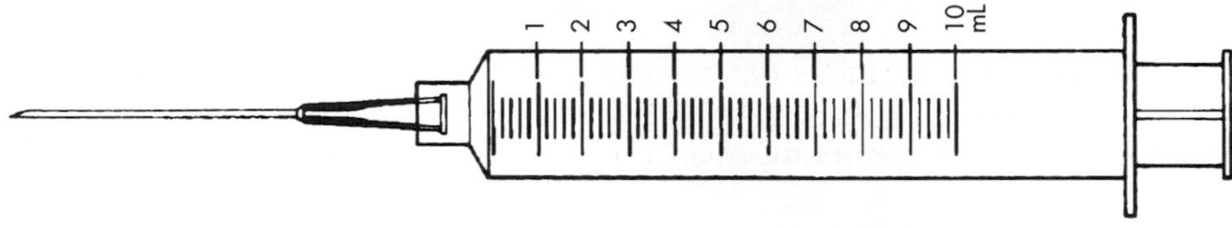

8. Indicate 1.8 mL.

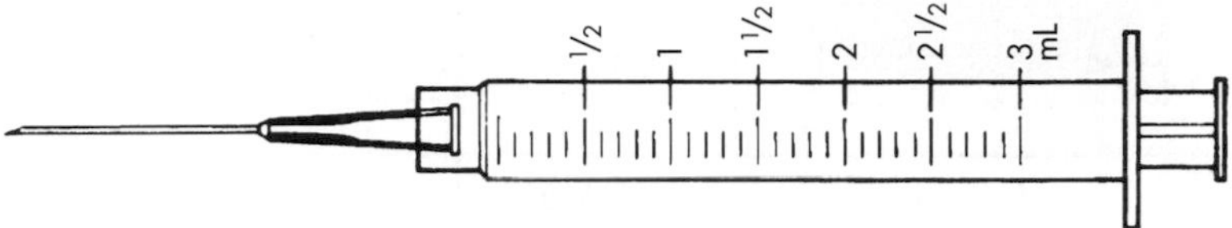

9. Indicate 3.4 mL.

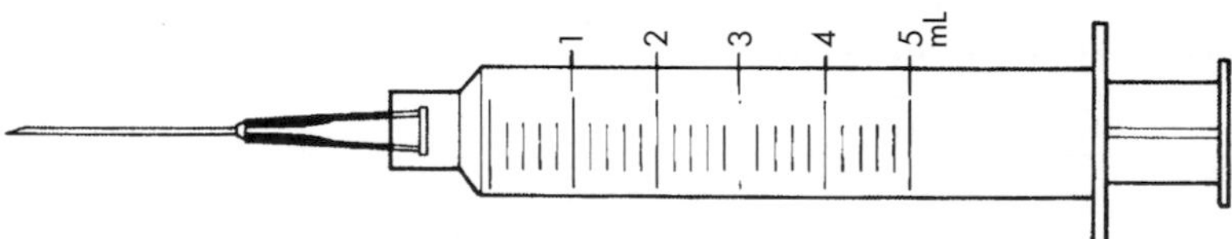

10. Indicate 8.6 mL.

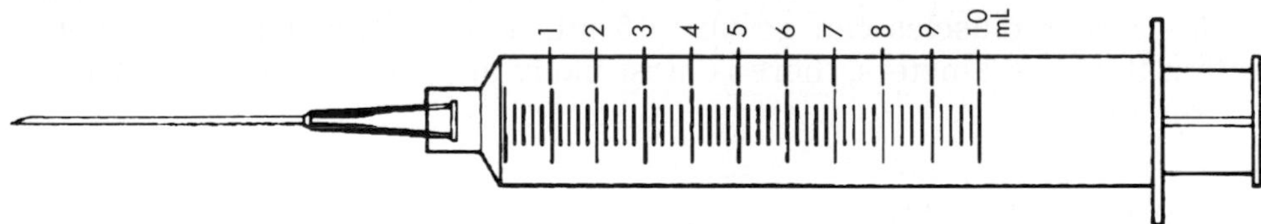

Ampules and Vials

Injectable medications are provided in vials or ampules (see Fig. 10.1). Some are also supplied in prefilled syringes. Ampules are sealed glass containers, which may only be used once because there is no way to ensure sterility after they have been opened. The use of a filter needle is required when withdrawing medication from ampules in case any glass shards enter the product when it is opened. The filter needle must be replaced with a regular needle before the medication is administered.

Vials have rubber stoppers. Multiple-dose vials contain preservatives so they can be used again, whereas single-dose vials do not. Single-dose vials and ampules are slightly overfilled, but the concentration is as written on the label. Powders for reconstitution are

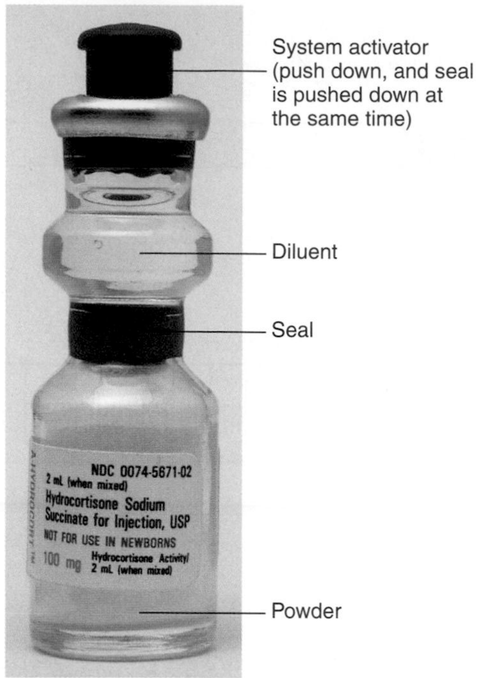

FIGURE 10.7 **An Act-O-Vial.**

supplied in multidose or single-dose vials or in Act-O-Vials (Fig. 10.7). Most sterile liquids used for reconstitution are also supplied in vials.

Amounts of Medicine

When calculating injectable doses, it is important to know the appropriate volumes for the various routes of administration. The intradermal injection limit is 0.1 mL. Medications given subcutaneously are usually less than 1 mL but may go as high as 2 mL in some instances. Small-volume intramuscular (IM) injections should be less than 3 mL but IM injections into larger muscles can go up to 5 mL. If your calculations do not yield an answer within these parameters, there is most likely an error in your calculations or the prescribed amount.

CALCULATING INJECTABLE MEDICATION DOSES

The rules for calculating injectable doses are the same as those for oral liquid medications. The same formulas are used, and the calculations are the same; however, the dose volume is generally smaller. If more than one strength of medication is available, the strength that requires the smallest volume of medication to be administered per dose should be chosen for subcutaneous or IM dosing, unless the medication is available in a strength that provides the dose to an exact marking on the syringe.

TECH NOTE

Many medications for IV use *may not* be given directly from the vial but require further dilution in IV fluid before administration.

EXAMPLE 10.1

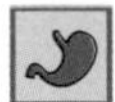

Medication order: Tagamet (cimetidine) 75 mg IM q6h

Stock available: cimetidine injection 300 mg/2 mL (8-mL multidose vial)

Interpret the order: Tagamet 75 mg intramuscularly every 6 hours

What volume of medication is needed for a single dose?

Ratio and proportion (R&P): $\frac{300\text{ mg}}{2\text{ mL}} = \frac{75\text{ mg}}{x}$ $300x = 150\text{ mL}$ $x = 0.5\text{ mL}$

OR

Dimensional analysis (DA): $\text{mL} = \frac{2\text{ mL}}{300\text{ mg}} \bullet \frac{75\text{ mg}}{1} = 0.5\text{ mL}$

This is an IM dose, and it is within the allowable volume range.

What is the appropriate size syringe for administering this dose? 1-mL TB syringe

EXAMPLE 10.2

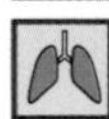

Order: aminophylline 125 mg IV q6h

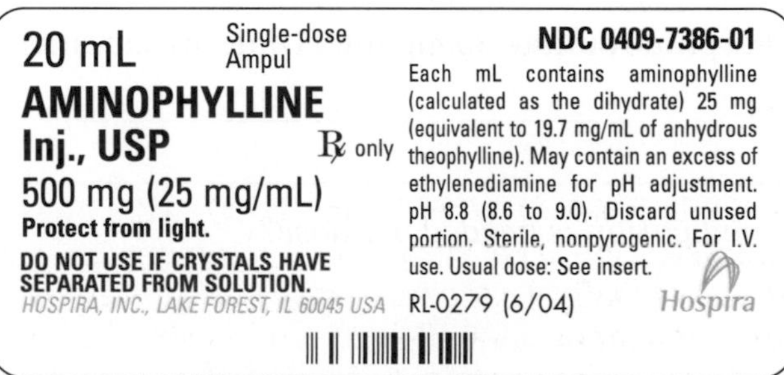

20 mL
Single-dose Ampul
AMINOPHYLLINE
Inj., USP
℞ only
500 mg (25 mg/mL)
Protect from light.
DO NOT USE IF CRYSTALS HAVE SEPARATED FROM SOLUTION.
HOSPIRA, INC., LAKE FOREST, IL 60045 USA
NDC 0409-7386-01
Each mL contains aminophylline (calculated as the dihydrate) 25 mg (equivalent to 19.7 mg/mL of anhydrous theophylline). May contain an excess of ethylenediamine for pH adjustment. pH 8.8 (8.6 to 9.0). Discard unused portion. Sterile, nonpyrogenic. For I.V. use. Usual dose: See insert.
RL-0279 (6/04)
Hospira

(© Pfizer. Used with permission.)

Interpret the order: aminophylline 125 mg intravenously every 6 hours

When interpreting this label, the strength of the medication can be read as 500 mg/20 mL or 25 mg/mL. These are equivalent fractions. The entire 20-mL ampule contains 500 mg, but only part of this is needed for each dose. Either strength designation may be used to calculate the dose, but smaller numbers make calculations easier. After reviewing the following examples, rework them replacing 500 mg/20 mL with 25 mg/mL to see that you reach the same answer.

What volume of medication is needed for a single dose?

R&P: $\frac{500\text{ mg}}{20\text{ mL}} = \frac{125\text{ mg}}{x}$ $500x = 2{,}500\text{ mL}$ $x = 5\text{ mL}$

OR

DA: $\text{mL} = \frac{20\text{ mL}}{500\text{ mg}} \bullet \frac{125\text{ mg}}{1} = 5\text{ mL}$

> **! TECH ALERT**
> If the answer to a calculation does not agree with the anticipated answer based on the amount of medication prescribed, the dose of medication on hand, or the intended route of administration, ALWAYS recalculate. Ask for assistance if necessary!

> **! TECH ALERT**
> An injectable dose less than 1 mL should be rounded to the nearest hundredth. If you have questions regarding acceptable rounding techniques, ask a pharmacist for assistance.

Some injectable doses require rounding to a measurable quantity. If an injectable dose is less than 1 mL, it should be rounded to the nearest hundredth. Once rounded, the dose should generally be within a 10% margin. Some medications require rounding to be within a much lower percentage of variation. This is due to the narrow **therapeutic range** between effectiveness and toxicity levels.

Practice Problems B

Use the method of calculation with which you are most comfortable to complete these problems. DA is best for multistep conversions, to keep track of units. Round answers less than 1 mL to the hundredths place and those greater than 1 mL to the tenths place.

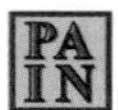

1. Medication order: morphine sulfate 15 mg IM q4h prn pain

   Stock strength: morphine sulfate 25 mg/mL (1-mL preservative-free vial)

   Interpret the order: ______________________________

   ____

   What volume of medication is needed per dose?

2. Medication order: prochlorperazine 10 mg IM q6h prn N&V

   Stock strength: prochlorperazine injection 5 mg/mL (2-mL vial)

   Interpret the order: ______________________________

   ____

   What volume of medication is needed for one dose?

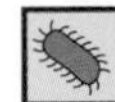

3. Medication order: Nebcin (tobramycin) 60 mg IM q8h

Tobramycin has a narrow therapeutic range and requires monitoring of medication levels.

Stock strength: tobramycin sulfate injection 80 mg/2 mL (2-mL vial)

Interpret the order:

What volume of medication is needed for one dose?

Indicate the correct amount of medication on the appropriate syringe.

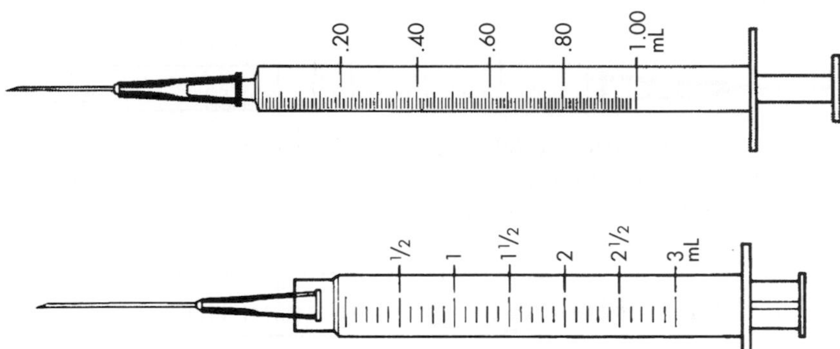

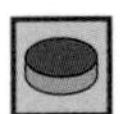

4. Medication order: vitamin B_{12} 1 mg IM qwk × 4 weeks

Stock strength: cyanocobalamin injection 1,000 mcg/mL (10-mL multidose vial)

Interpret the order:

What volume of medication is needed for one dose?

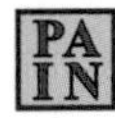

5. Medication order: meperidine 75 mg IM q4–6h prn pain

The following stock strengths are available:

A. meperidine injection 25 mg/mL (1-mL vial)

B. meperidine injection 50 mg/mL (1-mL vial)

C. meperidine injection 100 mg/mL (1-mL vial)

Interpret the order:____

____

Which strength should be used for this order? Hint: This is an IM injection. __________

Why did you choose this vial? ____

____

What volume of medication is needed per dose?

Indicate the correct amount of medication on the appropriate syringe.

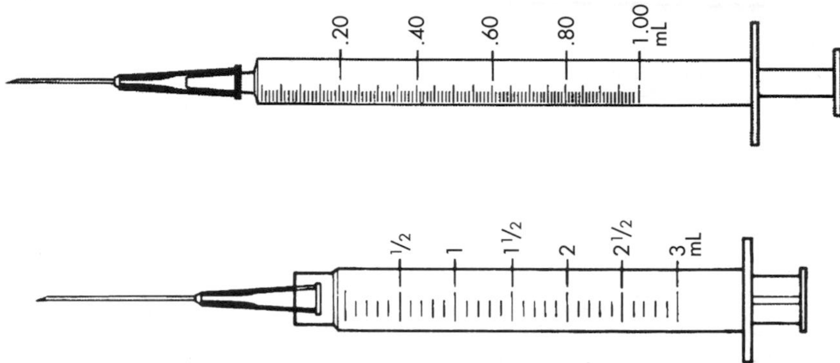

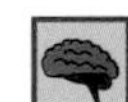

6. Medication order: Cogentin 1.5 mg IM daily

Stock strength: benztropine injection 2 mg/2 mL (2-mL single-dose vial)

Interpret the order:____

____

What volume of medication is needed per dose?

Indicate the correct amount of medication on the appropriate syringe.

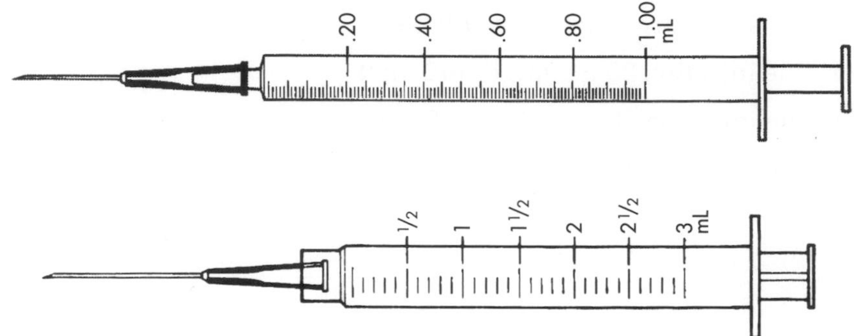

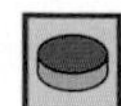

7. Medication order: vitamin K 2 mg IM stat

Stock strength: phytonadione injectable emulsion 10 mg/mL
(1-mL single-dose ampule)
Interpret the order: ____________________

____

What volume of medication is needed for the dose?

Indicate the correct amount of medication on the appropriate syringe.

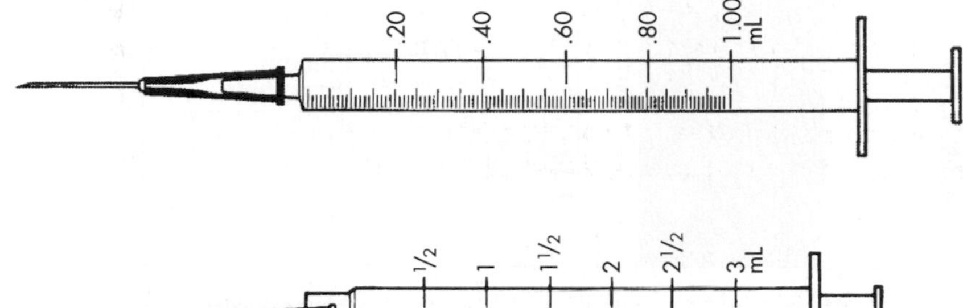

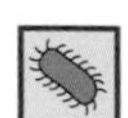

8. Medication order: amikacin 250 mg IM q8h

Stock strength: amikacin sulfate injection 500 mg/2 mL (2-mL vial)
Interpret the order: ____________________

____

What volume of medication is needed for one dose?

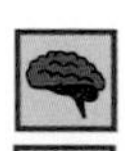
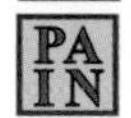

9. Medication order: hydroxyzine 75 mg and meperidine 50 mg IM stat

Stock strengths available:
hydroxyzine HCl injection 50 mg/mL (10-mL multidose vial for IM use only)
meperidine injection 100 mg/mL (1-mL ampule)
Interpret the order: ____________________

____

What volume of hydroxyzine is needed for this dose?

What volume of meperidine is needed for this dose?

Indicate the volume of *combined* medication needed on the syringe.

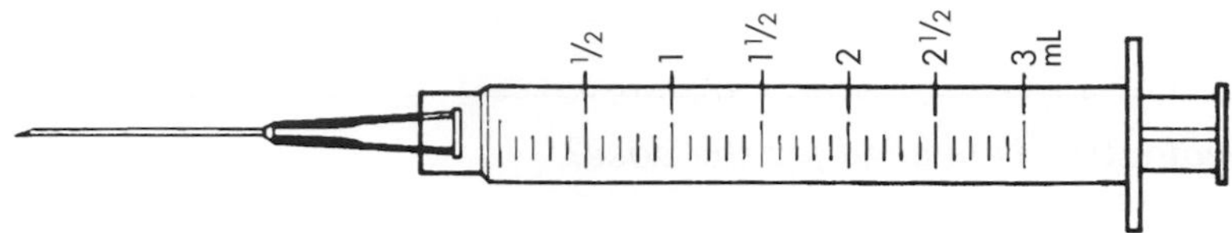

10. Medication order: Cleocin 0.25 g IM stat then q8h

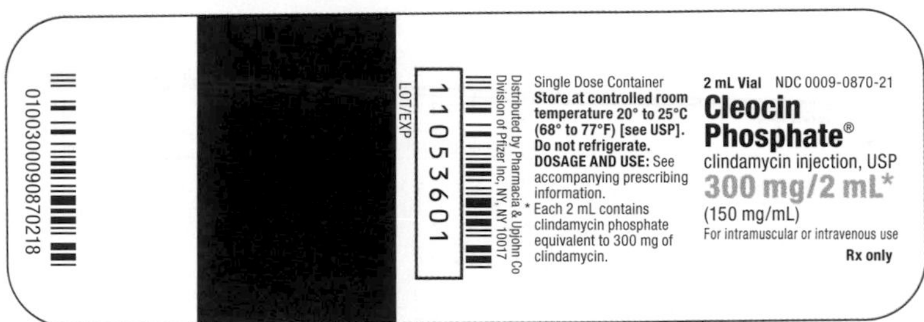

(© Pfizer. Used with permission.)

Interpret the order: ______________________________

____

What volume of medication is needed per dose?

Indicate the correct amount of medication on the appropriate syringe.

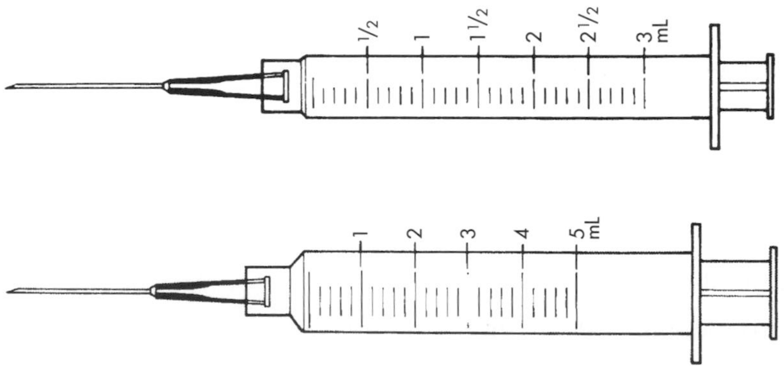

11. Medication order: lincomycin 0.45 g IM stat

Stock strength: lincomycin injection 300 mg/mL (2-mL vial)

Interpret the order: ______________________________

____

What volume of medication is needed for this dose?

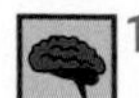 12. Prescribed: Dilantin (phenytoin) 0.1 g IV over 3 minutes

Stock Strength: phenytoin injection 250 mg/5 mL

What is the strength in mg/mL?

What volume of medication is needed for this dose?

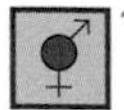 13. Order: Depo-Provera 0.3 g IM qmo

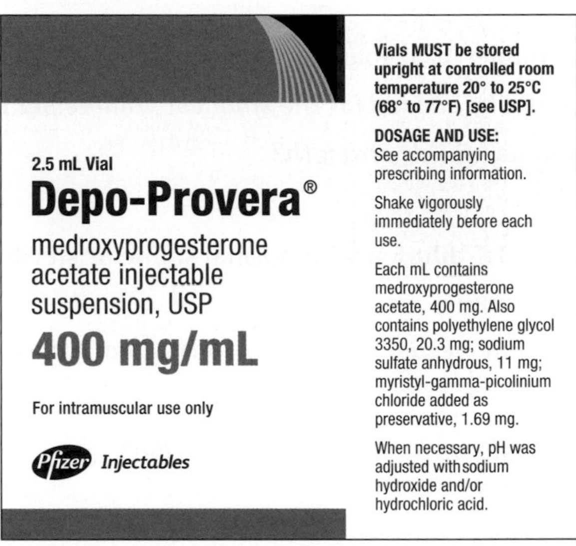

2.5 mL Vial
Depo-Provera®
medroxyprogesterone acetate injectable suspension, USP
400 mg/mL
For intramuscular use only
Pfizer Injectables
Vials MUST be stored upright at controlled room temperature 20° to 25°C (68° to 77°F) [see USP].
DOSAGE AND USE:
See accompanying prescribing information.
Shake vigorously immediately before each use.
Each mL contains medroxyprogesterone acetate, 400 mg. Also contains polyethylene glycol 3350, 20.3 mg; sodium sulfate anhydrous, 11 mg; myristyl-gamma-picolinium chloride added as preservative, 1.69 mg.
When necessary, pH was adjusted with sodium hydroxide and/or hydrochloric acid.

(© Pfizer. Used with permission.)

Interpret the order: ______________________________

What is the total amount of medication in the vial (g)? ____________

What volume of medication is needed for one dose?

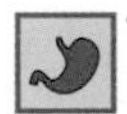 14. Medication order: prochlorperazine 6 mg IM

Stock strength: prochlorperazine injection 5 mg/mL

What volume of medication should be administered?

What size syringe should be used for administration? ____________

15. Medication order: aminophylline 65 mg IV

Stock strength: aminophylline 25 mg/mL injection

What volume of medication is needed?

What size syringe should be used for administration? ____________

16. Medication order: Ativan (lorazepam) 1 mg IM

Stock strengths available: lorazepam injection 2 mg/mL and 4 mg/mL

Which strength should be chosen for the smallest volume per dose? ____________

How much is needed using this strength?

Lorazepam requires a 1:1 dilution with normal saline or sterile water for injection to facilitate IM administration.

How much normal saline needs to be added to the above dose? ____________

What size syringe should be used for administration? ____________

17. Medication order: Lasix (furosemide) 10 mg IM

Stock strength: furosemide injection 40 mg/4 mL

What volume of medication should be administered?

What size syringe should be used for administration? ____________

18. Medication order: Lanoxin (digoxin) 0.125 mg IV

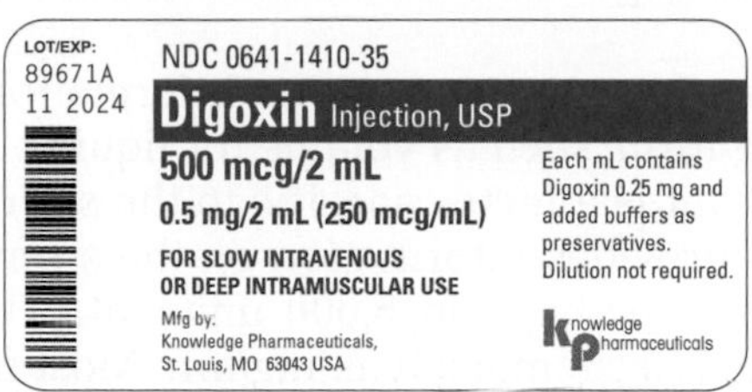

What volume of medication should be administered?

What size syringe should be used for administration? ____________

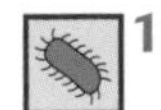

19. Medication order: gentamicin 5 mg IM

Stock strength: gentamicin 20 mg/2 mL injection

What volume of medication should be administered?

What size syringe should be used for administration? ____________

20. Medication order: diazepam 10 mg IM

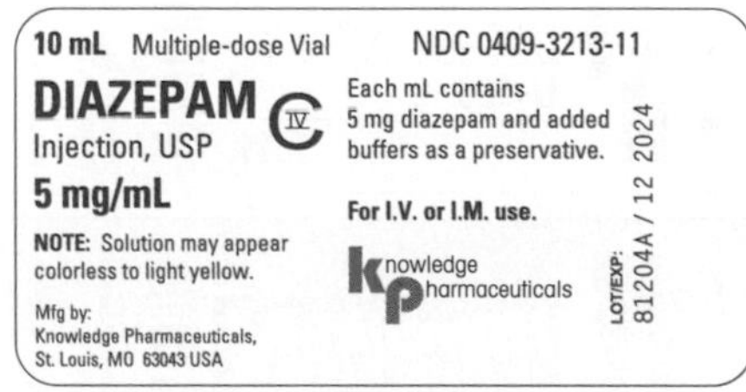

What volume of medication should be administered?

What size syringe should be used for administration? ____________

CALCULATIONS WITH INTERNATIONAL UNITS

Insulin, heparin, and penicillin are measured in **International Units**. Other, less common medications that are measured in units include fat-soluble vitamin E, some forms of vitamins A and D, and the topical antibiotic bacitracin. With injectable medications, the labels display the specific number of **units** per milliliter. Units *are not* interchangeable between different medications; rather, each medication unit is *specific* to the drug ordered and represents a standard amount of that particular medication that produces a desired biologic effect.

Insulin and heparin are considered **high-alert medications** on the ISMP List of High-Alert Medications. Another high-alert medication is potassium chloride injection, which is measured in mEq.

An International Unit measurement gives information concerning the strength of medication in a given drug form, such as volume for liquids. A conversion factor is not used because an International Unit is a factor specific to the strength of each particular medication. The medication label provides information on the strength of the medication, such as insulin U-100 (100 units/mL) or heparin 5,000 units/mL. These are similar to medication strengths found in the metric system such as mg/mL. Most important for a pharmacy technician is to be aware of the volume of the medication and strength for the dose as listed on medication labels. As with all medication calculations, reading a drug label accurately is of utmost importance and is the basis for correct preparation and administration of medication.

Insulin

Insulin is used to control type 1 diabetes mellitus and some stages of type 2 diabetes mellitus. The most common insulin strength is U-100, meaning that each milliliter of insulin contains 100 units of medication. Fig. 10.8 shows some different types of multiple-dose

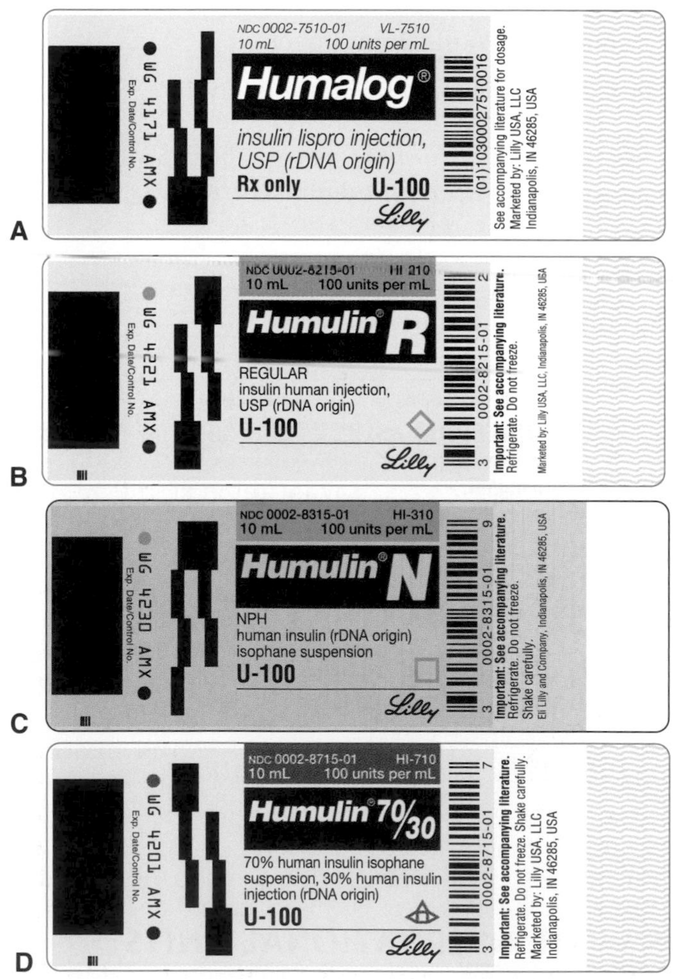

FIGURE 10.8 Labels for Some Different Types of Insulin Used on a Routine Basis. (A) Rapid-acting. (B) Short-acting. (C) Intermediate-acting. (D) Intermediate- and rapid-acting mixture. Not depicted are long-acting insulins. (© Eli Lilly and Company. All Rights Reserved. Used with Permission.)

TABLE 10.1 Approximate Action of Common Insulin Preparations

INSULIN TYPE	BRAND (GENERIC)	ONSET	PEAK	DURATION
RAPID-ACTING				
	Apidra (glulisine)	15 min	1 h	2–4 h
	Humalog (lispro)	15 min	1 h	2–4 h
	Novolog (aspart)	15 min	1 h	2–4 h
SHORT-ACTING REGULAR INSULINS				
	Humulin R	30 min	2–3 h	3–6 h
	Novolin R	30 min	2–3 h	3–6 h
INTERMEDIATE-ACTING NPH INSULINS				
	Humulin N	2–4 h	4–12 h	12–18 h
	Novolin N	2–4 h	4–12 h	12–18 h
LONG-ACTING				
	Lantus (glargine)	1–2 h	Considered no peak	24 h
	Levemir (detemir)	1–3 h	Considered no peak	24 h
ULTRA LONG-ACTING				
	Tresiba (degludec)	1 h	Considered no peak	up to 42 h or more
COMBINATION				
NPH/R	Humulin 50/50	30 min	2–6 h	16–24 h
	Humulin 70/30	30–60 min	2–12 h	18–24 h
	Novolin 70/30	30–60 min	2–12 h	18–24 h
NPH/aspart	Novolog 70/30	15 min	1–7 h	10–24 h
NPH/lispro	Humalog 75/25	15 min	1–7 h	10–18 h

insulin preparations. U-100 insulin syringes are used to administer U-100 insulin from these bottles; *no other syringe is based in units for U-100 insulin!* The design of the syringe helps ensure that the exact dose of medication is administered. Most insulin is available in pre-filled insulin syringes as well, to help avoid dosing errors.

Insulin preparations are labeled according to type. Each formulation has a specific onset, peak, and duration of action (Table 10.1). An abbreviation of "**R**" for regular insulin, *a clear solution,* indicates that the medication is short-acting. An abbreviation of "**N**" for NPH insulin, *a cloudy suspension,* indicates that it is an intermediate-acting insulin with a slower onset and longer duration of action. Manufacturers have placed large letters on these two types of vials, emphasizing the exact type of insulin. Other preparations include combinations of regular insulin and intermediate-acting insulin, and long-acting insulin.

Insulin syringes for U-100 insulin come in 30-unit, 50-unit, and 100-unit sizes (Fig. 10.9). Some of the 100-unit insulin syringes are marked in 2-unit increments, whereas others are marked in 1-unit increments with 2-unit increments of odd/even on each side of the syringe barrel. Note that 30-unit and 50-unit insulin syringes are calibrated in 1-unit increments and are therefore easier to see for patients with vision problems, a common complication of long-term or uncontrolled diabetes mellitus. All U-100 insulin contains 100 units/mL. U-100 insulin syringes are designed for this strength. A dose of 30 units or less should be measured in a 30-unit syringe, 31 to 50 units in a 50-unit syringe, and 51 to 100

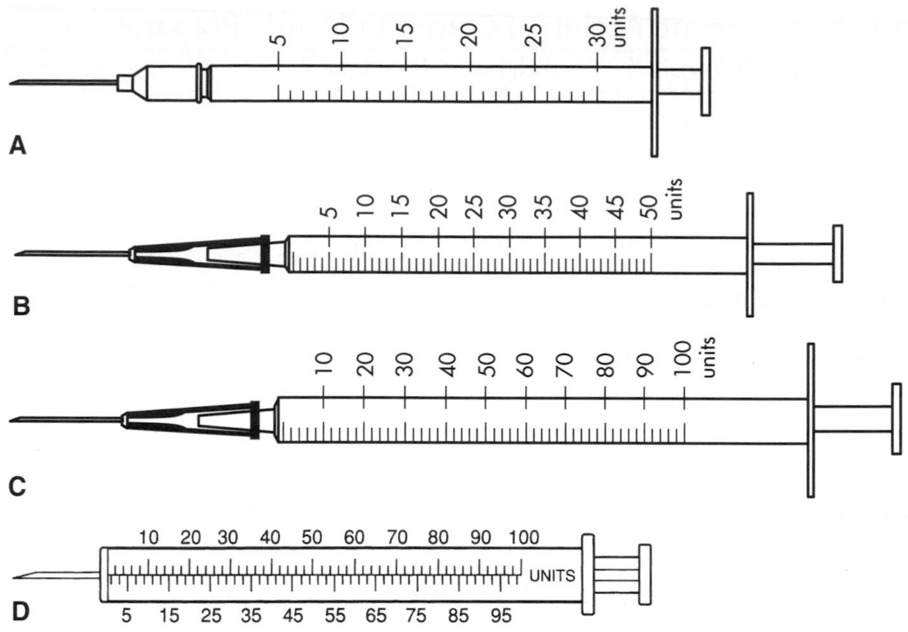

FIGURE 10.9 Insulin Syringes for Measuring 100-Unit/mL Strength Insulin. The 30-Unit insulin syringe (A) is recommended for measuring 30 Units or less; the 50-Unit syringe (B) should be used for measuring 31 to 50 Units; and the 100-Unit syringe (C) should be used for measuring 51 to 100 Units of insulin. (D) A 100-Unit insulin syringe depicts single Units on one syringe. (A–C, From Brown M, Mulholland JM: *Drug calculations: process and problems for clinical practice*, ed 8, St. Louis, Mosby, 2008. D, From Kee JL, Marshall SM: *Clinical calculations: with applications to general and specialty areas*, ed 8, St. Louis, Saunders, 2017.)

units in a 100-unit syringe for the greatest accuracy. These syringes *should not be used* for measuring *any* medication other than U-100 insulin.

> **!** TECH ALERT
>
> Always check the physician's insulin order with the insulin vial to be sure the correct type of insulin has been chosen. Do not confuse **R** and **N** on the labels.

All insulin formulations can be administered subcutaneously. ***Only*** **regular insulin is indicated for IV use**, which will be included in Chapter 15. When mixing a clear short- or rapid-acting solution and a cloudy longer-acting suspension in *one syringe* for subcutaneous administration, the rule is to draw up clear insulin before cloudy insulin, so regular insulin must be drawn up in a syringe before NPH, which is a suspension. If different *types* of insulin need to be administered at the same time, the same source of the insulin, such as DNA or recombinant sources, must be used together. Different *sources* of insulin cannot be mixed in the same syringe. Lantus and Levemir, two long-acting insulins, can ***never*** be mixed with *any* other type of insulin.

> **!** TECH ALERT
>
> Be sure the customer is aware that if their insulin prescription is changed, the newly ordered type cannot be combined with the old type in one syringe. Insulin from different sources or manufacturers may not be compatible. The old insulin should be discarded for patient safety.

TECH ALERT

Only regular insulin and some rapid-acting analogs may be administered by the IV route! It is most cost effective to use regular insulin when preparing IV formulations.

EXAMPLE 10.3

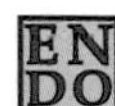

A physician orders 10 mL of Humulin N U-100, 12 units tid pc for an elderly patient.

What should the technician supply for the administration of this medication?

For maximum accuracy, provide 30-unit insulin syringes, because the dose is less than 30 units.

EXAMPLE 10.4

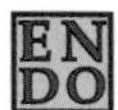

A physician orders Humulin 70/30 40 units qam.

Which U-100 syringe should be used to administer this medication? 50-unit syringe

70/30 means each dose contains 70% NPH insulin and 30% regular insulin.

How many units of NPH insulin would be received per dose?

40 units × 0.7 = 28 units

How many units of regular insulin would be received per dose?

40 units × 0.3 = 12 units

There are some more concentrated insulin products available as well, such as U-200, U-300, and U-500. These products are 2, 3, and 5 times as strong as U-100 insulin, containing 200 units/mL, 300 units/mL, and 500 units/mL respectively. This has added to the potential risk for errors. The ISMP recommends that, in a hospital setting, U-500 insulin should be dispensed from the pharmacy in patient-specific labeled pen devices or patient-specific pharmacy-prepared U-500 syringes. Insulin U-500 syringes hold up to 250 units and are specific for U-500 insulin. Unlike U-100 insulin products, which are stored on some nursing floors, *U-500 insulin vials and syringes are only stored in the pharmacy.* Other concentrated insulin products should be dispensed to the floor in patient-specific, labeled pen devices. *Extreme care* should be taken to verify the correct type and strength of insulin dispensed.

TECH ALERT

Technicians should be aware of stronger concentrations of insulin, such as Humulin R U-500 (500 Units/mL), TOUJEO U-300 (300 Units/mL), and Humalog U-200 (200 Units/mL). These formulations are more concentrated, allowing for more units to be delivered in a smaller volume than with U-100 insulin. This is important for diabetics requiring higher doses, to keep the volume small enough for subcutaneous injection. Specific attention is given to the U-500 insulin on the ISMP List of High-Alert Medications. It is five times more concentrated than U-100, and does come in a multidose vial, which has led to errors. U-500 insulin doses should be measured and administered using U-500 insulin syringes. Many pharmacies do not even store U-500 insulin near U-100 insulin to decrease the likelihood of dangerous errors.

> **! TECH ALERT**
> Only U-100 insulin should be measured in U-100 insulin syringes. Units are specific to the particular medication and strength.

Practice Problems C

Choose the correct label and indicate the correct dose on the appropriate syringe.

Types of Insulin:

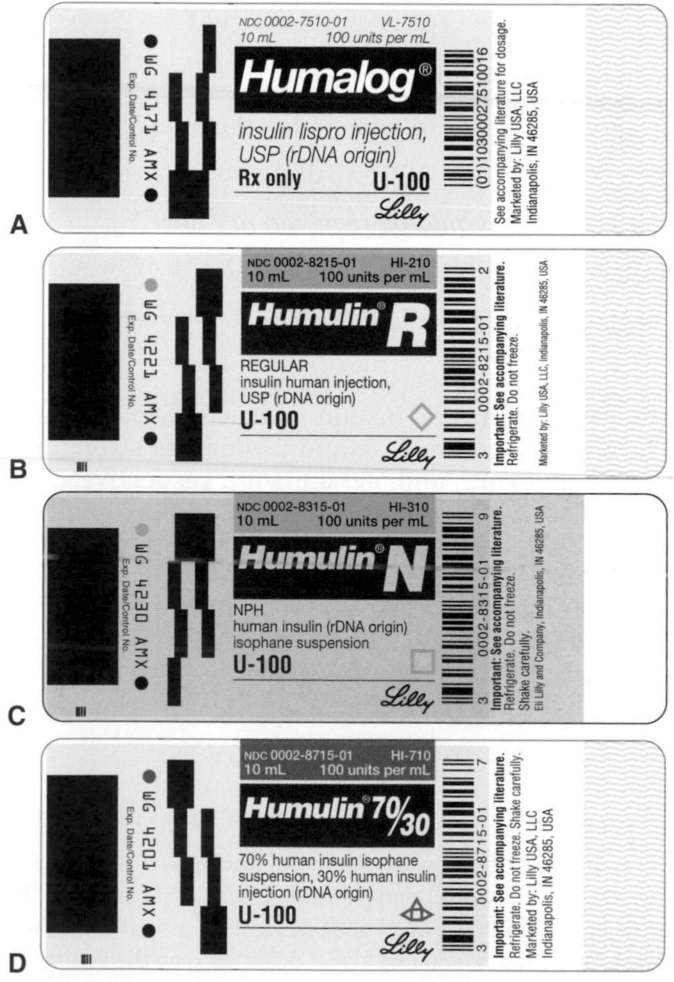

(© Eli Lilly and Company. All Rights Reserved. Used with Permission.)

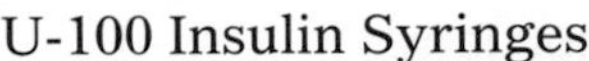

A.

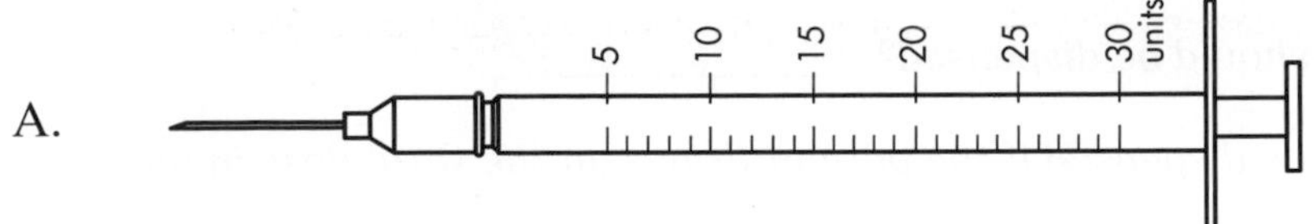

B.

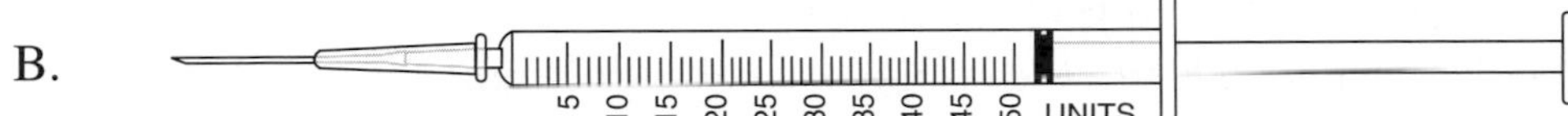

C.

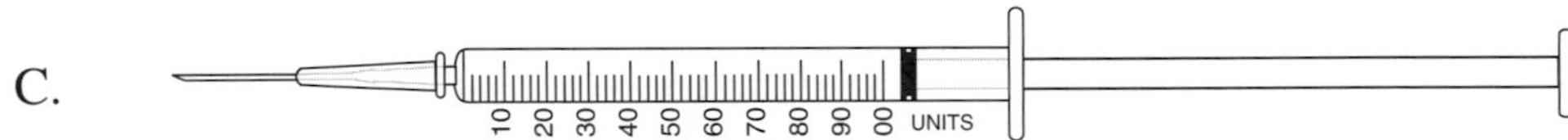

1. A physician orders Humulin N insulin 45 units subcutaneously to be given qam.

   Which vial of insulin should be dispensed for this prescription? ______________

   Which syringe should be used to supply the most accurate dose? ______________

2. A physician orders Humulin R 30 units subcutaneously 30 min ac for a person with poor eyesight.

   Which vial of insulin should be dispensed? ______________

   Which syringe should be used to supply the most accurate dose? ______________

3. A physician orders Humulin 70/30 42 units subcutaneously qam.

   Which vial of insulin should be dispensed? ______________

   Which syringe should be used to supply the most accurate dose? ______________

4. A physician orders Humalog 66 units subcutaneously ac.

   Which vial of insulin should be dispensed? ______________

   Which syringe should be used to supply the most accurate dose? ______________

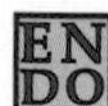

5. A physician orders Humulin N 28 units and Humulin R 36 units qam.

   Which vials of insulin should be dispensed? ______________

   Which syringe should be dispensed if the patient draws up the total dose in one syringe? ______________

   How should the patient draw this up in one syringe? __________________________

Calculating Anticoagulant Doses in Units

Heparin is an injectable anticoagulant medication that is measured in units. Heparin may be used as a flush for an IV injection site to keep it patent, as an IV infusion additive, or as a deep subcutaneous injection into fatty tissue. The doses for heparin are highly individualized based on body weight and blood coagulation laboratory values. Because heparin prolongs bleeding time, the time that it takes for blood to clot, accurate dosing is of the utmost importance. A dose that is larger than necessary may cause hemorrhage, whereas a dose that is insufficient may not produce the necessary results to prevent clot formation and possible thrombi (blood clots).

Heparin is available in 10 units/mL (pediatric heparin lock flush), 100 units/mL (heparin lock flush), 1,000 units/mL, 5,000 units/mL, 10,000 units/mL, and 20,000 units/mL strengths. It is ***essential*** to pay close attention to the strength of heparin chosen to provide the correct dose. Heparin doses should be measured using 1-mL tuberculin syringes for the greatest accuracy. Because no conversion factors are needed with unit calculations, they are performed easily with R&P, although DA can be used.

TECH ALERT

Heparin is ***never*** administered intramuscularly because of the danger of bleeding into the muscle tissue. It is given subcutaneously and by IV infusion as a therapeutic dose or as a means of maintaining patency of an IV line.

Some low-molecular-weight heparins, such as dalteparin sodium (Fragmin), are also measured in units, although some, such as enoxaparin (Lovenox), are measured on a milligram basis. The low-molecular-weight heparins do not have the short half-life of heparin, but they are also primarily administered subcutaneously.

EXAMPLE 10.5

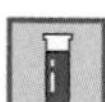

A physician orders heparin sodium 2,500 units subcutaneously stat.

The medication available is heparin sodium 5,000 units/mL.

How much should be administered?

$$\text{R\&P} \quad \frac{5{,}000\text{ units}}{1\text{ mL}} = \frac{2{,}500\text{ units}}{x}$$

$$5{,}000x = 2{,}500\text{ mL}$$

$$x = 0.5\text{ mL}$$

$$\text{DA} \quad \text{mL} = \frac{1\text{ mL}}{5{,}000\text{ units}} \times \frac{2{,}500\text{ units}}{1} = 0.5\text{ mL}$$

EXAMPLE 10.6

Order: heparin sodium 4,500 units subcut stat

What volume is needed using each of the following stock strengths?

1,000 units/mL: $\frac{1{,}000 \text{ units}}{\text{mL}} = \frac{4{,}500 \text{ units}}{x}$ $1{,}000x = 4{,}500 \text{ mL}$ $x = 4.5 \text{ mL}$

5,000 units/mL: $\frac{5{,}000 \text{ units}}{\text{mL}} = \frac{4{,}500 \text{ units}}{x}$ $5{,}000x = 4{,}500 \text{ mL}$ $x = 0.9 \text{ mL}$

10,000 units/mL: $\frac{10{,}000 \text{ units}}{\text{mL}} = \frac{4{,}500 \text{ units}}{x}$ $10{,}000x = 4{,}500 \text{ mL}$ $x = 0.45 \text{ mL}$

20,000 units/mL: $\frac{20{,}000 \text{ units}}{\text{mL}} = \frac{4{,}500 \text{ units}}{x}$ $20{,}000x = 4{,}500 \text{ mL}$ $x = 0.225 \text{ mL}$

What is the best choice for this dose?

Being that this is a subcutaneous dose, usually the smallest volume is best. However, heparin is a high-alert medication and in this case the smallest dose, 0.225 mL, would have to be rounded to the measurable dose of 0.23 mL, which is actually 4,600 units. Therefore, the best choice is the 0.45 mL dose, which is larger in volume but exact in dose. Use the 10,000-unit/mL vial.

Practice Problems D

Calculate the following medication orders using the labels provided. Round answers to hundredths for measurement on tuberculin syringes. Indicate the amount of medication on the syringe provided.

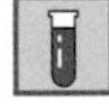

1. A physician orders heparin sodium 5,000 units subcutaneously.

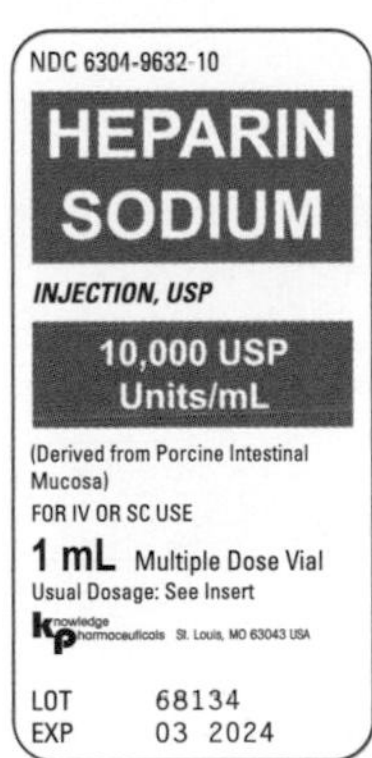

NDC 6304-9632-10
HEPARIN SODIUM
INJECTION, USP
10,000 USP Units/mL
(Derived from Porcine Intestinal Mucosa)
FOR IV OR SC USE
1 mL Multiple Dose Vial
Usual Dosage: See Insert
St. Louis, MO 63043 USA
LOT 68134
EXP 03 2024

What volume of medication should be given to the patient for this dose?

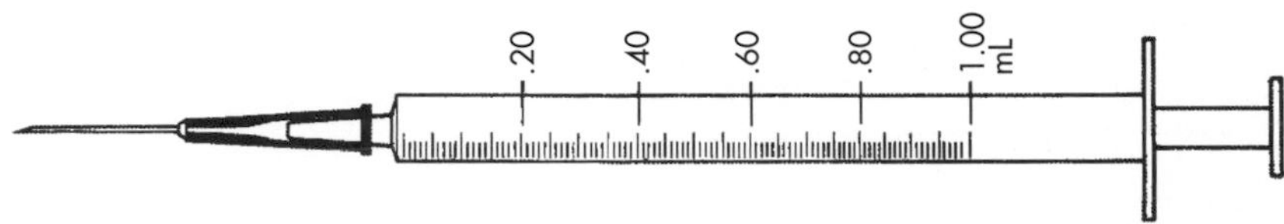

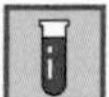

2. A physician orders heparin sodium 2,500 units subcutaneously stat.

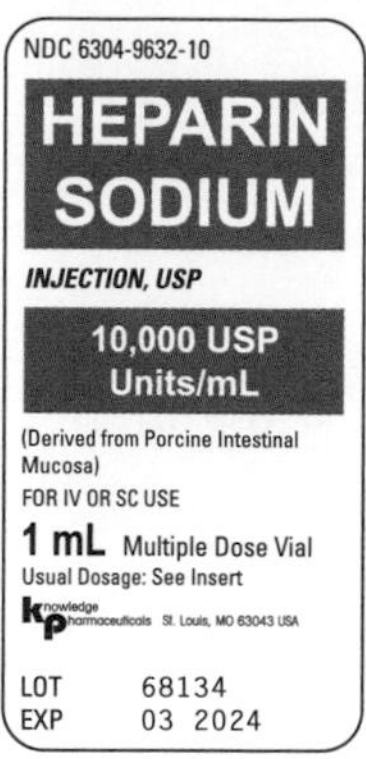

What volume of medication should be administered to this patient? ____________

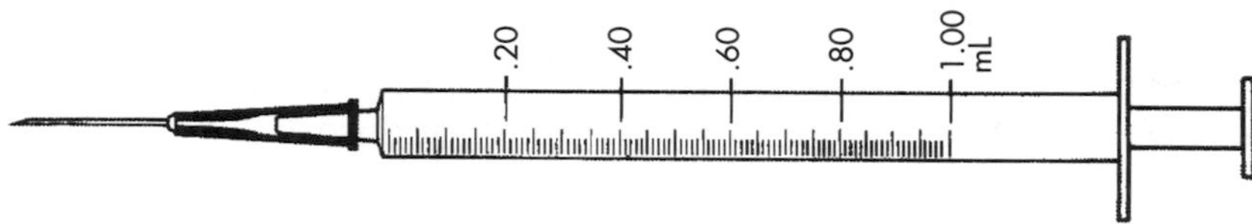

3. A physician orders heparin sodium 17,500 units subcutaneously stat.

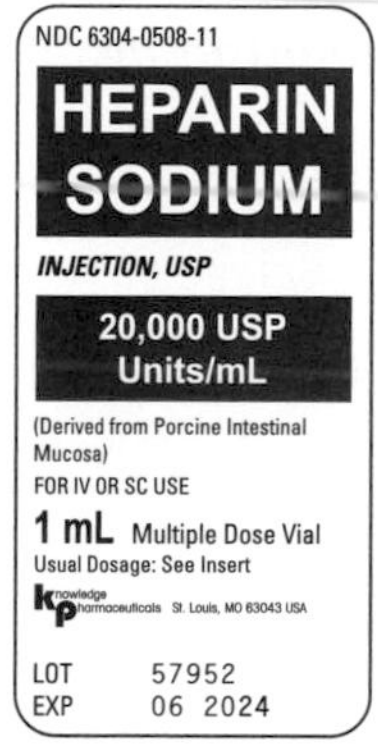

What volume of medication should be administered to the patient? ____________

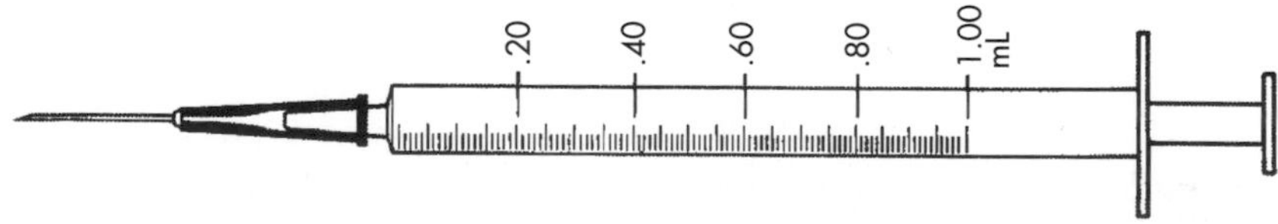

4. A physician orders heparin sodium 15,000 units subcutaneously.

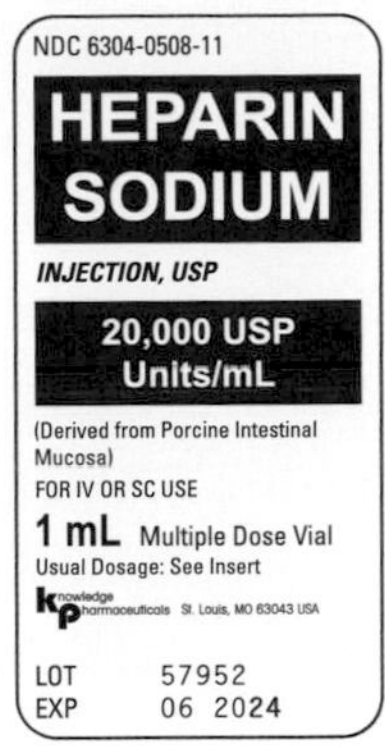

What volume of medication should be administered? ______________

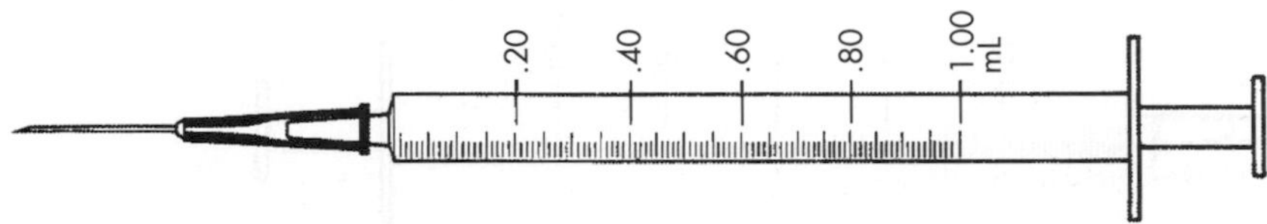

5. A physician orders heparin sodium 12,000 units subcutaneously.

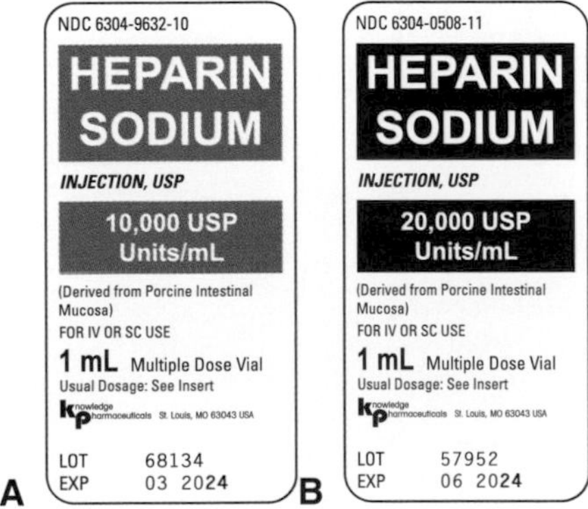

Which strength vial of medication is most appropriate for this dose? ______________

What volume of medication should be administered?

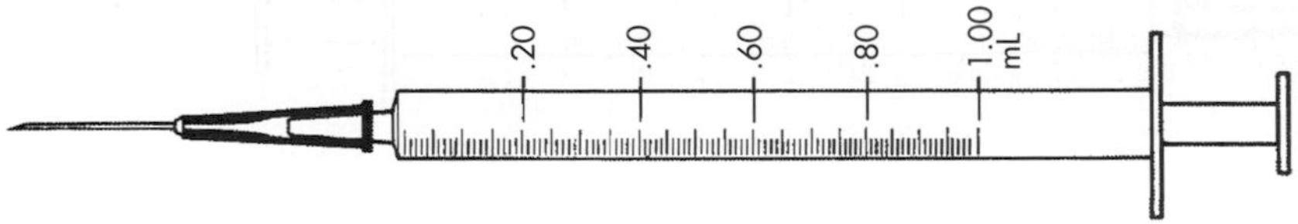

6. A physician orders heparin sodium flush 25 units.

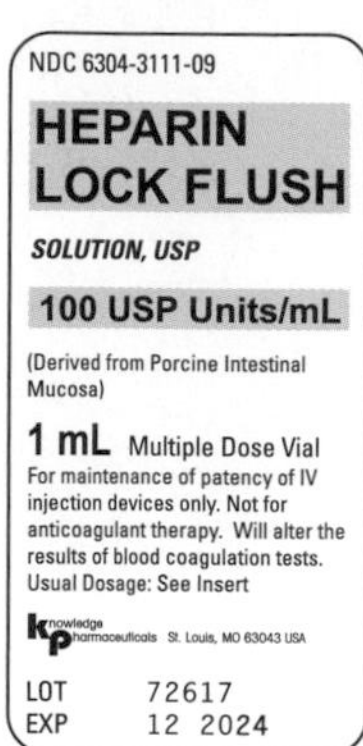

NDC 6304-3111-09
HEPARIN LOCK FLUSH
SOLUTION, USP
100 USP Units/mL
(Derived from Porcine Intestinal Mucosa)
1 mL Multiple Dose Vial
For maintenance of patency of IV injection devices only. Not for anticoagulant therapy. Will alter the results of blood coagulation tests.
Usual Dosage: See Insert
LOT 72617
EXP 12 2024

What volume of medication should be prepared for the flush?

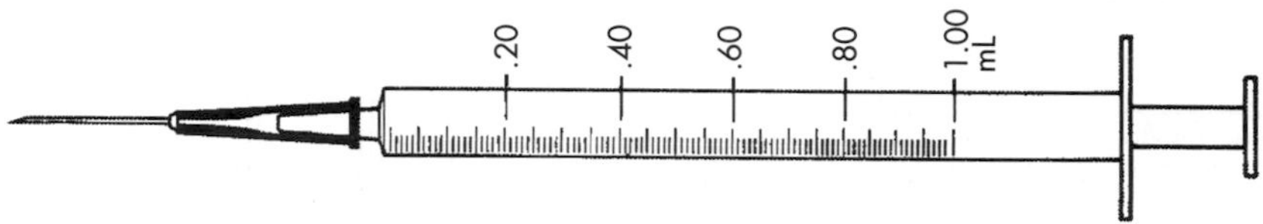

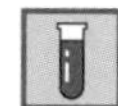

7. A physician orders heparin sodium 1,500 units subcutaneously daily.

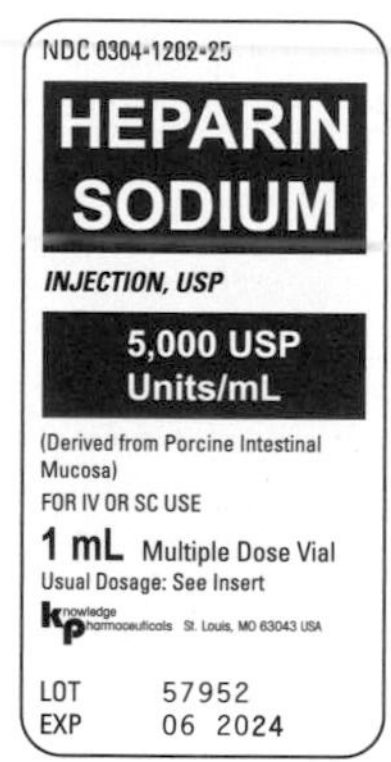

What volume of medication should be administered?

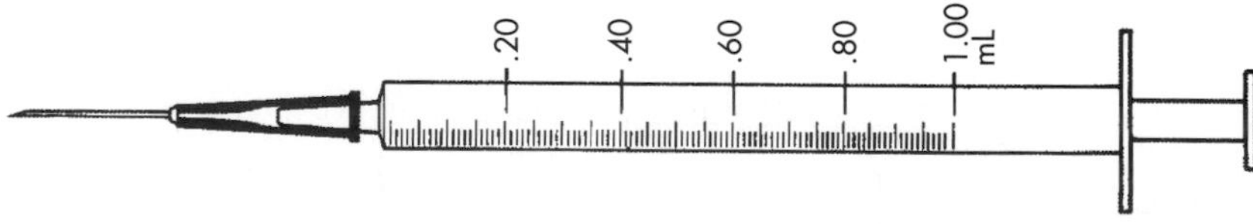

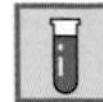

8. A physician orders heparin sodium 600 units subcutaneously stat.

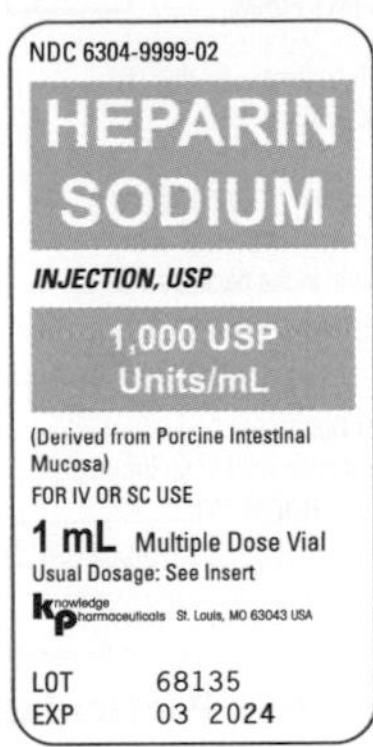

What volume of medication should be administered?

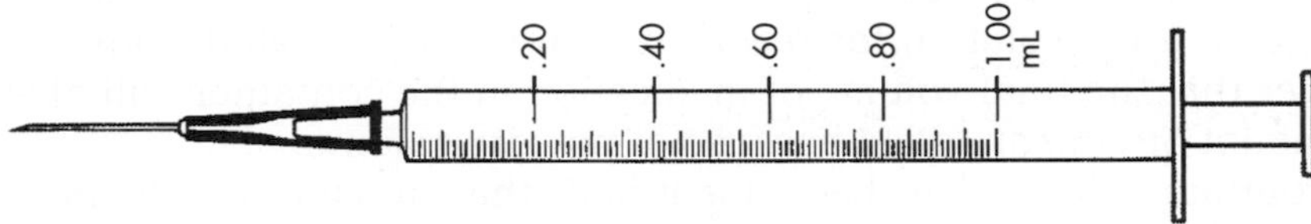

PHARMACY TECHNICIAN ROLE IN VACCINATION

Pharmacy technicians are now assisting pharmacists with vaccinations by helping to prepare vaccines in community and health-system pharmacies. Only a few states allow technicians to administer the vaccines, but this number should increase over time.

RECONSTITUTION

Parenteral medications that are unstable in liquid form for extended periods of time are manufactured in a powdered form for reconstitution before use. Most labels state the total quantity of drug in the container, the volume and type of diluent to use to attain the desired strength, the final strength of the medication after reconstitution, and the stability and storage requirements both before and after reconstitution. Sometimes, the package insert may need to be consulted for some of this information. To reconstitute a medication, follow the instructions on the medication label and package insert *exactly*. Before using, the powdered medication must be completely dissolved in the diluent.

TECH NOTE

The directions for reconstitution should be read **first** and followed **exactly** to prevent errors.

Some injectable powders are manufactured with the diluent and powder in two separate chambers, such as hydrocortisone sodium succinate (see Fig 10.7). This particular system is called the Act-O-Vial system. When the plunger is pushed down, the diluent drops from the upper chamber into the lower chamber, which contains the medication.

With injectable medications, the manufacturer may recommend the use of either sterile water for injection or sterile normal saline. Some drugs may require bacteriostatic water for IM injections or even require specific diluents, such as those with a small amount of anesthetic to prevent discomfort with IM administration. When a special diluent is

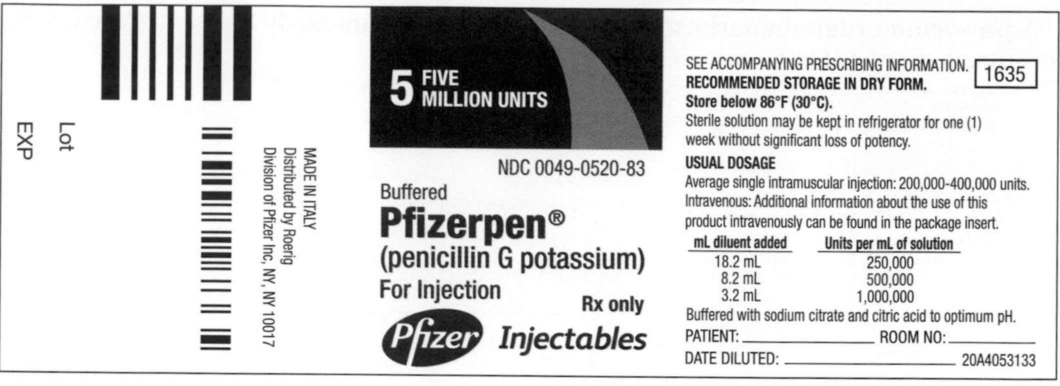
Lot
EXP
MADE IN ITALY
Distributed by Roerig
Division of Pfizer Inc, NY, NY 10017
5 FIVE MILLION UNITS
NDC 0049-0520-83
Buffered
Pfizerpen®
(penicillin G potassium)
For Injection
Rx only
Pfizer Injectables
SEE ACCOMPANYING PRESCRIBING INFORMATION.
1635
RECOMMENDED STORAGE IN DRY FORM.
Store below 86°F (30°C).
Sterile solution may be kept in refrigerator for one (1) week without significant loss of potency.
USUAL DOSAGE
Average single intramuscular injection: 200,000-400,000 units.
Intravenous: Additional information about the use of this product intravenously can be found in the package insert.
mL diluent added
Units per mL of solution
18.2 mL 250,000
8.2 mL 500,000
3.2 mL 1,000,000
Buffered with sodium citrate and citric acid to optimum pH.
PATIENT:
ROOM NO:
DATE DILUTED:
20A4053133

FIGURE 10.10 Label Showing the Volume of Diluent Necessary for Reconstituting to a Particular Strength When Multiple Doses Are a Possibility. (© Pfizer. Used with permission.)

necessary, this diluent may be packaged separately and supplied with the medication, as with some vaccinations. If the solution for reconstitution is not indicated, consult a drug reference. Remember that the final volume of medication in the container will always be greater than the amount of diluent added because of powder volume.

Once the appropriate diluent has been identified, the amount of diluent for the desired dose must be verified. Vials of some multidose parenteral drugs may be diluted with different volumes of diluent to attain different concentrations for different routes of administration, as shown on the Pfizerpen label in Fig. 10.10. Always check the possible concentrations or strengths for reconstitution because the desired diluent volume must match the intended route of administration. Decide on the amount of diluent to add and reconstitute.

TECH ALERT

Never assume the directions are the same as previously found on the same medication—READ the label directions every time medication is reconstituted.

TECH NOTE

The less diluent added, the more concentrated the medication. When reconstituting medications with multiple strengths possible, choose the strength closest to the physician's order that will provide a dose appropriate for the intended route of administration with the least chance for error.

In Fig. 10.11, the label reads to add 2.7 mL of Sterile Water for Injection, USP. After injecting diluent, the mixing process for an injectable medication is accomplished by inverting the container slowly, unless otherwise indicated by the manufacturer. Shaking the container may decrease the effectiveness of some medications and may cause the liquid to foam, which will make it difficult to withdraw the correct amount of medication. Note the length of time that the medication is stable and the directions for storage both before and after reconstitution. In Fig. 10.11, the directions for storage read: Discard solution after 3 days at room temperature or 7 days under refrigeration.

After a powder is reconstituted, the person who reconstituted it should write the following on the label if it is to be used again:

- Their initials
- The date and time prepared

- The beyond use date and time (For Fig. 10.11, calculate the BUD based on whether it is stored at room temperature or in the refrigerator)
- The strength to which it was reconstituted. (e.g., 500 mg/3 mL)

TECH NOTE

Patient safety is of utmost importance and should be safeguarded throughout each step of handling medications.

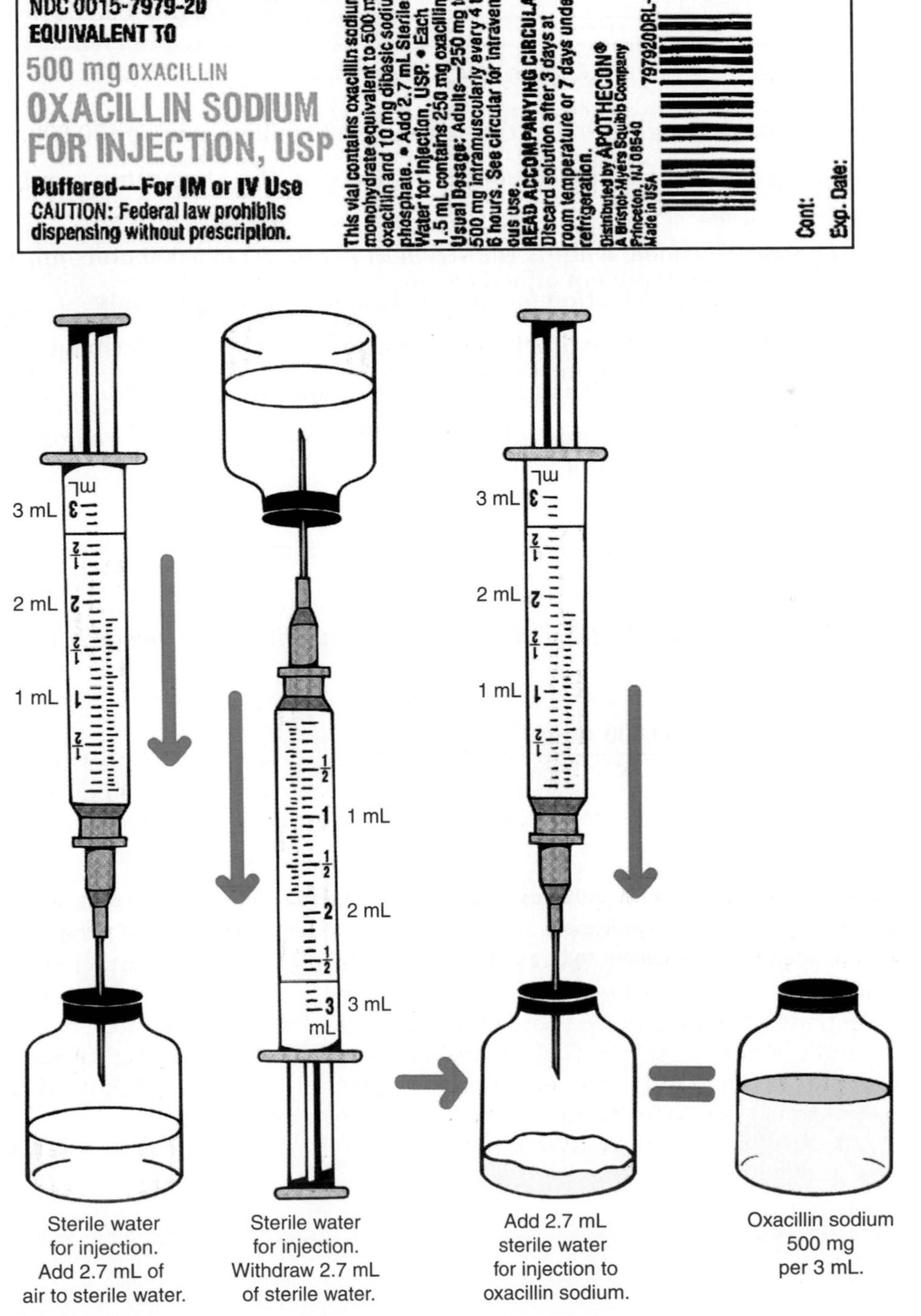

NDC 0015-7979-20
EQUIVALENT TO
500 mg OXACILLIN
OXACILLIN SODIUM
FOR INJECTION, USP
Buffered—For IM or IV Use
CAUTION: Federal law prohibits dispensing without prescription.
This vial contains oxacillin sodium monohydrate equivalent to 500 mg oxacillin and 10 mg dibasic sodium phosphate. • Add 2.7 mL Sterile Water for Injection, USP. • Each 1.5 mL contains 250 mg oxacillin.
Usual Dosage: Adults—250 mg to 500 mg intramuscularly every 4 to 6 hours. See circular for intravenous use.
READ ACCOMPANYING CIRCULAR
Discard solution after 3 days at room temperature or 7 days under refrigeration.
Distributed by APOTHECON®
A Bristol-Myers Squibb Company
Princeton, NJ 08540
Made in USA
797920DRL-1
Cont:
Exp. Date:
3 mL
2 mL
1 mL
1 mL
2 mL
3 mL
mL
Sterile water for injection. Add 2.7 mL of air to sterile water.
Sterile water for injection. Withdraw 2.7 mL of sterile water.
Add 2.7 mL sterile water for injection to oxacillin sodium.
Oxacillin sodium 500 mg per 3 mL.

FIGURE 10.11 Diluting Oxacillin Sodium in Sterile Water for Injection. (Brown M, Mulholland JM: *Drug calculations: process and problems for clinical practice*, ed 8, St. Louis, Mosby, 2008.)

EXAMPLE 10.7

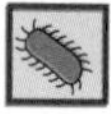

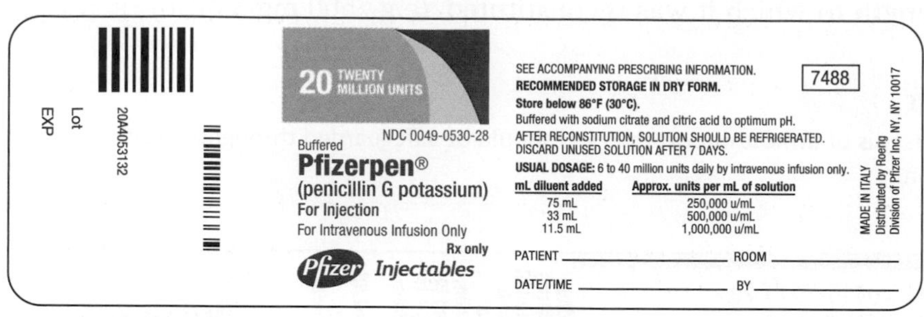

(© Pfizer. Used with permission.)

What is the total dosage found in the container? 20 million units or 20,000,000 units

If 75 mL of diluent is added to the container, what is the strength per mL? 250,000 units/mL

If 11.5 mL of diluent is added, what is the strength per mL? 1,000,000 units/mL

What is the route of administration for this medication? IV infusion only

What diluent is needed for reconstitution? Consult accompanying prescribing information

How long is the medication stable in the refrigerator after reconstitution? 7 days

If reconstituted to 250,000 units/mL, how many milliliters are needed for a dose of 375,000 units?

$$\frac{250{,}000}{1\text{ mL}} = \frac{375{,}000}{x} \quad 250{,}000x = 375{,}000\text{ mL} \quad x = 1.5\text{ mL}$$

If reconstituted to 1,000,000 units/mL, how many milliliters are needed for a dose of 2,500,000 units?

$$\frac{1{,}000{,}000\text{ units}}{1\text{ mL}} = \frac{2{,}500{,}000\text{ units}}{x} \quad x = 2.5\text{ mL}$$

TECH ALERT

Be aware that medications for IM and IV use are *not* interchangeable! The label on the medication will state its exact use. Some medications indicate that IM or IV use is acceptable but will show a difference in the amount of diluent to be added.

Practice Problems E

Answer the following questions and make necessary calculations as indicated.

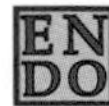

1. Prescribed: Solu-Cortef 125 mg IM stat

LOT/EXP
PAA045044

DOSAGE AND USE:
See accompanying prescribing information.
Lyophilized in container.
*Each 2 mL (when mixed) contains hydrocortisone sodium succinate equivalent to 250 mg of hydrocortisone.
Protect solution from light. Discard after 3 days.
Reconstituted ______
Distributed by Pharmacia & Upjohn Co
Division of Pfizer Inc, NY, NY 10017

Single-Dose Vial NDC 0009-0013-05
2 mL Act-O-Vial®
Solu-Cortef®
(hydrocortisone sodium succinate for injection, USP)
250 mg*
For IM or IV use
Preservative-Free **Rx only**

(© Pfizer. Used with permission.)

Interpret the order: ______

What is the strength of the medication after reconstitution? ______

How long is the medication safe to use after reconstitution? ______

What are the storage instructions? ______

What volume of medication is needed for this dose?

How many full doses are in this vial? ______

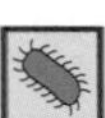

2.

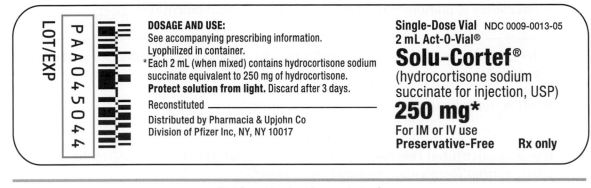

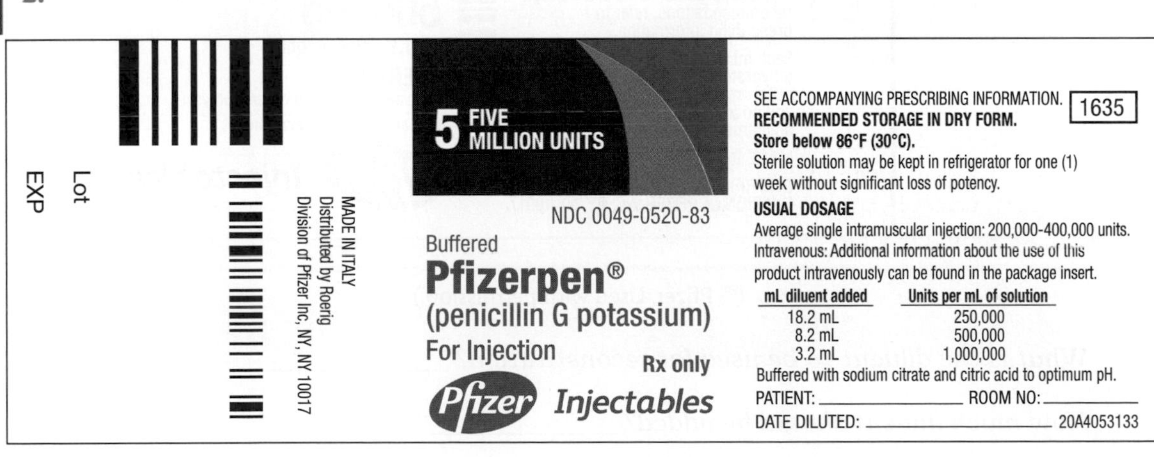

Lot
EXP
MADE IN ITALY
Distributed by Roerig
Division of Pfizer Inc, NY, NY 10017
5 FIVE MILLION UNITS
NDC 0049-0520-83
Buffered
Pfizerpen®
(penicillin G potassium)
For Injection
Rx only
Pfizer Injectables
SEE ACCOMPANYING PRESCRIBING INFORMATION.
1635
RECOMMENDED STORAGE IN DRY FORM.
Store below 86°F (30°C).
Sterile solution may be kept in refrigerator for one (1) week without significant loss of potency.
USUAL DOSAGE
Average single intramuscular injection: 200,000-400,000 units.
Intravenous: Additional information about the use of this product intravenously can be found in the package insert.
mL diluent added | Units per mL of solution
18.2 mL | 250,000
8.2 mL | 500,000
3.2 mL | 1,000,000
Buffered with sodium citrate and citric acid to optimum pH.
PATIENT: ROOM NO:
DATE DILUTED:
20A4053133

(© Pfizer. Used with permission.)

What is the total dosage of medication in this vial? ____________________

If 18.2 mL of diluent is added, what is the strength per milliliter? ____________________

If 8.2 mL of diluent is added, what is the strength per milliliter? ____________________

If 3.2 mL of diluent is added, what is the strength per milliliter? ____________________

What routes of administration can be used with this medication? ____________________

____

After dilution, how long can the medication be stored in the refrigerator without a loss of potency? ____________

What is the volume of the powder displacement?

If you reconstituted this medication on 9/20/2022 at 0130 with 8.2 mL of diluent, what information should you place on the label?

____

____

____

____

3.

Lot No./Exp. Date

12966300

Store at or below 86°F (30°C).

DOSAGE AND USE
See accompanying prescribing information.

Constitute to 100 mg/mL* with 4.8 mL of Sterile Water For Injection.

Must be further diluted before use. For appropriate diluents and storage recommendations, refer to prescribing information.

*Each mL contains azithromycin dihydrate equivalent to 100 mg of azithromycin, 76.9 mg of citric acid, and sodium hydroxide for pH adjustment.

MADE IN IRELAND

DISTRIBUTED BY PFIZER LABS
DIVISION OF PFIZER INC, NY, NY 10017

NDC 0069-3150-84 **Rx only**

Zithromax®
(azithromycin for injection)

500 mg

For **I.V.** infusion only

STERILE
equivalent to 500 mg of azithromycin

No Latex **No Preservative**

Pfizer *Injectables*

What is the diluent to be used for reconstitution? ____________

How much diluent should be added? ____________

What is the strength after reconstitution? ____________

What is the total volume of medication after reconstitution? ______________

What is the route of administration for this medication? ______________

What are the special administration instructions to follow after reconstitution?

____

What volume of medication is needed to provide 0.5 g?

What volume of medication is needed to provide 300 mg?

4. Medication order: streptomycin 300 mg IM daily.

Recommended Storage in dry form. Store below 86°F (30°C)
Sterile reconstituted solutions should be protected from light and may be stored at room temperature for four weeks without significant loss of potency.

Knowledge Pharmaceuticals
St. Louis, MO 63043

Streptomycin Sulfate, USP
Equivalent to 5.0 g of Streptomycin Base
5.0 g
For intramuscular use only

Usual Daily Dosage
Adults: Varies, consult package insert
Adult average single injection 0.5 – 1.0 g

mL diluent added	mg/mL of solution
9.0 mL	400 mg/mL

The dry powder is dissolved by adding Water for injection, USP or Sodium Chloride Injection, USP in an amount to yield the desired concentration.
Patient:________
Room No: ________
Date Diluted: ________

What volume of diluent should be added to the vial? ______________

What diluent should be used for this reconstitution? ______________

What is the strength of the medication following reconstitution?

____

What are the storage requirements following reconstitution?

____

____

What volume of medication should be administered per dose?

What syringe should be used for the administration? ______________________

REVIEW

Calculations with injectable medications can be performed with ratio and proportion or dimensional analysis for single-step calculations and DA for multistep calculations. Parenteral medications are supplied in single-dose vials, multidose vials, ampules, and prefilled syringes.

Insulin, anticoagulants, and some antimicrobial agents are supplied in units per milliliter. Insulin products are available in a variety of types, mainly in U-100 strength. Heparin is supplied in a wide variety of strengths. Read the label and physician's order carefully with both products to prepare the medication that has been ordered for administration in the proper strength/dosage.

TECH NOTE

The important key in working with units is the careful interpretation of the label to ensure that the *exact* amount per milliliter is known before preparation of the dose to be given.

! TECH ALERT

Injectable medications in units per milliliter are specific for each medication and are not interchangeable between units/mL of another medication.

Reconstitution is necessary when a medication is provided in powdered form due to instability in a liquid form. When medications are prepared for injectable routes, the required diluent may be sterile water for injection, bacteriostatic water for injection, 0.9% sodium chloride (normal saline) for injection, *or* a special solution provided with the medication by the manufacturer. After reconstitution, parenteral medications require special storage conditions and beyond use dates due to the instability of the liquid formulations. Some medications can be diluted to different strengths or concentrations as directed by the manufacturers, whereas others have only one dilution strength option. Always read directions carefully before preparing injectable products.

The necessary steps when reconstituting medications are as follows:

1. Read all of the directions on the medication label or package insert.
2. Tap the bottle to loosen the powder in the vial.
3. Use the diluent designated by the manufacturer in the amount appropriate for the strength of medication needed. If this information is not on the vial, use the package insert or drug reference to determine the appropriate diluent and amount.
4. After reconstitution of multidose vials, label the medication with the initials of the preparer, the date and time of reconstitution, the strength of the medication, and the beyond use date and time.

Posttest

Interpret the following orders and calculate the medication doses. Round the final answer to the nearest hundredth if less than 1 mL and the nearest tenth if over 1 mL.

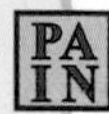

1. Medication order: Stadol (butorphanol) 1 mg IM stat for pain

   Stock strength: butorphanol injection 2 mg/mL (1 mL vial)

   Interpret the order: ______________________________

   ____

   What volume of medication is needed for the dose?

   Indicate the correct amount of medication on the appropriate syringe.

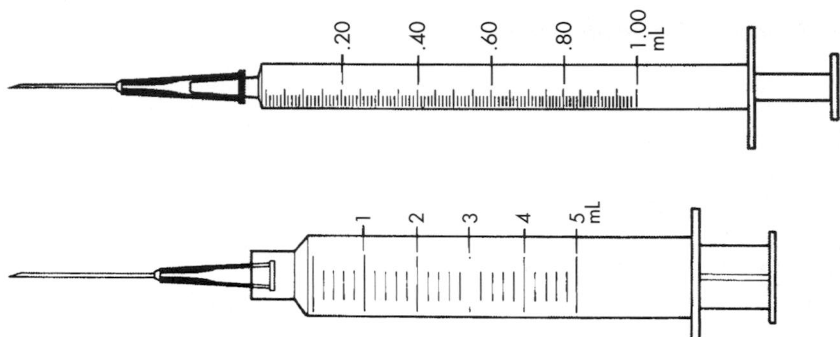

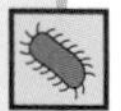

2. Medication order: Garamycin (gentamicin) 0.06 g IM q8h

   Stock strength: gentamicin injection 40 mg/mL

   Interpret the order: ______________________________

   ____

   What volume of medication is needed per dose?

   Indicate the correct amount of medication on the appropriate syringe.

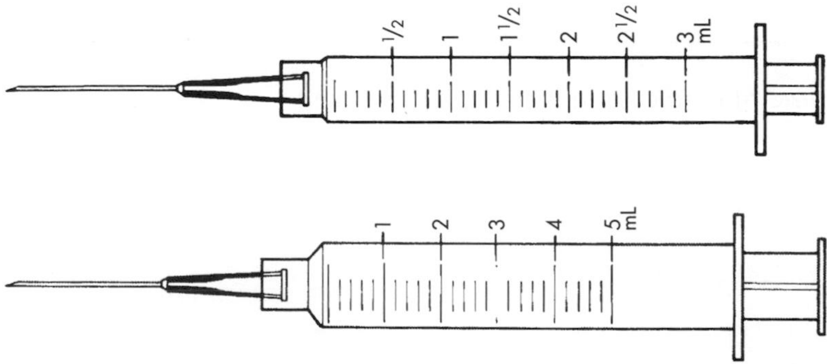

Continued

Posttest, cont.

3. Medication order: Solu-Medrol (methylprednisolone) 37.5 mg IM stat

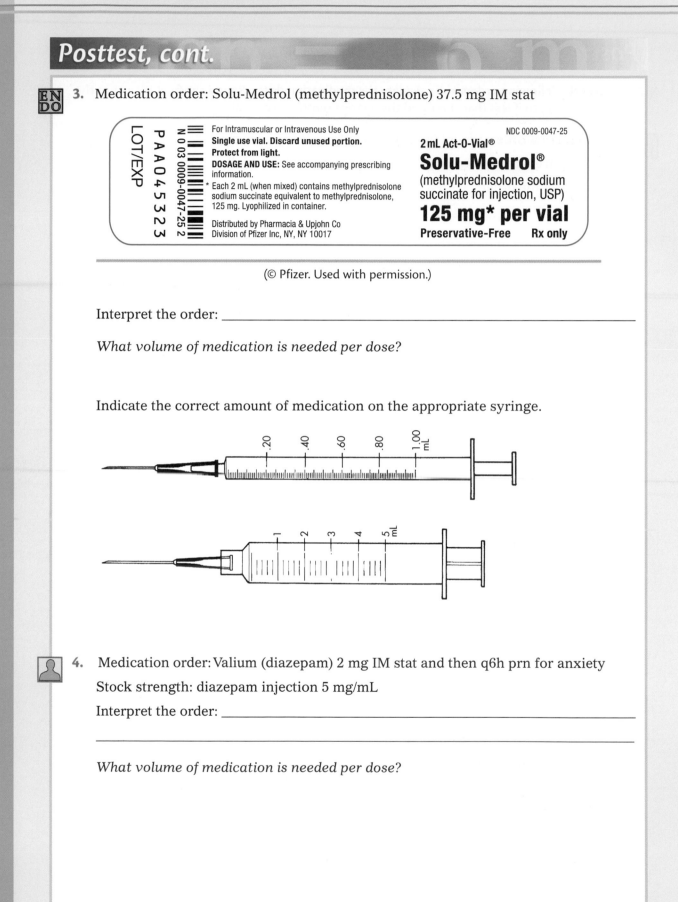

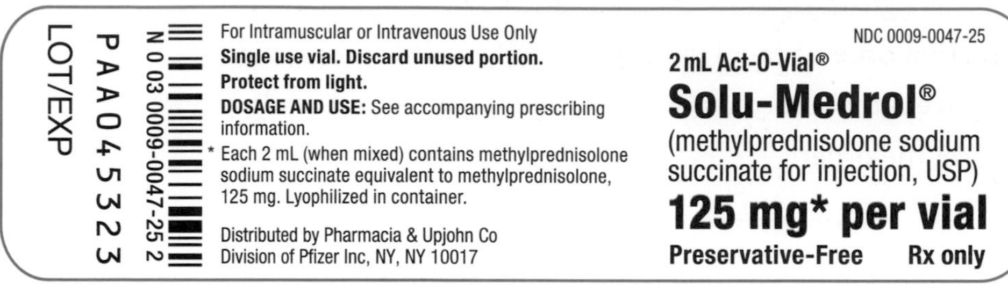

N 0 03 0009-0047-25 2
PAA045323
LOT/EXP
For Intramuscular or Intravenous Use Only
Single use vial. Discard unused portion.
Protect from light.
DOSAGE AND USE: See accompanying prescribing information.
* Each 2 mL (when mixed) contains methylprednisolone sodium succinate equivalent to methylprednisolone, 125 mg. Lyophilized in container.
Distributed by Pharmacia & Upjohn Co
Division of Pfizer Inc, NY, NY 10017
NDC 0009-0047-25
2 mL Act-O-Vial®
Solu-Medrol®
(methylprednisolone sodium succinate for injection, USP)
125 mg* per vial
Preservative-Free
Rx only

Interpret the order: ______________________________

What volume of medication is needed per dose?

Indicate the correct amount of medication on the appropriate syringe.

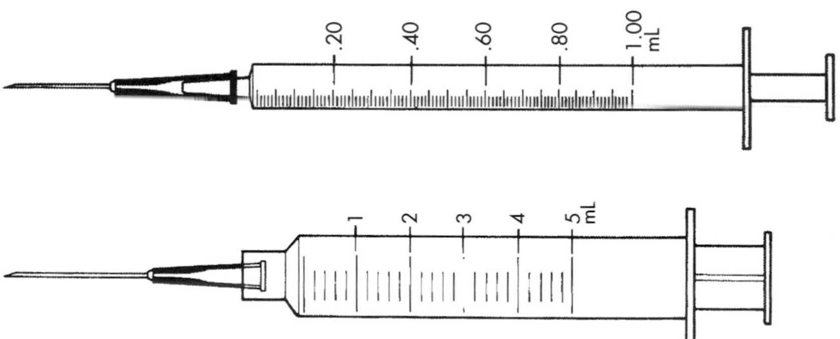

4. Medication order: Valium (diazepam) 2 mg IM stat and then q6h prn for anxiety

Stock strength: diazepam injection 5 mg/mL

Interpret the order: ______________________________

____

What volume of medication is needed per dose?

Posttest, cont.

5. Medication order: Dilaudid (hydromorphone) 500 mcg IM q4h prn severe pain

   Stock strength: hydromorphone injection 2 mg/mL (1 mL vial)

   Interpret the order: ____

   ____

   What volume of medication is needed per dose?

   Indicate the correct amount of medication on the appropriate syringe.

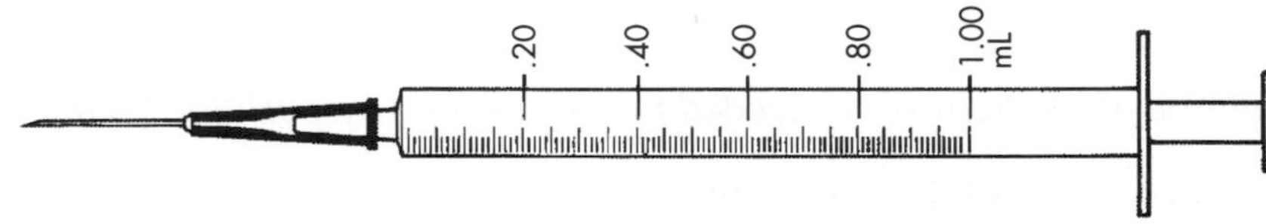

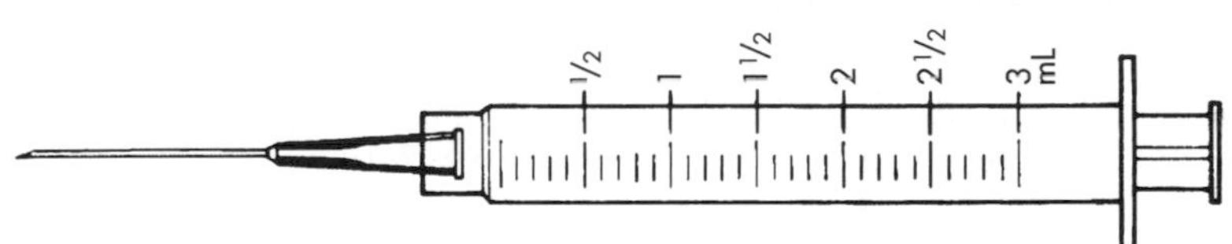

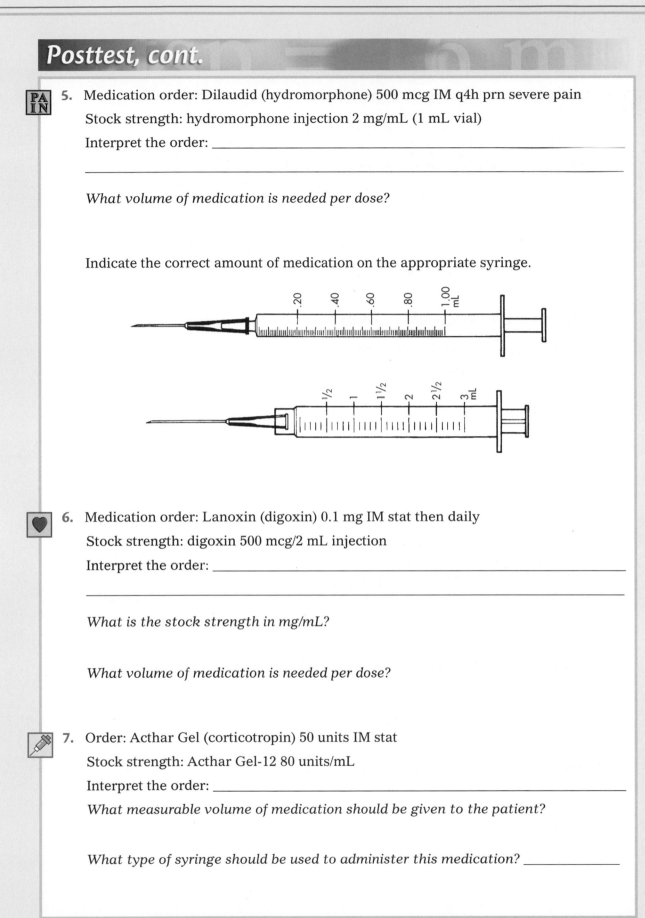

6. Medication order: Lanoxin (digoxin) 0.1 mg IM stat then daily

   Stock strength: digoxin 500 mcg/2 mL injection

   Interpret the order: ____

   ____

   What is the stock strength in mg/mL?

   What volume of medication is needed per dose?

7. Order: Acthar Gel (corticotropin) 50 units IM stat

   Stock strength: Acthar Gel-12 80 units/mL

   Interpret the order: ____

   What measurable volume of medication should be given to the patient?

   What type of syringe should be used to administer this medication? ______________

Continued

Posttest, cont.

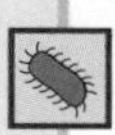

8. Medication order: Garamycin 30 mg IM q8h

Stock strength: gentamycin 40 mg/mL injection (20 mL multidose vial)

Interpret the order: ______________________________

What volume of medication is needed per dose?

9. Medication order: Demerol (meperidine) 50 mg IM q4h prn pain

Stock strengths available: meperidine 75 mg/mL and meperidine 100 mg/mL

Interpret the order: ______________________________

What volume of medication is needed per dose using meperidine 75 mg/mL?

What volume of medication is needed per dose using meperidine 100 mg/mL?

Which strength of meperidine would you choose to use for the IM dose?

____

10. A 37-lb child is prescribed induction doses of Humira (adalimumab) 80 mg on day 1 and 40 mg on day 15, and then maintenance doses of 20 mg every other week subcutaneously for Crohn disease. He will receive the first 3 doses at the physician's office before being supplied with a prescription for pre-filled pens.

Stock Injection: 40 mg/0.8 mL in a single-dose glass vial (institutional use only)

How many milliliters will be administered on day 1?

How many milliliters will be administered on day 15?

How many milliliters will be administered on day 29?

Posttest, cont.

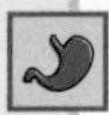

11. A patient is prescribed 10 mg Reglan (metoclopramide) IM at the end of surgery.

    Stock strength: metoclopramide IM Injection Solution 5 mg/mL

    How many milliliters should be administered?

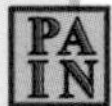

12. Medication order: Dilaudid 1-2 mg IM q 2-3h prn for severe pain

    Stock available: 1-mL ampules of hydromorphone injection in the following strengths: 1 mg/mL, 2 mg/mL, and 4 mg/mL

    Interpret the order:

    ____

    ____

    Dilaudid is a CII medication that requires documentation if any is wasted.

    Which ampule should be chosen for the 2 mg dose? ____________

    What volume is needed from this ampule for the 2 mg dose? ____________

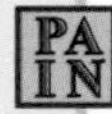

13. Medication order: Dilaudid 750 mcg IM stat

    Stock available: 1-mL ampules of hydromorphone injection in the following strengths: 1 mg/mL, 2 mg/mL, and 4 mg/mL

    What volume of medication would be administered using the 1 mg/mL strength?

    What volume of medication would be administered using the 2 mg/mL strength?

    What volume of medication would be administered using the 4 mg/mL strength?

    Which of the above strengths will provide a dose that is most exact (does not require rounding to a measurable dose or wasting)? ____________

    How many mcg would each of the other strengths provide once rounded to a measurable dose?

Continued

Posttest, cont.

EN DO **14.** Medication order: Solu-Medrol 75 mg IM stat

Stock available: Solu-Medrol (methylprednisolone sodium succinate) 125 mg/2 mL Inj

What volume of medication should be administered?

What size syringe should be used for administration? ____________

15. Medication order: Valium (diazepam) 3 mg IM

Stock available: diazepam injection 5 mg/mL

What volume of medication should be administered?

What size syringe should be used for administration? ____________

16. Medication order: Vitamin B-12 0.25 mg subcut

Stock strength: cyanocobalamin (B-12) 10,000 mcg/10 mL.

What volume of medication should be administered?

What syringe should be used for the administration? ____________

EN DO **17.** Prescription: 18 units of regular insulin and 37 units of NPH subcut qam

Strengths available: U-100

What size U-100 insulin syringe must be used to draw them up as a single injection?

____

Posttest, cont.

18. A physician orders Humulin 70/30 60 units subcut qam

How many units of regular insulin does the patient receive per day?

How many units of NPH insulin does the patient receive per day?

19. Medication order: heparin 350 units subcut

Stock strength: heparin sodium 1,000 USP units/mL

What is the volume of the dose to be given?

20. Medication order: Zithromax 500 mg IV qd × 2 days

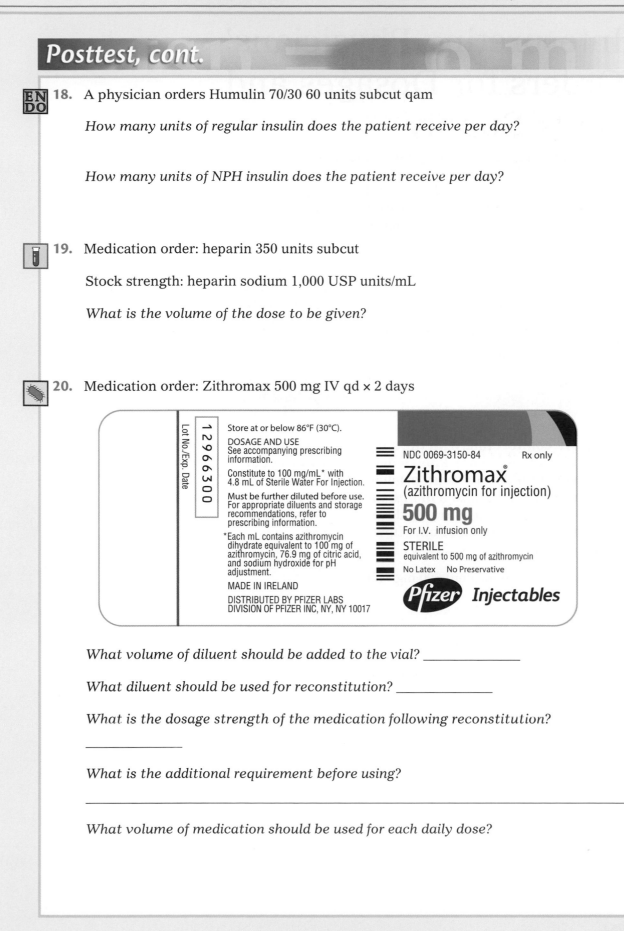

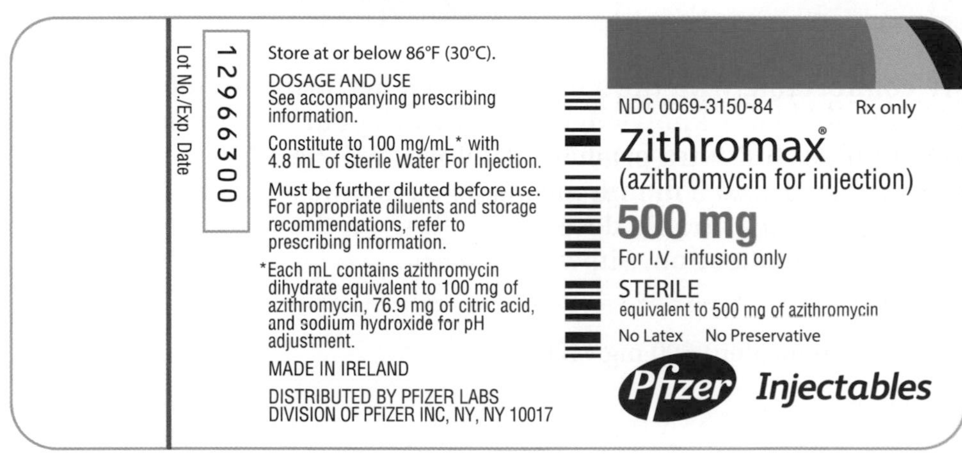
Lot No./Exp. Date
12966300
Store at or below 86°F (30°C).
DOSAGE AND USE
See accompanying prescribing information.
Constitute to 100 mg/mL* with 4.8 mL of Sterile Water For Injection.
Must be further diluted before use. For appropriate diluents and storage recommendations, refer to prescribing information.
*Each mL contains azithromycin dihydrate equivalent to 100 mg of azithromycin, 76.9 mg of citric acid, and sodium hydroxide for pH adjustment.
MADE IN IRELAND
DISTRIBUTED BY PFIZER LABS
DIVISION OF PFIZER INC, NY, NY 10017
NDC 0069-3150-84
Rx only
Zithromax®
(azithromycin for injection)
500 mg
For I.V. infusion only
STERILE
equivalent to 500 mg of azithromycin
No Latex No Preservative
Pfizer Injectables

What volume of diluent should be added to the vial? ______________

What diluent should be used for reconstitution? ______________

What is the dosage strength of the medication following reconstitution?

____

What is the additional requirement before using?

____

What volume of medication should be used for each daily dose?

Interpreting Physicians' Orders for Dosages and Days' Supply

OBJECTIVES

1. Calculate the amount of medication needed when quantity is not indicated.
2. Calculate the number of doses of medication in a container.
3. Calculate the length of time a prescription will last.

KEY WORDS

Days' supply Number of days a prescription will last; important to input for insurance reimbursement

Inhaler A device used to deliver medicine by breathing it in through the mouth or nose

Nebulizer A device used to produce a fine spray of medication for inhalation

Pretest

If you are comfortable with the subject matter, perform the following calculations to test your knowledge. If not, work your way through the chapter and return to them for extra practice. All doses will be administered on the first day as ordered, and a month means 30 days unless otherwise stated. Round answers to measurable doses depending on the utensil to be used or the available form of medication. Show your work.

PA IN

1. Rx: Motrin (ibuprofen) 600 mg #120
   Sig: i q6h with food

   Days' supply: ____________

2. Rx: Xanax (alprazolam) 0.25 mg #60
   Sig: i to ii tabs bid prn anxiety

   Days' supply: ____________

Pretest, cont.

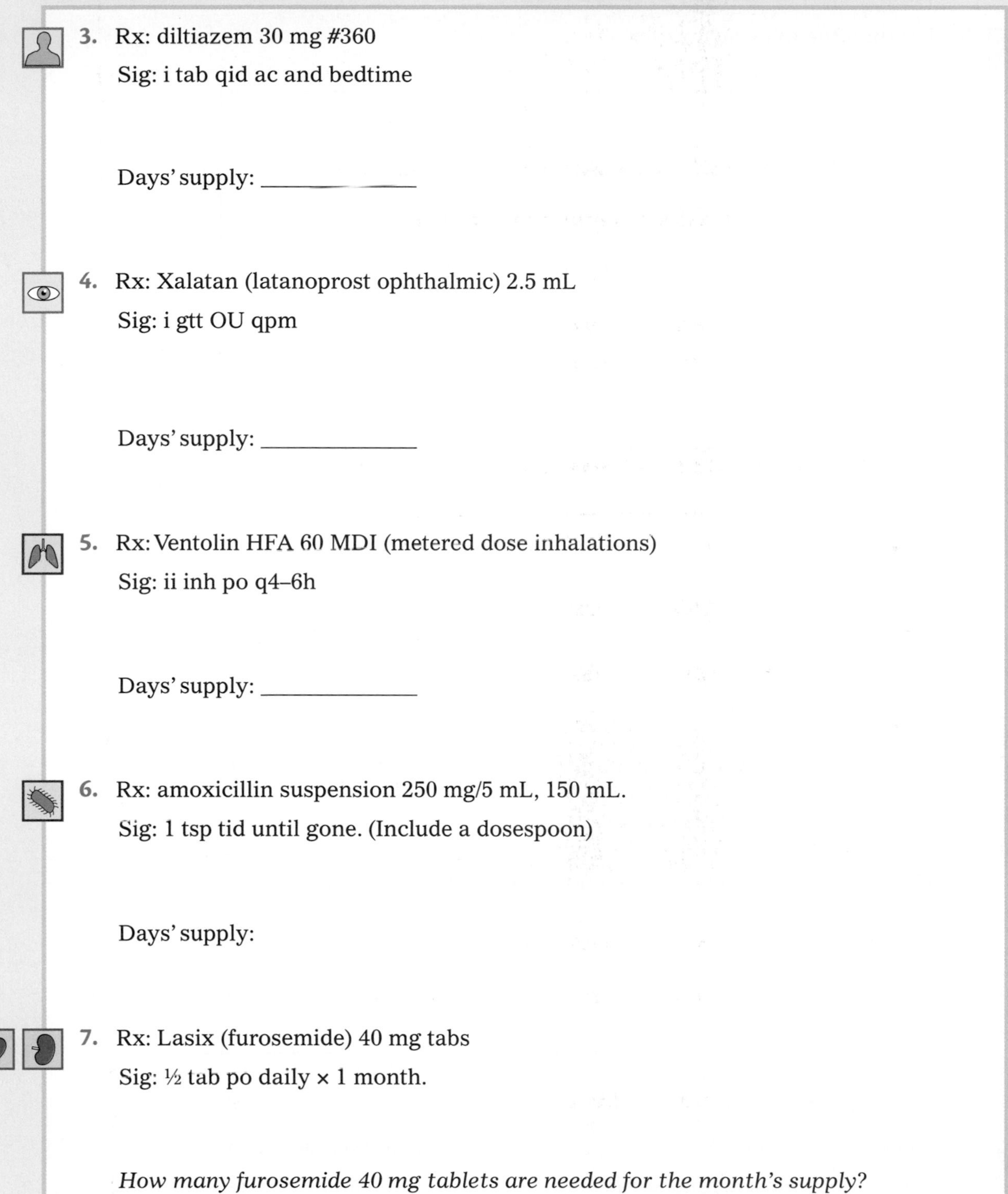

3. Rx: diltiazem 30 mg #360
   Sig: i tab qid ac and bedtime

   Days' supply: ____________

4. Rx: Xalatan (latanoprost ophthalmic) 2.5 mL
   Sig: i gtt OU qpm

   Days' supply: ____________

5. Rx: Ventolin HFA 60 MDI (metered dose inhalations)
   Sig: ii inh po q4–6h

   Days' supply: ____________

6. Rx: amoxicillin suspension 250 mg/5 mL, 150 mL.
   Sig: 1 tsp tid until gone. (Include a dosespoon)

   Days' supply:

7. Rx: Lasix (furosemide) 40 mg tabs
   Sig: ½ tab po daily × 1 month.

   How many furosemide 40 mg tablets are needed for the month's supply?

Continued

Pretest, cont.

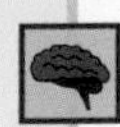

8. Interpret the following prescription:

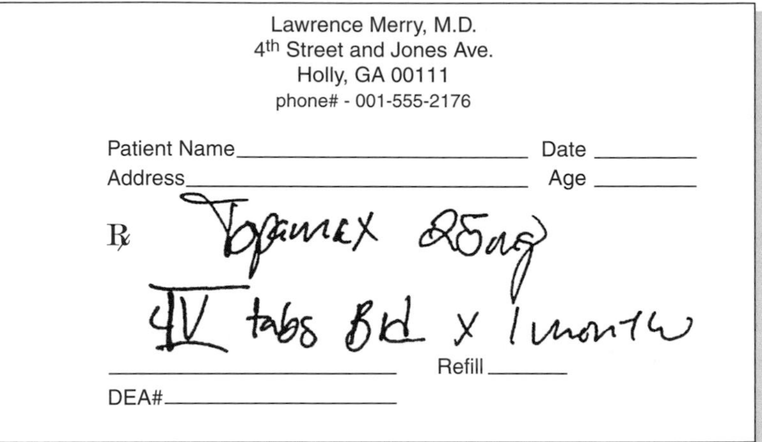

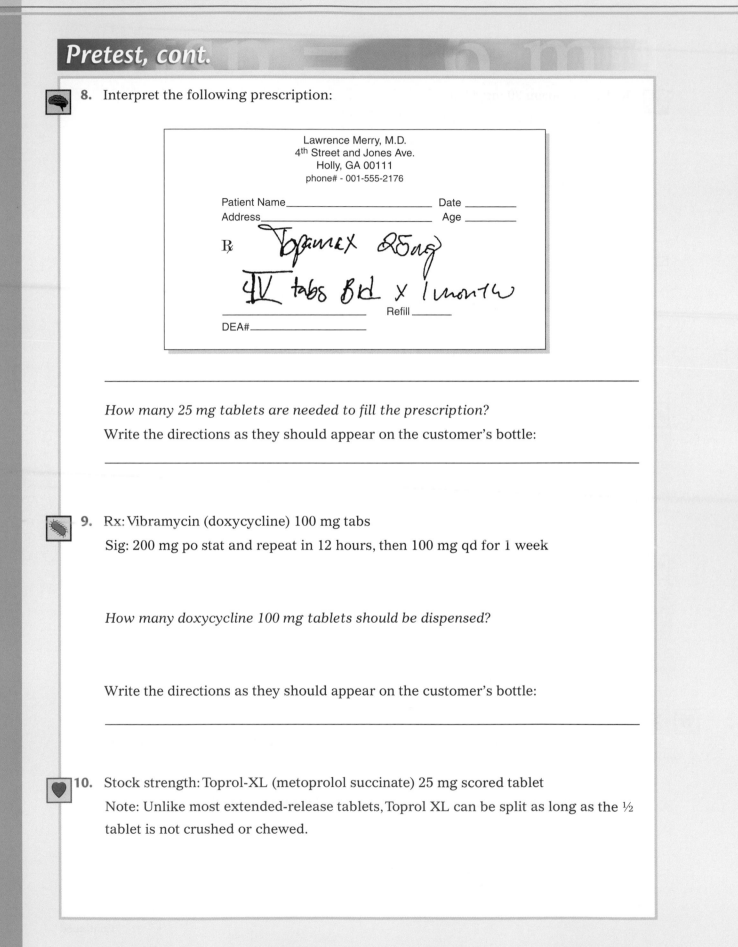

Lawrence Merry, M.D.
4th Street and Jones Ave.
Holly, GA 00111
phone# - 001-555-2176

Patient Name________ Date ______
Address________ Age ______

℞ Topamax 25mg
IV tabs Bid x 1 month

________ Refill ______
DEA#________

____

How many 25 mg tablets are needed to fill the prescription?

Write the directions as they should appear on the customer's bottle:

____

9. Rx: Vibramycin (doxycycline) 100 mg tabs
   Sig: 200 mg po stat and repeat in 12 hours, then 100 mg qd for 1 week

   How many doxycycline 100 mg tablets should be dispensed?

   Write the directions as they should appear on the customer's bottle:

   ____

10. Stock strength: Toprol-XL (metoprolol succinate) 25 mg scored tablet
    Note: Unlike most extended-release tablets, Toprol XL can be split as long as the ½ tablet is not crushed or chewed.

Pretest, cont.

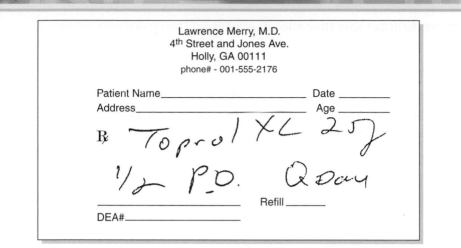

Lawrence Merry, M.D.
4th Street and Jones Ave.
Holly, GA 00111
phone# - 001-555-2176

Patient Name__________ Date _____
Address__________ Age _____

℞ Toprol XL 25 mg
1/2 P.O. Q Day

__________ Refill _____
DEA#__________

How many tablets are needed to fill the prescription for a month's supply?

How many mg will the patient receive per dose?

Write the directions as they should appear on the customer's bottle:

____

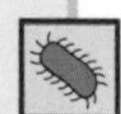

11. Rx: amoxicillin 125 mg/5 mL
Sig: 62.5 mg po tid for 10 days

What quantity of medication should the parents give per dose?

Amoxicillin 125 mg/5 mL suspension is available in 100-mL and 150-mL bottles

Which size bottle should be dispensed?

How much medication would be discarded if the order was followed correctly?

Continued

Pretest, cont.

Write the directions as they should appear on the customer's bottle:

____

12. A patient without insurance presents the following prescription for 40 mg capsules and only wants a 2-week supply.

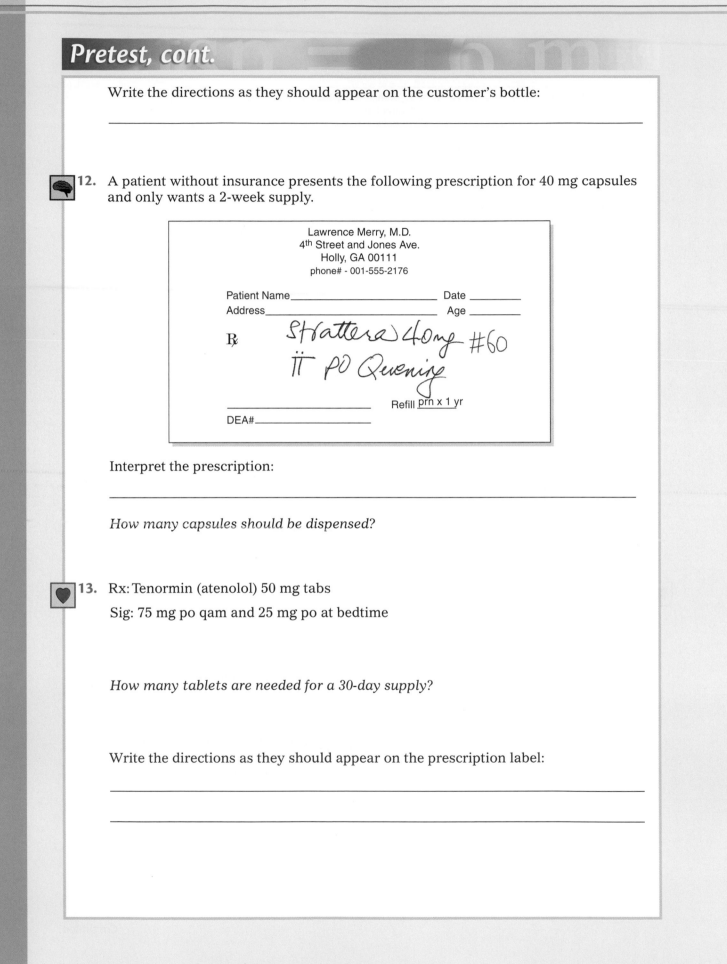

Lawrence Merry, M.D.
4th Street and Jones Ave.
Holly, GA 00111
phone# - 001-555-2176

Patient Name__________________ Date ________
Address__________________ Age ________

℞ Strattera 40mg #60
ii po Qevening

__________________ Refill prn x 1 yr
DEA#__________________

Interpret the prescription:

____

How many capsules should be dispensed?

13. Rx: Tenormin (atenolol) 50 mg tabs

Sig: 75 mg po qam and 25 mg po at bedtime

How many tablets are needed for a 30-day supply?

Write the directions as they should appear on the prescription label:

____

____

Pretest, cont.

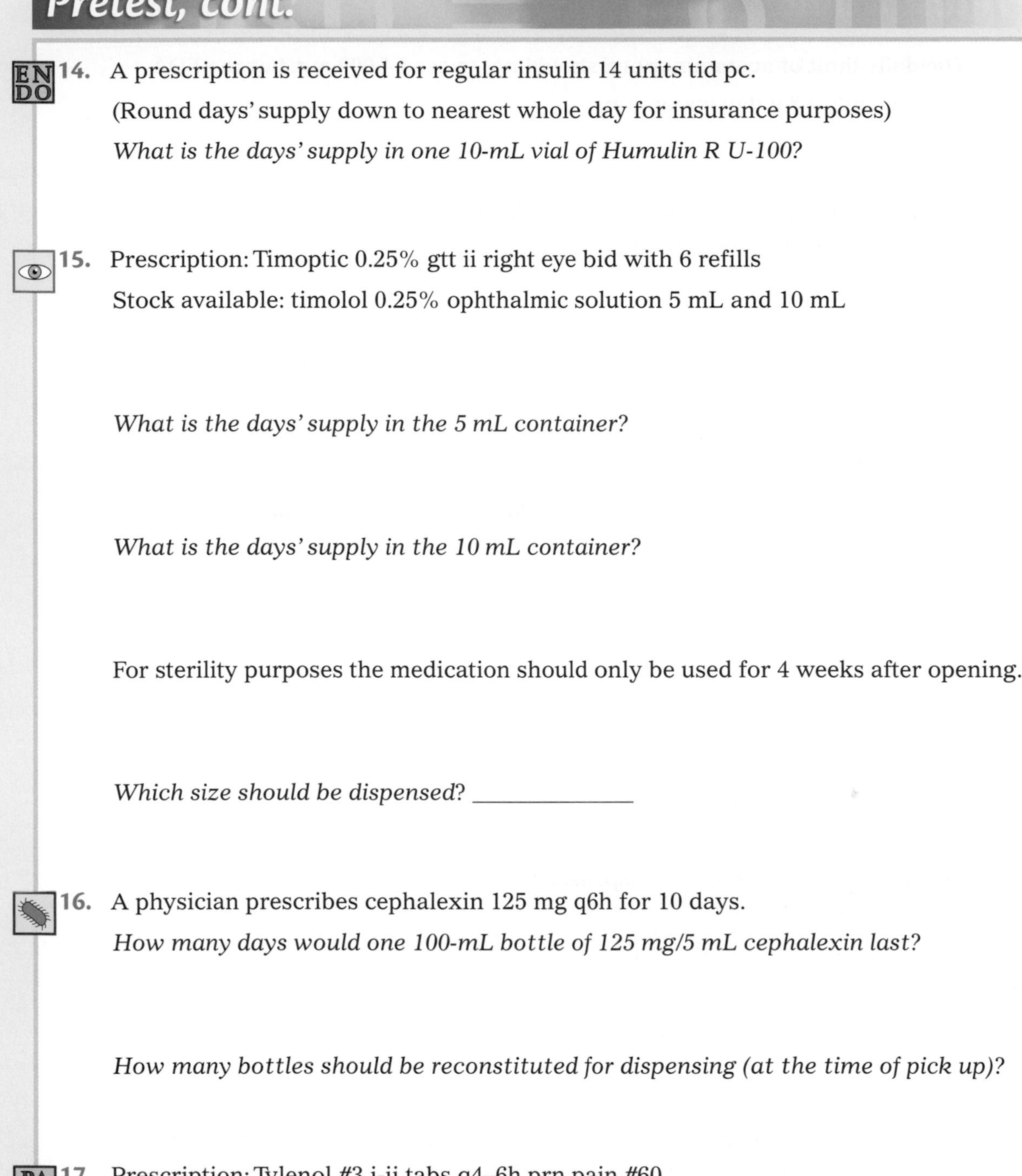

14. A prescription is received for regular insulin 14 units tid pc.
    (Round days' supply down to nearest whole day for insurance purposes)
    What is the days' supply in one 10-mL vial of Humulin R U-100?

15. Prescription: Timoptic 0.25% gtt ii right eye bid with 6 refills
    Stock available: timolol 0.25% ophthalmic solution 5 mL and 10 mL

    What is the days' supply in the 5 mL container?

    What is the days' supply in the 10 mL container?

    For sterility purposes the medication should only be used for 4 weeks after opening.

    Which size should be dispensed? ______________

16. A physician prescribes cephalexin 125 mg q6h for 10 days.
    How many days would one 100-mL bottle of 125 mg/5 mL cephalexin last?

    How many bottles should be reconstituted for dispensing (at the time of pick up)?

17. Prescription: Tylenol #3 i-ii tabs q4–6h prn pain #60
    Stock available: Tylenol #3: acetaminophen 300 mg and codeine 30 mg/tablet

    What is the days' supply if the maximum amount is taken daily?

Continued

Pretest, cont.

The daily limit of acetaminophen should not exceed 4,000 mg, but the FDA recommends a 3 g/day maximum.

What amount of acetaminophen would this patient receive in 1 day at the maximum dosage for the prescription?

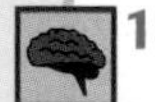

18. A consumer purchases Benadryl (diphenhydramine) elixir over the counter. The strength is 12.5 mg diphenhydramine/5 mL.

How long will the 4-ounce bottle last if she takes 25 mg every night?

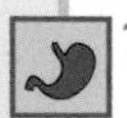

19. Rx: Protonix (pantoprazole) 20 mg tabs
Sig: 1 bid

Insurance allows a 90-day supply.

How many tablets should be dispensed?

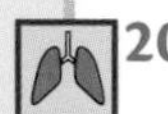

20. Rx: Spiriva (tiotropium) Respimat 1.25 mcg/actuation
Sig: 2 inhalations po qd for asthma maintenance

Stock available: Spiriva Respimat Inhalation Spray 1.25 mcg/actuation 60 metered actuations

How many oral inhaler cartridges should be dispensed for a 90-day supply?

INTRODUCTION

The objective of this chapter is to bring together mathematical skills learned in previous chapters to accurately prepare medication for dispensing, given the information provided on a prescription. In some instances, the medical professional omits the number of doses of medication necessary or the dose to be given from a total dosage. In many instances, because only one element is missing, pharmacy staff can make the necessary calculation from the prescription without contacting the physician. This chapter provides the knowledge base needed for making accurate decisions for doses and dosages.

Determining the Appropriate Quantity for Dispensing (Dosage)

As long as the physician provides a time frame for a prescription, the pharmacy staff is responsible for ensuring that the patient has sufficient medication to complete the desired medication cycle. Basically, the total dosage needed is the number of doses needed per day times the total number of days prescribed. This can be calculated with dimensional analysis (DA) or, in the case of solid medications, ratio and proportion (R&P).

EXAMPLE 11.1

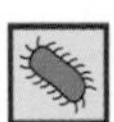

Rx: amoxicillin 500 mg caps

Sig: 1 tid × 10 days

Dispense amoxicillin 500 mg capsules to be taken three times a day for 10 days.

Three capsules per day × 10 days = 30 capsules.

The pharmacy technician in a retail pharmacy would prepare 30 capsules for the pharmacist to check for dispensing. In an inpatient setting, such as a nursing home, the date of the order and the ending date would be noted, so the medication would be discontinued 10 days later.

This example essentially involves applying R&P or DA as follows:

$$\frac{3\text{ caps}}{1\text{ day}} = \frac{x\text{ caps}}{10\text{ days}} \quad x = 30\text{ caps} \quad \text{or} \quad \text{caps} = \frac{3\text{ caps}}{1\text{ day}} \bullet \frac{10\text{ days}}{1} = 30\text{ caps}$$

With prescriptions such as this, most pharmacists will expect a quick mental calculation of the answer because it is simple multiplication. Never forget to use common sense when looking at an answer. If a prescription is written for 4 capsules a day for 7 days, simple multiplication gives you the answer of 28 capsules. You are using the process of DA or R&P mentally.

EXAMPLE 11.2

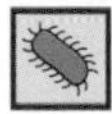

Rx: cefdinir 125 mg/5 mL

Sig: 125 mg bid × 10 days

How many mL are needed for the entire course of therapy?

Using DA will help keep track of the units.

$$\text{total mL required} = \frac{5\text{ mL}}{125\text{ mg}} \bullet \frac{125\text{ mg}}{1\text{ dose}} \bullet \frac{2\text{ doses}}{1\text{ day}} \bullet \frac{10\text{ days}}{1} = 100\text{ mL}$$

EXAMPLE 11.3

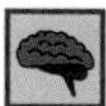

A physician prescribes phenobarbital gr i po q6h for epilepsy. Provide a month's supply.

Stock strength: phenobarbital 30 mg tablets (Use gr i = 60 mg)

How many tablets should be provided to fill the prescription?

$$\text{tablets} = \frac{1\text{ tablet}}{30\text{ mg}} \bullet \frac{60\text{ mg}}{\text{gr i}} \bullet \frac{\text{gr i}}{\text{dose}} \bullet \frac{4\text{ doses}}{\text{day}} \bullet \frac{30\text{ days}}{1} = 240\text{ tablets}$$

How many tablets are needed for a single dose?

$$\text{tablets} = \frac{1\text{ tablet}}{30\text{ mg}} \bullet \frac{60\text{ mg}}{\text{gr i}} \bullet \frac{\text{gr i}}{\text{dose}} = 2\text{ tablets}$$

What is the dose in milligrams?

Write the directions as they would appear on the customer's bottle:

Take two tablets by mouth every 6 hours for epilepsy.

EXAMPLE 11.4

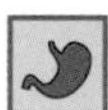

On Friday a doctor orders Tagamet (cimetidine) 300 mg IM q6h to be sent to the hospital floor for the weekend.

Stock strength: cimetidine 300 mg/2 mL injection in 8 mL multidose vials

How many vials should be sent for Friday noon through the weekend, with a sufficient amount to provide the medication on Monday 6 a.m.?

The medication will be administered every 6 hours or 1200, 1800, 0000, 0600

Friday: 2 doses 1200 and 1800

Saturday: 4 doses

Sunday: 4 doses

Monday: 2 doses 0000 and 0600

Total doses = 12

$$\text{vials} = \frac{1\text{ vial}}{8\text{ mL}} \bullet \frac{2\text{ mL}}{300\text{ mg}} \bullet \frac{300\text{ mg}}{1\text{ dose}} \bullet \frac{12\text{ doses}}{1} = 3\text{ vials}$$

EXAMPLE 11.5

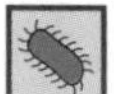

After adding 5.7 mL of sterile water for injection (SWI) to a vial of powdered oxacillin 1 g for injection, the resulting strength is oxacillin 250 mg/1.5 mL.

How many vials are needed to prepare a 24-hour supply of an order for 750 mg IM q6h?

$$\#\text{ vials} = \frac{1\text{ vial}}{1\text{ g}} \bullet \frac{1\text{ g}}{1{,}000\text{ mg}} \bullet \frac{750\text{ mg}}{\text{dose}} \bullet \frac{4\text{ doses}}{\text{day}} = 3\text{ vials}$$

Practice Problems A

Show your calculations. A month means 30 days unless otherwise stated.

1. Rx: Lasix (furosemide) 20 mg tabs

   Sig: 1 qam

   How many tablets are needed for a 1-month supply?

2. Rx: Valium (diazepam) 5 mg tablets

   Sig: 7.5 mg at bedtime.

   How many tablets are needed for a 1-month supply?

3. EN DO Rx: Actos (pioglitazone) 15 mg tabs

   Sig: 30 mg qd

   How many tablets are needed for a 90-day supply?

4. Rx: Prozac (fluoxetine) 20 mg caps

   Sig: 60 mg qd

   How many capsules are needed for a 90-day supply?

5. Rx: methylphenidate solution 10 mg/5 mL

   Sig: 5 mg bid ac breakfast and lunch for ADHD

   How much is needed for a 30-day supply?

6. Rx: cephalexin 125 mg/5 mL 200 mL

   Sig: 175 mg po q6h × 7 day

   How many mL are needed for the entire ***dosage****?*

7. Rx: amoxicillin 250 mg caps

Sig: 1 po qid × 7 days

How many capsules are needed to fill this prescription?

8. Rx: Amoxil (amoxicillin) 250 mg/5 mL

Sig: 500 mg four times a day for 7 days

How many mL are needed to fill this prescription?

9. Rx: Voltaren (diclofenac) 50 mg tabs

Sig: 1 po tid with meals or snack

How many tablets are needed to fill this prescription for 1 month?

Write the directions as they should appear on the customer's bottle:

____

10. Rx: Keflex (cephalexin) 125 mg/5 mL

Sig: 62.5 mg po q6h × 10 days

How many milliliters are needed for the entire course of therapy?

How many 60 mL bottles need to be dispensed for this prescription?

How many milliliters should be remaining after 10 days?

What volume of medication should be administered with each dose?

What is the dose in household measurements?

Write the directions as they should appear on the customer's bottle:

____

11. Rx: nitrofurantoin 50 mg capsules

Sig: 0.1 g po qid × 7 days for a urinary tract infection

How many capsules are needed to fill this prescription?

Write the directions as they should appear on the customer's bottle:

____

12. Interpret the following prescription:

____

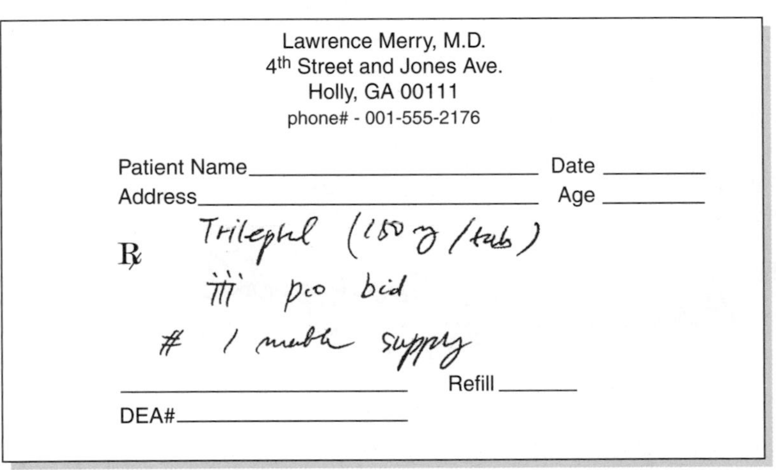

Lawrence Merry, M.D.
4th Street and Jones Ave.
Holly, GA 00111
phone# - 001-555-2176

Patient Name________ Date ________
Address________ Age ________

℞ Trileptal (150 mg/tab)
iii po bid
1 month supply

________ Refill ________
DEA#________

____

How many tablets are needed to fill the prescription?

13. *What volume of medication is needed to fill the following prescription?*

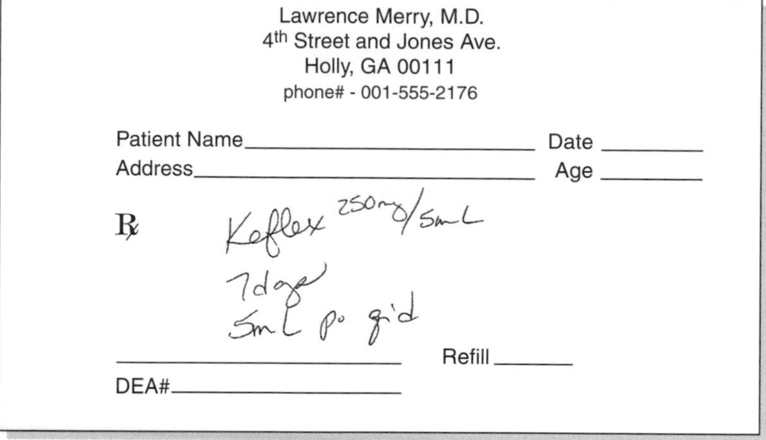

Lawrence Merry, M.D.
4th Street and Jones Ave.
Holly, GA 00111
phone# - 001-555-2176

Patient Name__________________ Date _______
Address______________________ Age _______

℞ Keflex 250mg/5mL
7days
5mL po qid

__________________ Refill ______
DEA#__________________

Write the directions as they should appear on the customer's bottle:

____

14. During a severe influenza epidemic, a physician writes the following prescription as a prophylaxis against a secondary bacterial infection in an older adult with COPD.

Lawrence Merry, M.D.
4th Street and Jones Ave.
Holly, GA 00111
phone# - 001-555-2176

Patient Name__________________ Date _______
Address______________________ Age _______

℞ Amoxicillin 500 mg bid
x 10 days.

__________________ Refill ______
DEA#__________________

Interpret the order:

____

The amoxicillin in stock is 250 mg/capsule.

How many capsules should be dispensed to the patient to complete this order?

Write the directions as they should appear on the customer's bottle:

____

15. A patient presents the following prescription:

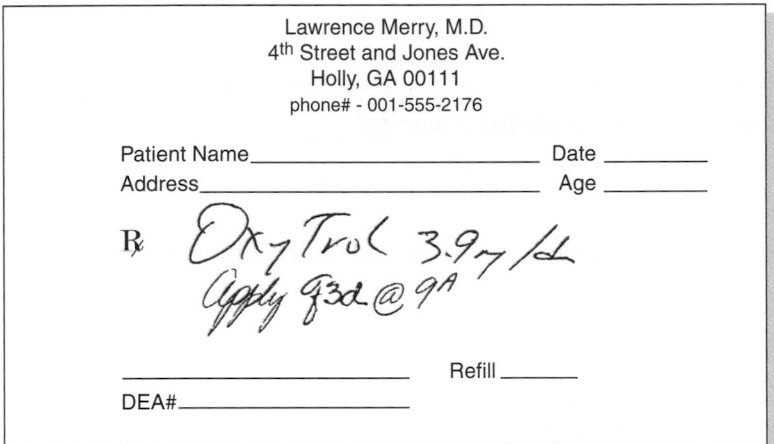

Lawrence Merry, M.D.
4th Street and Jones Ave.
Holly, GA 00111
phone# - 001-555-2176

Patient Name________________ Date ________
Address________________ Age ________

℞ OxyTrol 3.9mg/d
Apply q3d @ 9A

________________ Refill ______
DEA#________________

How many patches does the patient need for 1 month's supply?

Write the directions as they should appear on the customer's box:

____

16. A physician orders Solu-Cortef 150 mg IM q8h for a patient with allergic dermatitis.

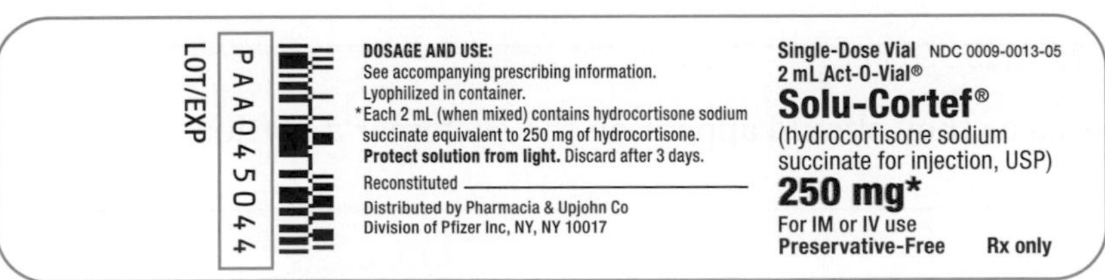

LOT/EXP
PAA045044
DOSAGE AND USE:
See accompanying prescribing information.
Lyophilized in container.
*Each 2 mL (when mixed) contains hydrocortisone sodium succinate equivalent to 250 mg of hydrocortisone.
Protect solution from light. Discard after 3 days.
Reconstituted
Distributed by Pharmacia & Upjohn Co
Division of Pfizer Inc, NY, NY 10017
Single-Dose Vial NDC 0009-0013-05
2 mL Act-O-Vial®
Solu-Cortef®
(hydrocortisone sodium succinate for injection, USP)
250 mg*
For IM or IV use
Preservative-Free
Rx only

How many vials should be sent to the hospital floor for a 24-hour period?

17. Rx: cyanocobalamin 1,000 mcg/mL inj, 10 mL multidose vial

Sig: 1.5 mg subcut two times a week for 4 weeks

How many milliliters are needed for one dose?

How many vials of cyanocobalamin are needed to fill this order?

18. Rx: cephalexin 500 mg caps

Sig: 1 po qid × 2 weeks

How many capsules should be supplied for 2 weeks?

Write the directions as they should appear on the customer's bottle:

___

19. How many 20 mg tablets are needed for a 14-day supply?

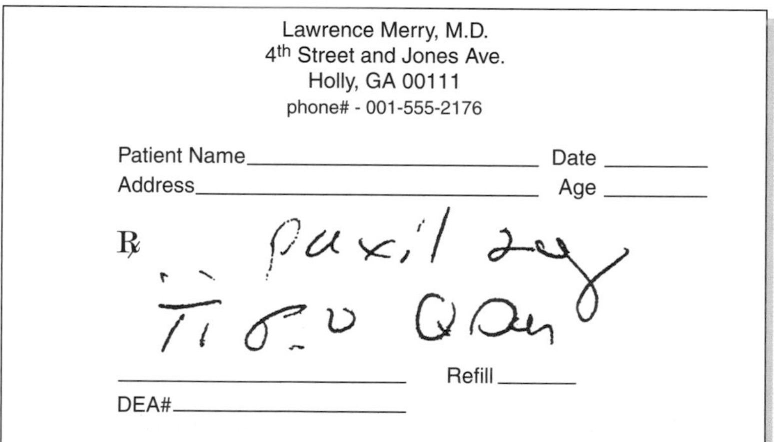

Lawrence Merry, M.D.
4th Street and Jones Ave.
Holly, GA 00111
phone# - 001-555-2176

Patient Name________ Date ________
Address________ Age ________

℞

________ Refill ______
DEA#________

Write the directions as they should appear on the customer's bottle:

___

20. Rx: Lasix (furosemide) 40 mg tablets

Sig: 80 mg po stat, then Lasix 40 mg po qd.

How many tablets are needed for the first month's supply?

Write the directions as they should appear on the customer's bottle:

____

Determining the Number of Doses in a Container

If the size and frequency of the dose and the amount of medication in a container are known, the number of doses in the container can be calculated to ensure that the patient has a sufficient amount of medication for the expected time of administration. Basically, the number of doses in a container is the total amount of medication divided by the dose size.

EXAMPLE 11.6

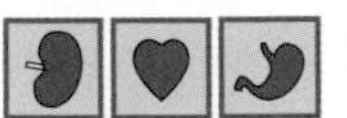

Prescription: furosemide 80 mg po daily for 1 month

How many doses are in a 100-count stock bottle of 40 mg tablets?

$$\text{doses} = \frac{1 \text{ dose}}{80 \text{ mg}} \bullet \frac{40 \text{ mg}}{\text{tablet}} \bullet \frac{100 \text{ tabs}}{1} = 50 \text{ doses}$$

Write the directions as they should appear on the customer's bottle:

Take 2 tablets by mouth daily.

How many tablets are needed to fill this order?

$$\frac{2 \text{ tabs}}{1 \text{ day}} = \frac{x}{30 \text{ days}} \qquad x = 60 \text{ tabs for a 1-month supply}$$

EXAMPLE 11.7

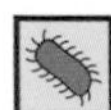

Rx: Keflex (cephalexin) suspension 125 mg/5 mL

Sig: 125 mg q6h for 10 days

How many doses are in one 60 mL bottle?

$$\text{doses} = \frac{1 \text{ dose}}{125 \text{ mg}} \bullet \frac{125 \text{ mg}}{5 \text{ mL}} \bullet \frac{60 \text{ mL}}{1} = 12 \text{ doses}$$

Will one 60 mL bottle be sufficient for the prescription?

No, 4 doses are needed per day for 10 days so 40 doses are needed.

How many 60 mL bottles of cephalexin 125 mg/5 mL would be needed?

$$\text{bottles} = \frac{1 \text{ bottle}}{12 \text{ doses}} \bullet \frac{40 \text{ doses}}{1} = 3.3 \text{ bottles}$$

Dispense four bottles to cover the entire length of therapy. Remember they should only be reconstituted once the customer comes in to pick up the prescription since the medication begins to degrade once water is added.

Write the directions as they should appear on the customer's bottle:

Take 5 mL every 6 hours for 10 days.

Practice Problems B

Determine the number of doses in the container. Note that a month means 30 days unless otherwise stated. Show your work.

1. Rx: E.E.S. (erythromycin ethylsuccinate) 400 mg/5 mL

Sig: 200 mg po qid × 10d for bronchitis

How many doses are in one 60-mL bottle?

For how many days would this container provide the necessary medication?

How many containers would be needed for 10 days of therapy?

Write the directions as they should appear on the customer's bottle:

____

2. Rx: Halcion (triazolam) 0.125 mg tabs

Sig: 1-2 tabs at bedtime prn sleep

How many doses are in one 10-tablet stock bottle? (base on maximum use)

Write the directions as they should appear on the customer's bottle:

____

3. Rx: Rifadin (rifampin) 150 mg caps

Sig: 600 mg qd 1 hour ac for tuberculosis

*How many **full** doses of medication are in one 30-capsule stock bottle?*

Write the directions as they should appear on the customer's bottle:

____

4. One 10-mL multidose vial of Compazine (prochlorperazine) 5 mg/mL has been provided to the medical floor for a patient with postoperative emesis.

How many 10 mg doses can be administered from this vial?

5. PA IN Demerol (meperidine) 50 mg has been given to four patients over the past 24 hours from the box of 25 ampules in the narcotic floor stock. Each 1-mL ampule contains 75 mg of meperidine.

How many ampules should be left in the box if the floor stock supply has only been used for these injections?

Explain your answer.

____

____

6. PA IN Rx: Motrin (ibuprofen) 400 mg tabs

Sig: 0.8 g tid pc for osteoarthritis

How many full ***doses*** *are in one 100-tablet bottle of ibuprofen 400 mg tablets?*

Write the directions as they should appear on the customer's bottle:

____

7. A physician orders lincomycin 0.6 g IM q12h. Stock available: 10-mL vial of lincomycin 300 mg/mL injection

How many doses of medication are in this vial?

8. A patient is prescribed cephalexin 62.5 mg qid.

Stock available: 60-mL bottles of cephalexin oral suspension 125 mg/5 mL

How many doses of medication are in one 60-mL bottle?

9. A vaccine contains 2 units/0.5 mL.

How many 2-unit doses are available in one 5-mL multi-dose vial?

10. A physician orders phenobarbital elixir gr ½ tid

The available medication strength is phenobarbital elixir 20 mg/5 mL.

How many doses are in a 480 mL stock bottle? **(use gr i = 60 mg)**

Determining the Length of Time a Prescription Will Last—Days' Supply

It is important to know how to calculate the length of time a prescription will last according to the directions, which is called the **days' supply**. Pharmacists use this information to monitor patients' compliance with their medications. Additionally, care must be taken to input the correct days' supply in the computer for insurance purposes. One of the common reasons claims are rejected is for incorrect days' supply. Also, refills are only approved after a specified period of time has passed based on the days' supply. If an attempt is made to refill too soon, the claim will be rejected.

! TECH ALERT

If the proper length of time between prescription refills is inappropriate, the pharmacist should be notified and will consult with the patient and the physician for clarification.

TECH NOTE

When calculating days' supply for insurance purposes, always **round down** to the closest whole number if you calculate a partial day. This will help avoid "Refill too soon" responses.

Determining days' supply for tablets and capsules is the simplest of these calculations. Oral and IV liquids, insulin, eye and ear drops, and inhaler calculations require more steps. Labels for **inhalers** will state how many inhalations are present in each container. Some medications intended for inhalation need to be placed in a **nebulizer**, which is a device used to produce a fine spray of medication. These calculations will depend on whether the medication is supplied in single or multidose containers.

EXAMPLE 11.8

A physician orders 60 tablets of antibiotic to be administered qid. What is the days' supply?

$$\text{R\&P} \quad \frac{4 \text{ tablets}}{1 \text{ day}} = \frac{60 \text{ tablets}}{x \text{ days}}$$

$$4x = 60 \text{ days}$$

$$x = 15 \text{ days}$$

$$\text{DA days} = \frac{1 \text{ days}}{4 \text{ tablets}} \bullet \frac{60 \text{ tablets}}{1} = 15 \text{ days}$$

This is basically dividing the total amount of medication by the number of doses to be administered per day.

TECH NOTE

Use 20 gtt = 1 mL for calculating days' supply of ophthalmic and otic medications for insurance purposes unless your pharmacy specifies something different.

EXAMPLE 11.9

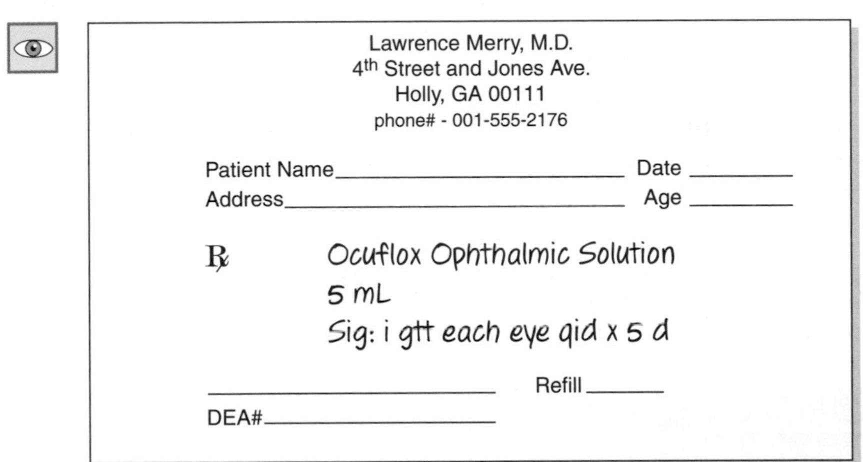

Lawrence Merry, M.D.
4th Street and Jones Ave.
Holly, GA 00111
phone# - 001-555-2176

Patient Name________ Date ______
Address________ Age ______

℞ Ocuflox Ophthalmic Solution
5 mL
Sig: i gtt each eye qid x 5 d

________ Refill ______
DEA# ________

What is the days' supply? Use 2 gtt per dose because the prescription is written for *both* eyes.

$$\text{days} = \frac{1 \text{ day}}{4 \text{ doses}} \bullet \frac{1 \text{ dose}}{2 \text{ gtt}} \bullet \frac{20 \text{ gtt}}{1 \text{ mL}} \bullet \frac{5 \text{ mL}}{1} = 12.5 \text{ days}$$

Days' supply would be 12 full days.

Even though the medication is only ordered for 5 days, it is best to enter the actual days' supply in the computer for insurance purposes.

TECH NOTE

Pay close attention to whether directions are for one or both eyes/ears when interpreting prescriptions for ophthalmic and otic medications.

EXAMPLE 11.10

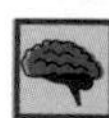

ALWAYS DISPENSE WITH MEDICATION GUIDE

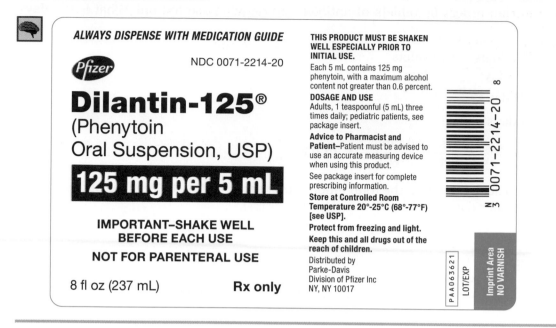

NDC 0071-2214-20

Dilantin-125®
(Phenytoin
Oral Suspension, USP)

125 mg per 5 mL

IMPORTANT–SHAKE WELL BEFORE EACH USE

NOT FOR PARENTERAL USE

8 fl oz (237 mL) **Rx only**

THIS PRODUCT MUST BE SHAKEN WELL ESPECIALLY PRIOR TO INITIAL USE.
Each 5 mL contains 125 mg phenytoin, with a maximum alcohol content not greater than 0.6 percent.
DOSAGE AND USE
Adults, 1 teaspoonful (5 mL) three times daily; pediatric patients, see package insert.
Advice to Pharmacist and Patient–Patient must be advised to use an accurate measuring device when using this product.
See package insert for complete prescribing information.
Store at Controlled Room Temperature 20°-25°C (68°-77°F) [see USP].
Protect from freezing and light.
Keep this and all drugs out of the reach of children.
Distributed by
Parke-Davis
Division of Pfizer Inc
NY, NY 10017

PAA063621
LOT/EXP
Imprint Area
NO VARNISH

(© Pfizer. Used with permission.)

Rx: Dilantin-125 Susp

Sig: 100 mg tid

How many *full* days should this bottle of medication last?

$$\text{days} = \frac{1\text{ day}}{3\text{ doses}} \bullet \frac{1\text{ dose}}{100\text{ mg}} \bullet \frac{125\text{ mg}}{5\text{ mL}} \bullet \frac{237\text{ mL}}{1} = 19.75\text{ days} = 19\text{ days}$$

Indicate the prescription label directions: Take 4 mL three times a day.

EXAMPLE 11.11

EN DO

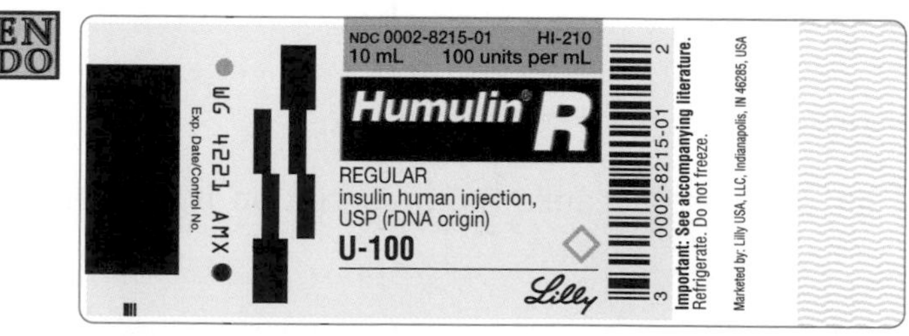

(© Eli Lilly and Company. All Rights Reserved. Used with Permission.)

Rx: Humulin R 10 mL

Sig: 50 units subcut at breakfast and 40 units subcut before the evening meal

How many *full* days should this vial last?

$$\text{days} = \frac{1\text{ day}}{90\text{ units}} \bullet \frac{100\text{ units}}{1\text{ mL}} \bullet \frac{10\text{ mL}}{1} = 11.1\text{ days}$$

Days' supply for one vial is 11.

How many 10-mL vials of Humulin R should be dispensed for a month's supply?

$$\#\text{ vials} = \frac{1\text{ vial}}{10\text{ mL}} \bullet \frac{1\text{ mL}}{100\text{ units}} \bullet \frac{90\text{ units}}{\text{day}} \bullet \frac{30\text{ days}}{1} = 2.7\text{ vials}$$

Three vials are needed for a 1-month supply.

TECH NOTE

Always round the days' supply of insulin **down** to the whole number of days and the needed amount of vials **up** to the next whole number.

EXAMPLE 11.12

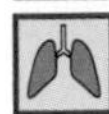
Rx: Proventil (albuterol) inhaler, 17 g

Sig: 2 puffs qid

Stock: albuterol inhaler 200 metered inhalations/17 g (a "puff" is equal to an inhalation)

What is the days' supply in one inhaler?

$$\text{days} = \frac{1\text{ day}}{4\text{ doses}} \bullet \frac{1\text{ dose}}{2\text{ inh}} \bullet \frac{200\text{ inh}}{1} = 25\text{ days}$$

EXAMPLE 11.13

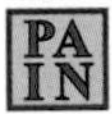

Rx: acetaminophen with codeine elixir, 120 mL

Sig: 5 to 10 mL q4–6h prn pain

What is the days' supply for the following prescription?

When calculating days' supply for insurance purposes, base it on the maximum possible dose. The patient *may* take a maximum of 10 mL six times a day, or 60 mL.

The 120 mL bottle is a 2-day supply.

TECH NOTE

Never enter a days' supply that exceeds the beyond use date of a medication.

For example, if the days' supply for one vial of Lantus insulin is calculated to be 45 days, it needs to be reduced to 28 days.

Days' supply for topical medications is not an exact process. Generally, 1 g of cream is considered to be an amount that would cover four flat hands of area. This requires knowing how much of an area is to be covered, which could be an uncomfortable question. Most pharmacies have general guidelines to follow for days' supply of creams, ointments, and lotions.

Practice Problems C

Complete the following, showing calculations. A month means 30 days unless otherwise stated.

1. Interpret the prescription for Zaroxolyn (metolazone) tablets.

____

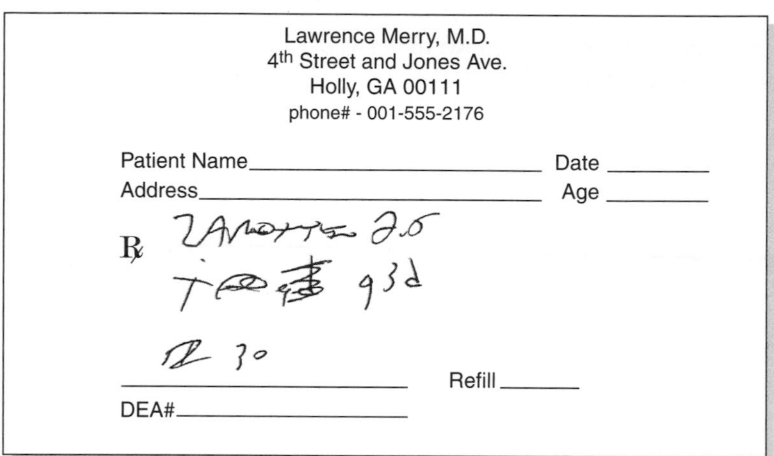

Lawrence Merry, M.D.
4th Street and Jones Ave.
Holly, GA 00111
phone# - 001-555-2176

Patient Name________________ Date ______
Address________________ Age ______

℞

Refill ______

DEA#________________

What is the days' supply?

2. How long would the medication in this prescription last?

Lawrence Merry, M.D.
4th Street and Jones Ave.
Holly, GA 00111
phone# - 001-555-2176

Patient Name________________ Date ______
Address________________ Age ______

℞

AllegraD ī bid # 30

Refill ______

DEA#________________

Write the directions as they should appear on the customer's bottle:

____

3. Rx: minoxidil 10 mg tablets #40

Sig: 0.04 g po qd

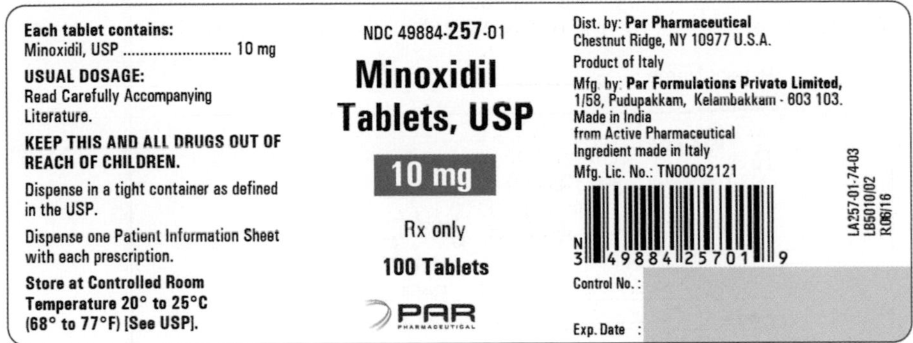

Each tablet contains:
Minoxidil, USP .... 10 mg
USUAL DOSAGE:
Read Carefully Accompanying Literature.
KEEP THIS AND ALL DRUGS OUT OF REACH OF CHILDREN.
Dispense in a tight container as defined in the USP.
Dispense one Patient Information Sheet with each prescription.
Store at Controlled Room Temperature 20° to 25°C (68° to 77°F) [See USP].
NDC 49884-257-01
Minoxidil Tablets, USP
10 mg
Rx only
100 Tablets
PAR
Dist. by: Par Pharmaceutical
Chestnut Ridge, NY 10977 U.S.A.
Product of Italy
Mfg. by: Par Formulations Private Limited, 1/58, Pudupakkam, Kelambakkam - 603 103.
Made in India
from Active Pharmaceutical Ingredient made in Italy
Mfg. Lic. No.: TN00002121
N 3 49884 25701 9
Control No. :
Exp. Date :
LA257-01-74-03
LB5010/02
R06/16

(Reprinted with permission of Endo/Par Pharmaceutical)

How many days would this prescription last?

How many tablets are needed for a 1-month supply?

Write the directions as they should appear on the customer's bottle:

____

4. Rx: Lanoxin (digoxin) 0.125 mg tablets #40

Sig: 0.5 mg stat, 0.375 mg in a.m., then tab i qam

*How long would this prescription last **after** the two initial doses?*

Write the directions as they should appear on the customer's bottle:

____

5. *What is the days' supply for the following prescription?*

Lawrence Merry, M.D.
4th Street and Jones Ave.
Holly, GA 00111
phone# - 001-555-2176

Patient Name__________ Date ______
Address__________ Age ______

℞

__________ Refill ______
DEA#__________

Write the directions as they should appear on the customer's bottle:

____

6. *What is the days' supply for the following prescription of Altace (ramipril)?*

Lawrence Merry, M.D.
4th Street and Jones Ave.
Holly, GA 00111
phone# - 001-555-2176

Patient Name__________ Date ______
Address__________ Age ______

℞

__________ Refill ______
DEA#__________

Interpret the prescription:

____

7. Rx: erythromycin ethylsuccinate 200 mg/5 mL, 200 mL

Sig: 200 mg tid,

Stock available: erythromycin ethylsuccinate for oral suspension 200 mg/5 mL when reconstituted/200-mL bottles

How many full days should the medication last?

How many doses of medication are available in the container?

Indicate the prescription label directions.

____

8. Interpret the following prescription:

____

Lawrence Merry, M.D.
4th Street and Jones Ave.
Holly, GA 00111
phone# - 001-555-2176

Patient Name______________ Date ________
Address______________ Age ________

℞ Pepcid 20mg
Sig: i po BID
Disp: #20

______________ Refill ______
DEA#______________

What is the days' supply?

Write the directions as they should appear on the customer's bottle:

____

9. *What is the days' supply?*

Lawrence Merry, M.D.
4th Street and Jones Ave.
Holly, GA 00111
phone# - 001-555-2176

Patient Name__________ Date _____
Address__________ Age _____

℞ Pen VK 500 mg
Disp: 28
Sig: i tab qid until gone

__________ Refill _____
DEA#__________

Write the directions as they should appear on the customer's bottle:

____

10. Interpret the following prescription:

____

Lawrence Merry, M.D.
4th Street and Jones Ave.
Holly, GA 00111
phone# - 001-555-2176

Patient Name__________ Date _____
Address__________ Age _____

℞ Urocit. K 10 mEq (1080 mg)
#540
Sig: ii po TID

__________ Refill _____
DEA#__________

What is the days' supply?

Write the directions as they should appear on the customer's bottle:

____

11. Medication order: pen G potassium 5,000,000 units in 1 L of fluid to be delivered over 12 hours (q12h) × 7 days. The vial has been reconstituted with 11.5 mL of diluent.

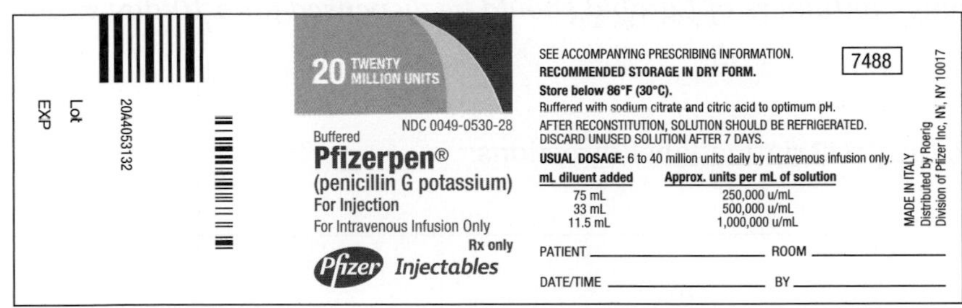

Lot
EXP
20A4053132
20 TWENTY MILLION UNITS
NDC 0049-0530-28
Buffered
Pfizerpen®
(penicillin G potassium)
For Injection
For Intravenous Infusion Only
Rx only
Pfizer Injectables
SEE ACCOMPANYING PRESCRIBING INFORMATION.
7488
RECOMMENDED STORAGE IN DRY FORM.
Store below 86°F (30°C).
Buffered with sodium citrate and citric acid to optimum pH.
AFTER RECONSTITUTION, SOLUTION SHOULD BE REFRIGERATED.
DISCARD UNUSED SOLUTION AFTER 7 DAYS.
USUAL DOSAGE: 6 to 40 million units daily by intravenous infusion only.
mL diluent added Approx. units per mL of solution
75 mL 250,000 u/mL
33 mL 500,000 u/mL
11.5 mL 1,000,000 u/mL
PATIENT ROOM
DATE/TIME BY
MADE IN ITALY
Distributed by Roerig
Division of Pfizer Inc, NY, NY 10017

How many doses can be prepared from one vial of medication?

What is the days' supply from one vial?

What volume of medication should be added to each liter of fluid?

What three pieces of information should be written on the vial at the time of reconstitution if it is to be saved for future doses?

____

____

____

12. Rx: Lorabid (loracarbef) Oral Suspension

Sig: 200 mg po bid × 10 days

Stock available: loracarbef for oral suspension 100 mg/5 mL once reconstituted, 50-mL

How many full days would a 50-mL bottle last?

How many containers of Lorabid should be dispensed for a 10-day supply?

Indicate the prescription label directions:

____

13. Rx: Dilantin 100 mg #100

Sig: 300 mg po qam and Dilantin 100 mg po at bedtime for epilepsy

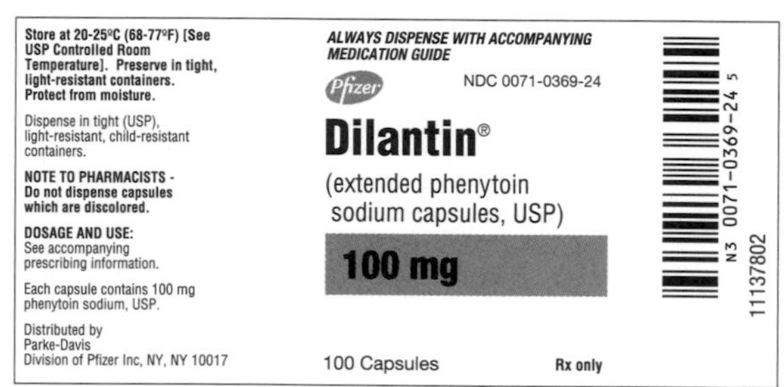
Store at 20-25°C (68-77°F) [See USP Controlled Room Temperature]. Preserve in tight, light-resistant containers. Protect from moisture.
Dispense in tight (USP), light-resistant, child-resistant containers.
NOTE TO PHARMACISTS - Do not dispense capsules which are discolored.
DOSAGE AND USE: See accompanying prescribing information.
Each capsule contains 100 mg phenytoin sodium, USP.
Distributed by Parke-Davis Division of Pfizer Inc, NY, NY 10017
ALWAYS DISPENSE WITH ACCOMPANYING MEDICATION GUIDE
Pfizer
NDC 0071-0369-24
Dilantin®
(extended phenytoin sodium capsules, USP)
100 mg
100 Capsules
Rx only
N3 0071-0369-24 5
11137802

(© Pfizer. Used with permission.)

How many days would this container of medication last?

How many extra capsules are needed for a 1-month supply?

Write the directions as they should appear on the customer's bottle:

____

____

14. Rx: Prozac (fluoxetine) Liquid, 120 mL

Sig: 40 mg po qam

Stock available: fluoxetine oral solution 20 mg/5 mL

What is the days' supply?

Write the directions as they should appear on the customer's bottle:

____

15. Rx: Benadryl (diphenhydramine) elixir, 4 oz

Sig: 18.75 mg po q6h prn

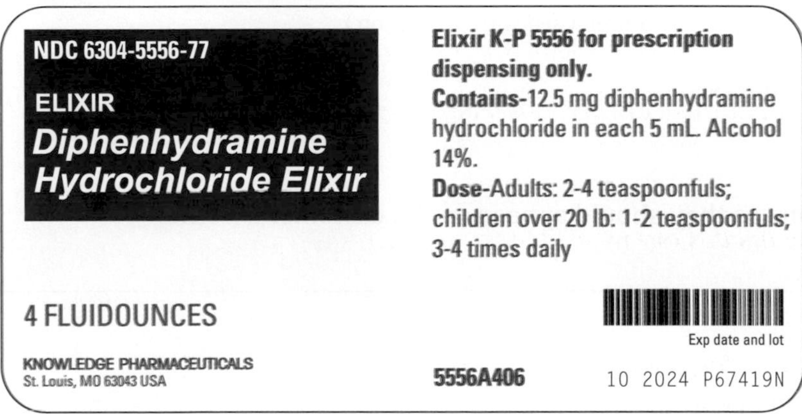

NDC 6304-5556-77
ELIXIR
Diphenhydramine Hydrochloride Elixir
4 FLUIDOUNCES
KNOWLEDGE PHARMACEUTICALS
St. Louis, MO 63043 USA
Elixir K-P 5556 for prescription dispensing only.
Contains-12.5 mg diphenhydramine hydrochloride in each 5 mL. Alcohol 14%.
Dose-Adults: 2-4 teaspoonfuls; children over 20 lb: 1-2 teaspoonfuls; 3-4 times daily
Exp date and lot
5556A406
10 2024 P67419N

How many mL are needed for one dose?

How many doses are in this bottle?

What is the days' supply for insurance purposes?

16. Rx: Cortisporin Otic, 10 mL

Sig: 2 gtt au tid × 10 days

What is the days' supply? (Remember to round down to a whole number.)

17. Rx: Xalatan, 2.5 mL

Sig:1 gtt ou qpm

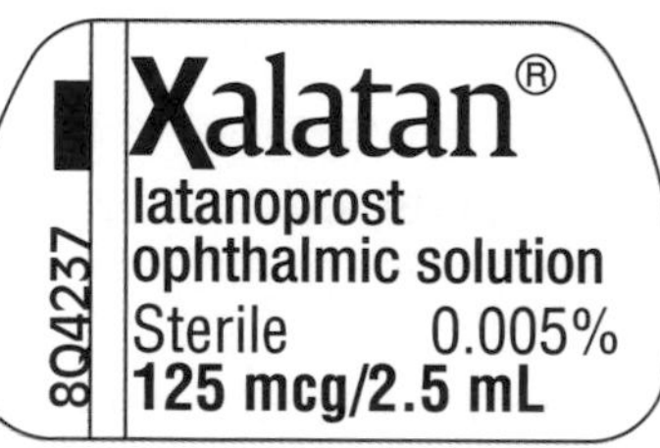

(© Pfizer. Used with permission.)

What is the days' supply?

Write the directions as they should appear on the customer's bottle:

____

18. Rx: Lopid 600 mg, #135

Sig: 600 mg qam and 300 mg qpm

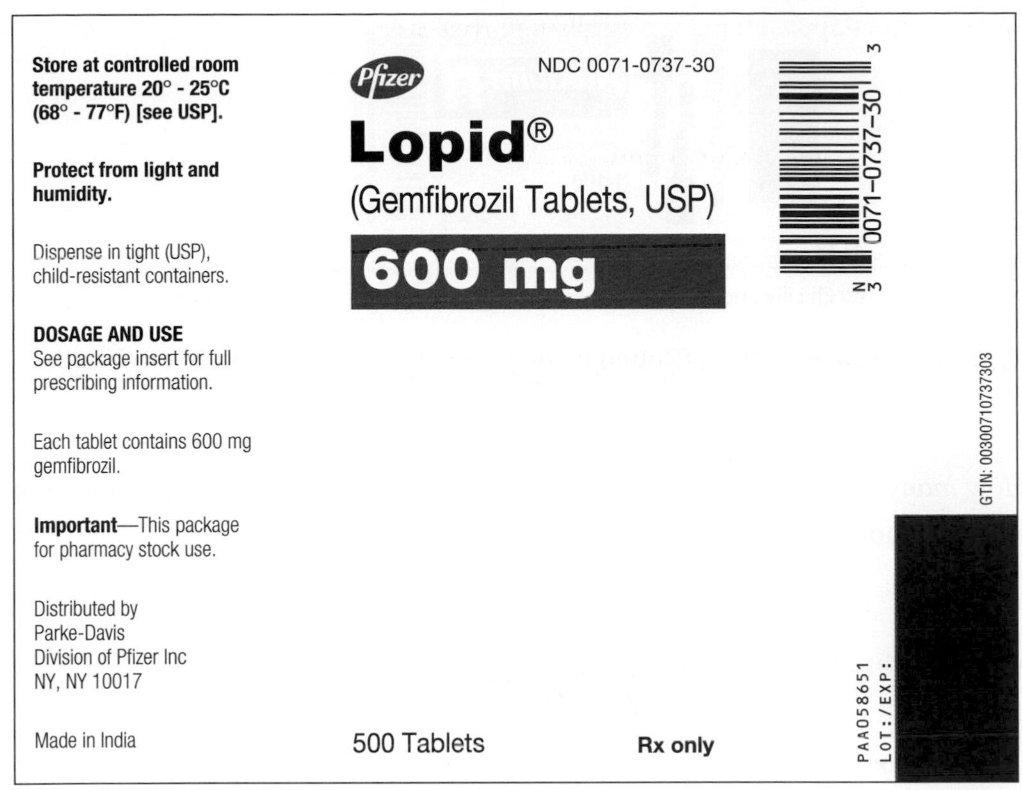
Store at controlled room temperature 20° - 25°C (68° - 77°F) [see USP].
Protect from light and humidity.
Dispense in tight (USP), child-resistant containers.
DOSAGE AND USE
See package insert for full prescribing information.
Each tablet contains 600 mg gemfibrozil.
Important—This package for pharmacy stock use.
Distributed by
Parke-Davis
Division of Pfizer Inc
NY, NY 10017
Made in India
Pfizer
NDC 0071-0737-30
Lopid®
(Gemfibrozil Tablets, USP)
600 mg
500 Tablets
Rx only
3 0071-0737-30 3
GTIN: 00300710737303
PAA058651
LOT:/EXP:

(© Pfizer. Used with permission.)

What is the days' supply?

If the insurance company only pays for a 30-day supply each time, how many should be dispensed?

Write the directions as they should appear on the customer's bottle:

____

19. ENDO Rx: Humulin R, 10 mL

Sig: 14 units subcut tid 30 min ac

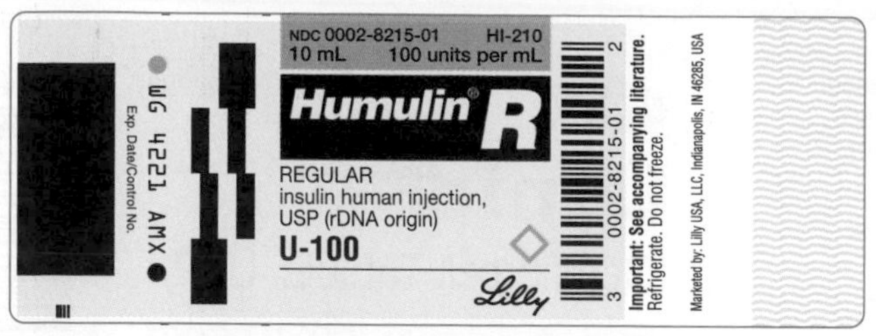

(© Eli Lilly and Company. All Rights Reserved. Used with Permission.)

What is the days' supply? (Round down to the nearest whole number.)

How many vials of Humulin R are needed for a 90-day supply? (Round up to the nearest whole number.)

Write the directions as they should appear on the prescription label:

____

20. ENDO Rx: Humulin R, 10 mL

Sig: 10 units tid pc and 25 units at bedtime

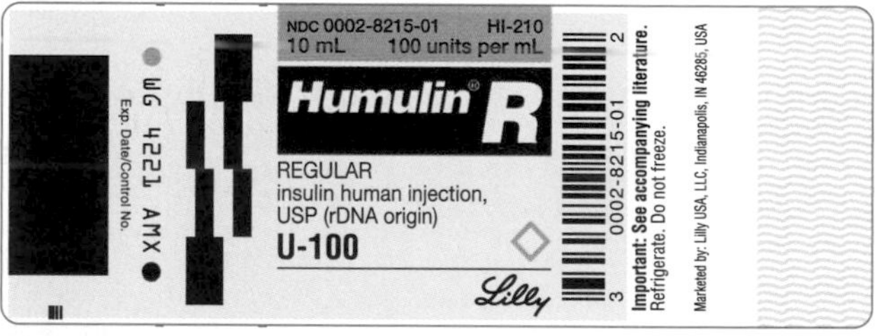

(© Eli Lilly and Company. All Rights Reserved. Used with Permission.)

What is the days' supply?

How many vials of Humulin R are needed for a 30-day supply?

Write the directions as they should appear on the prescription label:

____

REVIEW

In some cases, pharmacy technicians may be asked to calculate the amount of medication to be dispensed when the number of doses per day and the number of days for treatment is known. On other occasions, the calculation of the number of doses of medication in a container may be necessary to ensure the patient has adequate medication to complete the prescription or physician's order. Finally, for determining days' supply for insurance purposes, for monitoring refills to assess patient compliance, and for meeting insurance companies' regulations regarding restrictions on the amount of medication that can be dispensed at a given time, pharmacy staff will be required to determine how long the medication should last if taken according to the directions. All of these skills may be needed to accurately dispense medications.

Posttest

Complete the following calculations. A month is 30 days unless otherwise stated. Show your calculations. All calculations should be for full days.

1. Interpret the prescription.

____

____

Lawrence Merry, M.D.
4th Street and Jones Ave.
Holly, GA 00111
phone# - 001-555-2176

Patient Name________________ Date ________
Address________________ Age ________

℞ Trazodone 100mg
1 mo supply
1/2 tab po qam
1/2 tab qpm
1 1/2 po q hs*

________________ Refill ______
DEA#________________

How many 100 mg tablets are needed to fill this prescription?

*Note: "hs" is an abbreviation found in the ISMP's List of Error-Prone Abbreviations, Symbols, and Dose Designations. It should never be used when communicating dose information but is still seen on some prescriptions. The phrase "at bedtime" is preferred.

Continued

Posttest, cont.

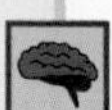

2. Interpret the following Neurontin (gabapentin) prescription.

____

____

Lawrence Merry, M.D.
4th Street and Jones Ave.
Holly, GA 00111
phone# - 001-555-2176

Patient Name________________ Date ________
Address________________ Age ________

℞ Neurontin 300mg
#
88 1 tab po daily
x 3 days then
1 tab bid x 3 days
then 1 tab po tid
thereafter.

________________ Refill ______
DEA#________________

How many tablets are needed to fill this prescription for 30 days?

3. How many Alora (estradiol) patches can be dispensed for a 1-month supply?

Lawrence Merry, M.D.
4th Street and Jones Ave.
Holly, GA 00111
phone# - 001-555-2176

Patient Name________________ Date ________
Address________________ Age ________

℞ Alora 0.1
#
S. i Twice weekly

________________ Refill ______
DEA#________________

Indicate the prescription label directions.

____

Posttest, cont.

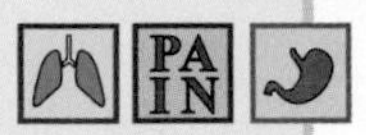

4. A physician writes a prescription for a 1:1:1 proportion of the following:
   Benadryl
   Lidocaine 1% viscous
   Maalox

   What is the amount of each component necessary to make 180 mL?

   How many doses of medication are available if the patient swishes and spits 5 mL q4h?

5. Rx: Decadron (dexamethasone) taper, 0.5 mg tablets
   Sig: 1 po qid × 2 days, 1 tid × 2 days, 1 bid × 2 days, and 1 daily × 4 days.

   How many tablets are needed to fill this prescription?

   How many milligrams of dexamethasone would the patient receive on each day?

   Days 1 and 2:

   Days 3 and 4:

   Days 5 and 6:

   Days 7 to 10:

   Indicate the prescription label directions.

   ____

   ____

   ____

Continued

Posttest, cont.

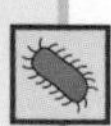

6. Interpret the prescription.

____

Lawrence Merry, M.D.
4th Street and Jones Ave.
Holly, GA 00111
phone# - 001-555-2176

Patient Name________________________ Date ________
Address____________________________ Age ________

℞ Cipro 500
20
i bid

________________________ Refill ______
DEA#____________________

What is the days' supply?

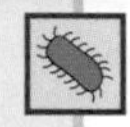

7. A physician orders erythromycin ethylsuccinate 300 mg po tid for 10 days.
Stock supply: 200 mL bottles of erythromycin ethylsuccinate for oral suspension 200 mg/5 mL when reconstituted

How many milliliters of medication are needed per dose?

What total volume of medication is needed to fill the prescription?

8. Rx: Voltaren (diclofenac) 50 mg
Sig: 1 tab bid with food for 7 days then decrease to qd

How many diclofenac 50 mg tablets are needed for the initial 30-day supply?

Write the directions as they should appear on the customer's bottle:

____

Posttest, cont.

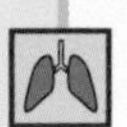

9.

Lawrence Merry, M.D.
4th Street and Jones Ave.
Holly, GA 00111
phone# - 001-555-2176

Patient Name__________ Date ______
Address__________ Age ______

℞ Albuterol Unit Dose 2.5/3ml
Disp 25
SG Use in Jet Neb Q8° prn cap

__________ Refill ______
DEA#__________

What is the days' supply?

10. *How many capsules are needed for a 3-month supply?*

Lawrence Merry, M.D.
4th Street and Jones Ave.
Holly, GA 00111
phone# - 001-555-2176

Patient Name__________ Date ______
Address__________ Age ______

℞ HCTZ 12.5mg cap
i po daily

__________ Refill ______
DEA#__________

Interpret the order as written.

____

11. Rx: Coumadin (warfarin) 2.5 mg tabs

Sig: 5 mg po Sunday, Tuesday, Wednesday, Friday, and Saturday and 7.5 mg po Monday and Thursday.

How many tablets are needed for a 1-week supply?

Continued

Posttest, cont.

How many milligrams will be taken in 1 week?

Write the directions as they should appear on the customer's bottle:

____

____

12. *What is the days' supply for this prescription?*

Lawrence Merry, M.D.
4th Street and Jones Ave.
Holly, GA 00111
phone# - 001-555-2176

Patient Name________________ Date ______
Address________________ Age ______

℞ Amoxicillin 500mg #30
Sig: 1 BID for infection

________________ Refill ______
DEA#________________

13. A prescription for Acular (ketorolac) is dispensed as a 5-mL bottle.

Lawrence Merry, M.D.
4th Street and Jones Ave.
Holly, GA 00111
phone# - 001-555-2176

Patient Name________________ Date ______
Address________________ Age ______

℞ Acular Opthalmic 0.5%
i drop left eye tid

________________ Refill ______
DEA#________________

What is the calculated days' supply?

Posttest, cont.

Note: Acular ophthalmic is only good for 4 weeks after opening, so it should be entered in the computer as a 28-day supply even if the calculated value is greater than 28.

Write the directions as they should appear on the customer's bottle:

____

PA IN **14.** How many 6 mL doses are in 4 oz?

Lawrence Merry, M.D.
4th Street and Jones Ave.
Holly, GA 00111
phone# - 001-555-2176

Patient Name______________ Date ________
Address______________ Age ________

℞ Motrin 100mg/5cc 4oz
6cc PO Q8° PRN

______________ Refill ______
DEA#______________

What weight in mg of Motrin (ibuprofen) per dose?

Interpret the prescription.

____

____

Write the directions as they should appear on the customer's bottle:

____

Continued

Posttest, cont.

15. Rx: Dilantin 100 mg caps

Sig: 200 mg po bid for 14 days

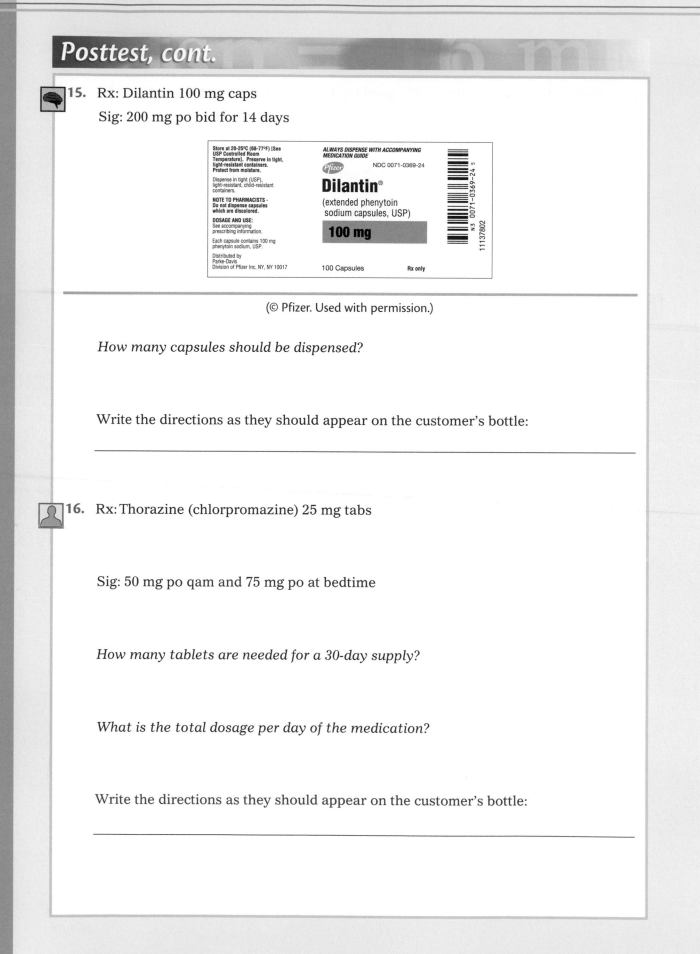

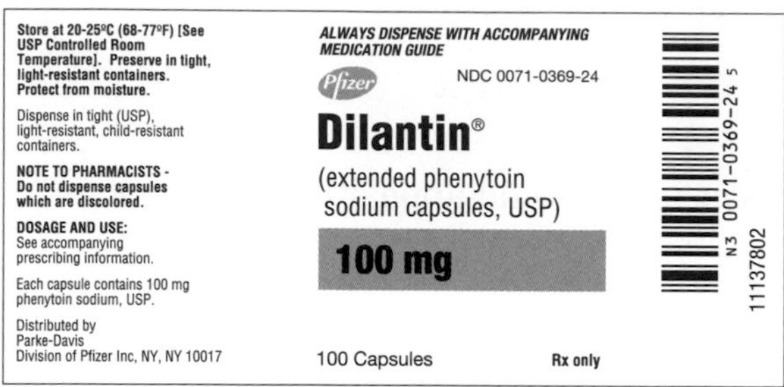

Store at 20-25ºC (68-77ºF) [See USP Controlled Room Temperature]. Preserve in tight, light-resistant containers. Protect from moisture.
Dispense in tight (USP), light-resistant, child-resistant containers.
NOTE TO PHARMACISTS - Do not dispense capsules which are discolored.
DOSAGE AND USE: See accompanying prescribing information.
Each capsule contains 100 mg phenytoin sodium, USP.
Distributed by Parke-Davis Division of Pfizer Inc, NY, NY 10017
ALWAYS DISPENSE WITH ACCOMPANYING MEDICATION GUIDE
Pfizer
NDC 0071-0369-24
Dilantin®
(extended phenytoin sodium capsules, USP)
100 mg
100 Capsules
Rx only
N3 0071-0369-24 5
11137802

(© Pfizer. Used with permission.)

How many capsules should be dispensed?

Write the directions as they should appear on the customer's bottle:

___

16. Rx: Thorazine (chlorpromazine) 25 mg tabs

Sig: 50 mg po qam and 75 mg po at bedtime

How many tablets are needed for a 30-day supply?

What is the total dosage per day of the medication?

Write the directions as they should appear on the customer's bottle:

___

Posttest, cont.

17. *What is the days' supply in the following prescription?*

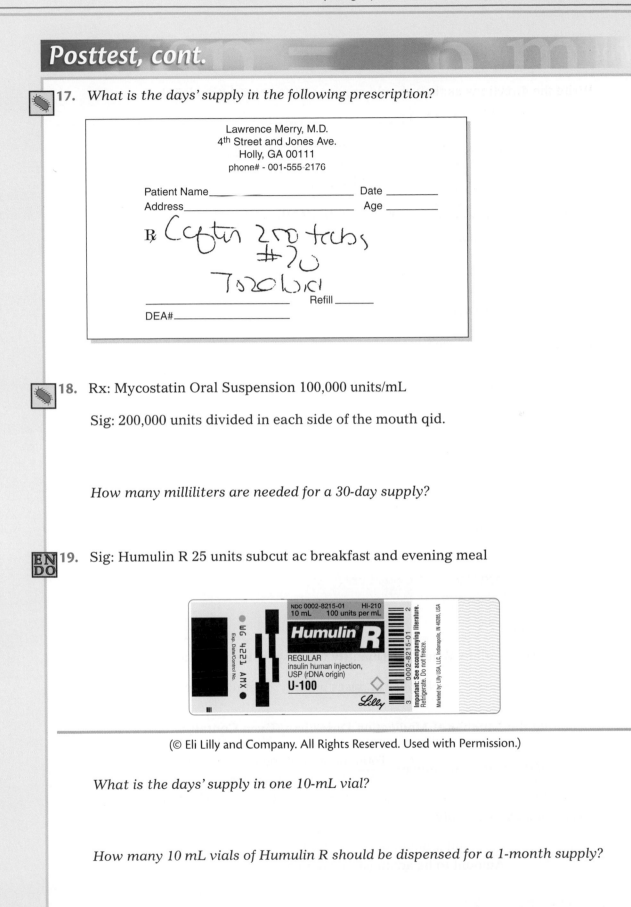

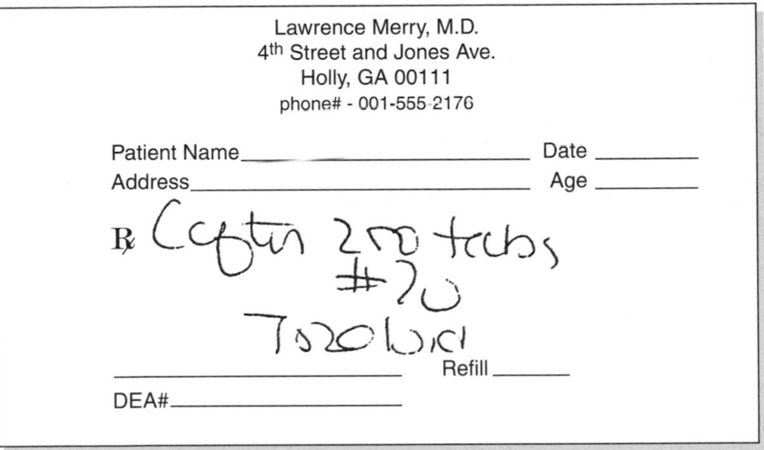
Lawrence Merry, M.D.
4th Street and Jones Ave.
Holly, GA 00111
phone# - 001-555-2176

Patient Name________ Date ________
Address________ Age ________

℞ Ceftin 250 tabs
#20
T po bid

________ Refill ________
DEA#________

18. Rx: Mycostatin Oral Suspension 100,000 units/mL

Sig: 200,000 units divided in each side of the mouth qid.

How many milliliters are needed for a 30-day supply?

19. Sig: Humulin R 25 units subcut ac breakfast and evening meal

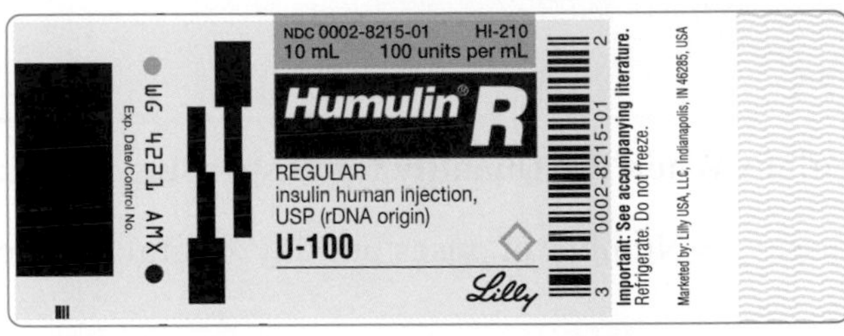

(© Eli Lilly and Company. All Rights Reserved. Used with Permission.)

What is the days' supply in one 10-mL vial?

How many 10 mL vials of Humulin R should be dispensed for a 1-month supply?

Continued

Posttest, cont.

Write the directions as they should appear on the prescription label:

____

____

ENDO 20. Rx: Lantus (insulin glargine) 100 units/mL, 10-mL vial
Sig: 35 units subcut qam

What is the days' supply in one 10-mL vial?

How many vials of Lantus are needed for a 1-month supply?

How many vials of medication would be needed for a 90-day supply?

Write the directions as they should appear on the prescription label:

____

REVIEW OF RULES

- **Preparing Medications When the Quantity for Dispensing Is Unknown**

  Total dosage necessary = Number of doses per day × Total number of days

- **Calculating the Number of Medication Doses in a Given Container**

  $$\text{Number of doses in a container} = \frac{\text{Total amount of medication in container}}{\text{Dose size}}$$

- **Determining Days' Supply**

  $$\text{Days' Supply} = \frac{\text{Total amount of medication}}{\text{Amount to be administered per day}}$$

IN SECTION IV

SECTION IV
Special Medication Calculations

CHAPTER 12

Calculation of Doses by Age, Body Weight, and Body Surface Area

OBJECTIVES

1. Calculate doses of medications for children and adults using body weight.
2. Calculate doses of medications for children using Clark's rule.
3. Calculate doses of medication for special populations based on body surface area.
4. Calculate doses of medication for neonates and infants using Fried's rule.
5. Calculate doses of medication for children using Young's rule.

KEY WORDS

Adolescent 12 through 21 years of age[a]

Body surface area (BSA) Measurement of total body area exposed to the environment; calculated from weight and height and expressed in square meters (m^2); used as a basis for calculating some medication doses

Child 2 to less than 12 years of age[a]

Clark's rule Means of calculating a dose of medication for a child from an adult dose using weight in pounds

Fried's rule Means of calculating a dose of medication for a neonate or infant from an adult dose using age in months

Infant 29 days to less than 2 years[a]

Neonate From birth through the first 28 days of life[a]

Nomogram A chart on which height and weight are plotted to determine BSA

Pharmacokinetics Movement of drugs through the body; absorption, distribution, metabolism, and excretion (ADME)

Young's rule Means of calculating a dose of medication for a child from an adult dose based on age in years

[a]According to the U.S. FDA (https://www.fda.gov/medical-devices/products-and-medical-procedures/pediatric-medical-devices).

Pretest

If you are already comfortable with the subject matter, complete the Pretest to test your knowledge. If not, work your way through the chapter and return to it for extra practice. Show your calculations. Round your answers to tenths if greater than 1, and hundredths if less than 1. Be sure your answer is a measurable dose.

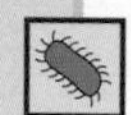

1. The adult dose of amoxicillin is 500 mg tid.

   What is the approximate dose for a child who is 2 years old?

2. The adult dose for Augmentin is 500 mg tid.

   What is the approximate dose for a 9-month-old infant?

3. A child weighing 55 lb is to take phenobarbital. The physician orders 1 mg/kg tid.

   What is the dose to be given?

   What is the dosage? ____________

4. A child weighs 55 lb and has an order for acetaminophen. The adult dose is 325 mg.

   What is the approximate dose for the child?

5. A child has an order for digoxin based on 8 mcg/kg of body weight. The child weighs 35 lb. Stock strength: Lanoxin (digoxin) 50 mcg (0.05 mg)/mL

   How many mcg of Lanoxin should be administered to the child?

   What is the volume needed for one dose?

Pretest, cont.

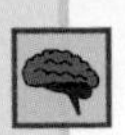

6. An 8-year-old child is ordered phenobarbital, and the adult dose is phenobarbital gr $\overline{ss}$.

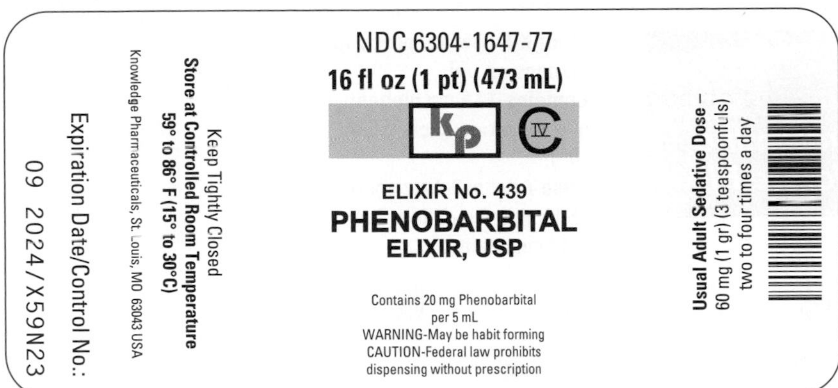

NDC 6304-1647-77
16 fl oz (1 pt) (473 mL)
kp
IV
ELIXIR No. 439
PHENOBARBITAL
ELIXIR, USP
Contains 20 mg Phenobarbital per 5 mL
WARNING-May be habit forming
CAUTION-Federal law prohibits dispensing without prescription
Keep Tightly Closed
Store at Controlled Room Temperature
59° to 86° F (15° to 30°C)
Knowledge Pharmaceuticals, St. Louis, MO 63043 USA
Expiration Date/Control No.:
09 2024/X59N23
Usual Adult Sedative Dose –
60 mg (1 gr) (3 teaspoonfuls)
two to four times a day

What is the child's dose in milligrams?

Using the label shown, what volume of medication would the child receive?

Show the correct dose of medication to be provided on the oral syringe.

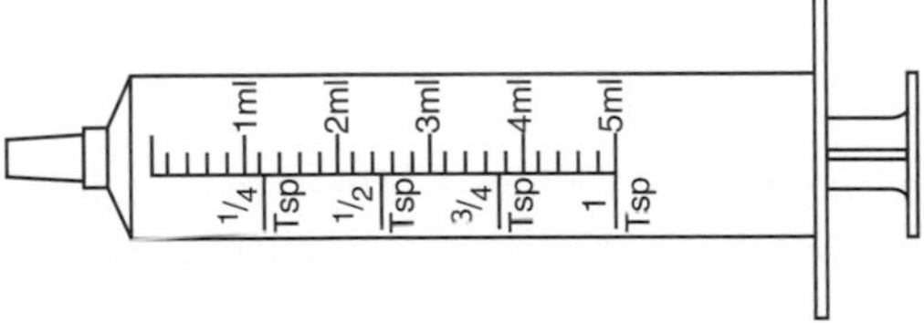

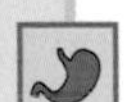

7. A physician orders Zantac syrup for a 10-month-old child. The adult dose is 150 mg bid. Stock strength: Zantac (ranitidine) syrup 15 mg/mL

What is the approximate dose for the child in milligrams?

What volume of medication should be given to the child per dose?

Continued

Pretest, cont.

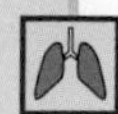

8. A child weighs 66 lb. The physician orders Benadryl (diphenhydramine) elixir. The adult dose is 50 mg q6–8h prn.

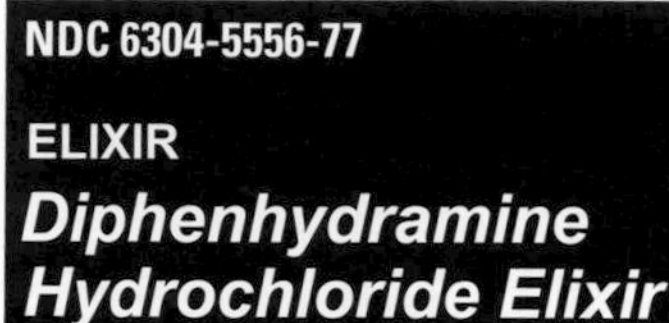

NDC 6304-5556-77
ELIXIR
Diphenhydramine
Hydrochloride Elixir

Elixir K-P 5556 for prescription dispensing only.
Contains-12.5 mg diphenhydramine hydrochloride in each 5 mL. Alcohol 14%.
Dose-Adults: 2-4 teaspoonfuls; children over 20 lb: 1-2 teaspoonfuls; 3-4 times daily

4 FLUIDOUNCES

Exp date and lot

KNOWLEDGE PHARMACEUTICALS
St. Louis, MO 63043 USA

5556A406 10 2024 P67419N

What is the approximate dose for the child in milligrams?

What is the measurable volume to be given per dose using the provided label?

Is this within the normal range for a child of this weight? ______________

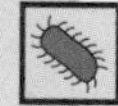

9. A 10-year-old child has bronchitis, and the physician orders Keflex suspension. The normal adult dose is 500 mg bid. Stock strength: Keflex (cephalexin) 125 mg/5 mL

What is the approximate dose for the child in milligrams?

What volume of medication should be given per dose?

Pretest, cont.

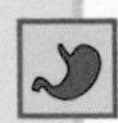

10. A 5-year-old child is ordered Colace (docusate sodium) syrup for constipation. The adult dose is Colace 100 mg. Stock strength: docusate sodium 20 mg/5 mL

What is the approximate dose for the child in milligrams?

What is the volume of medication to be given?

What is the measurable dose volume in household measurements?

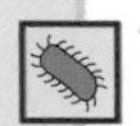

11. A child weighs 83 lb. The physician orders Biaxin oral suspension 10 mg/kg bid.

Stock strength: Biaxin (clarithromycin) 125 mg/5 mL when reconstituted

What volume of medication should be given to the child per dose?

What is the measurable volume of medication in each of the following systems?

Metric: ______________ *Household:* ______________

Show the *measurable* volume of medication to be provided on the measuring devices.

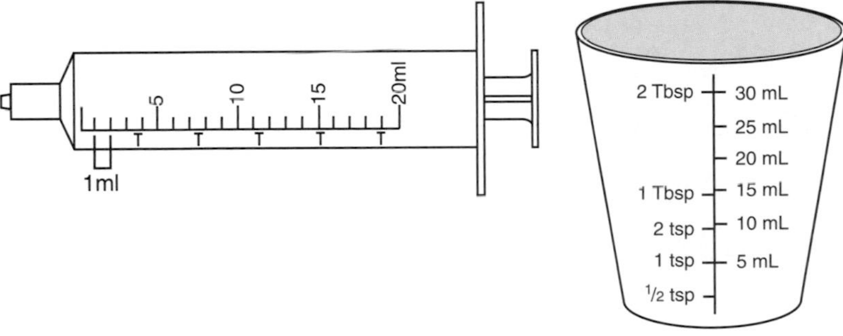

Continued

Pretest, cont.

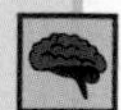

12. A 10-year-old child weighs 56 lb and is 40″ tall. He has been diagnosed with epilepsy.

The physician orders Dilantin suspension for this child based on BSA. The normal adult dose is Dilantin 300 mg/day in three divided doses (100 mg/dose).

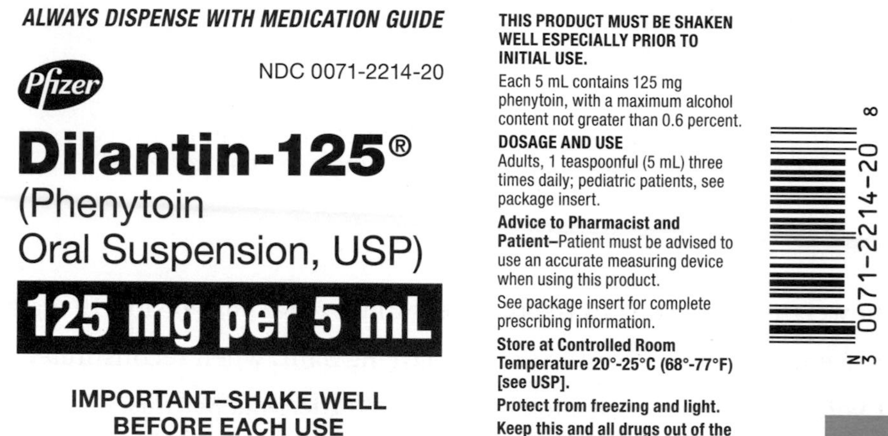

What is the child's BSA according to the nomogram on page 321 ______________?

What is the dose in milligrams to be given with each administration?

What is the volume of medication to be given for this dose?

Pretest, cont.

What is the approximate dose in mg using only the child's body weight and average adult dose?

What is the approximate dose in mg using only the child's age and average adult dose?

Considering that BSA calculation is most accurate, are the last two very accurate methods of approximating doses? ____________

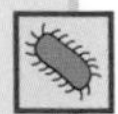

13. A 75-pound child has otitis media. The physician orders Keflex tid.

Stock strength: Keflex (cephalexin) 250 mg capsules

What is the dose to be administered if the adult dose is 500 mg?

How many capsules should be given to the child per dose?

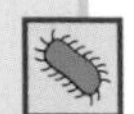

14. A 45-pound child is prescribed Lorabid (loracarbef) 15 mg/kg per *day* in divided doses bid.

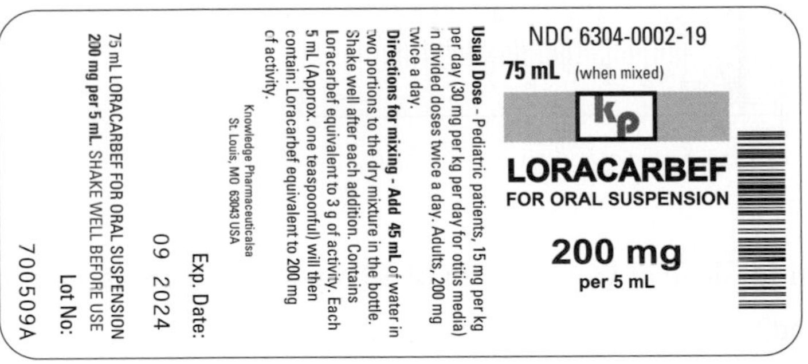

NDC 6304-0002-19
75 mL (when mixed)
kp
LORACARBEF
FOR ORAL SUSPENSION
200 mg
per 5 mL
Usual Dose - Pediatric patients, 15 mg per kg per day (30 mg per kg per day for otitis media) in divided doses twice a day. Adults, 200 mg twice a day.
Directions for mixing - Add 45 mL of water in two portions to the dry mixture in the bottle. Shake well after each addition. Contains Loracarbef equivalent to 3 g of activity. Each 5 mL (Approx. one teaspoonful) will then contain: Loracarbef equivalent to 200 mg of activity.
Knowledge Pharmaceuticalsa
St. Louis, MO 63043 USA
Exp. Date:
09 2024
75 mL LORACARBEF FOR ORAL SUSPENSION
200 mg per 5 mL. SHAKE WELL BEFORE USE
Lot No:
700509A

What is the strength per ***dose*** *for the child using the label shown?*

What is the measurable volume per ***dose*** *of medication for administration?*

What is the total dosage of loracarbef in milligrams per ***day****?*

Continued

Pretest, cont.

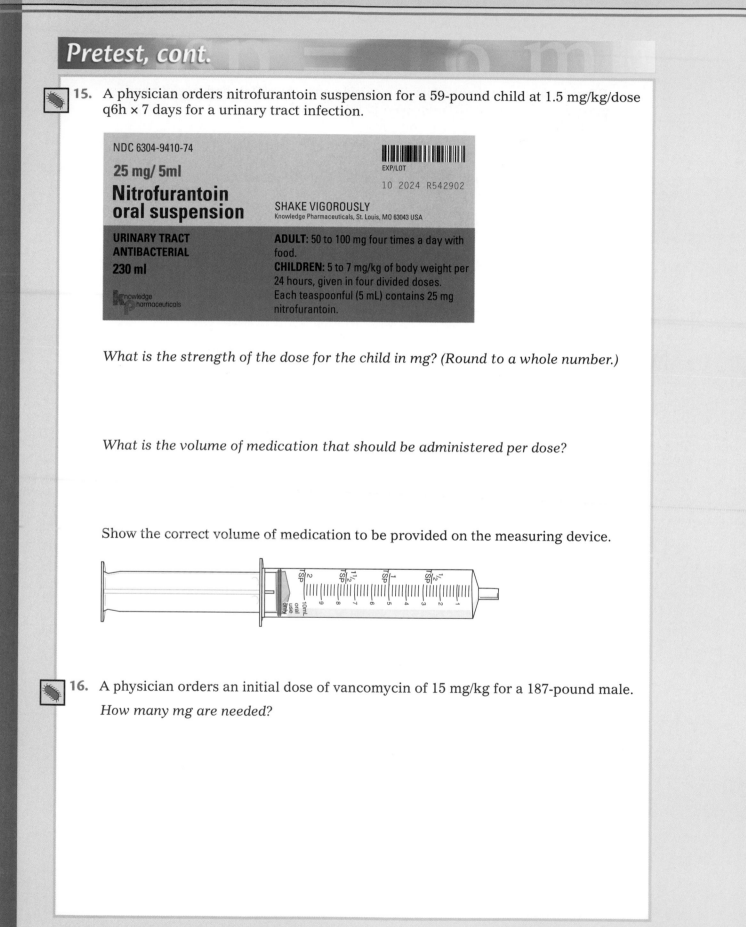

15. A physician orders nitrofurantoin suspension for a 59-pound child at 1.5 mg/kg/dose q6h × 7 days for a urinary tract infection.

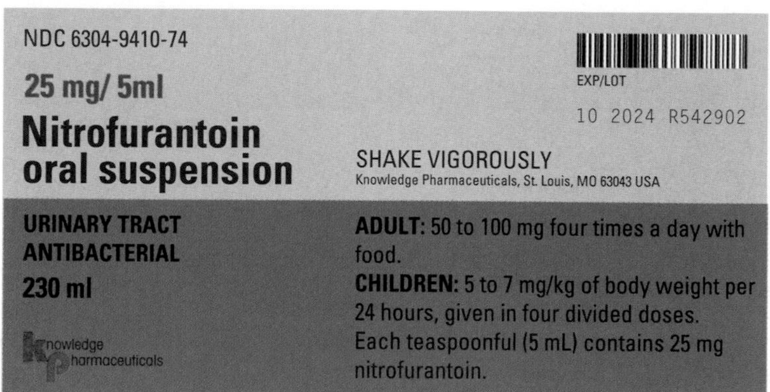

NDC 6304-9410-74
25 mg/ 5ml
Nitrofurantoin oral suspension
EXP/LOT
10 2024 R542902
SHAKE VIGOROUSLY
Knowledge Pharmaceuticals, St. Louis, MO 63043 USA
URINARY TRACT ANTIBACTERIAL
230 ml
Knowledge Pharmaceuticals
ADULT: 50 to 100 mg four times a day with food.
CHILDREN: 5 to 7 mg/kg of body weight per 24 hours, given in four divided doses.
Each teaspoonful (5 mL) contains 25 mg nitrofurantoin.

What is the strength of the dose for the child in mg? (Round to a whole number.)

What is the volume of medication that should be administered per dose?

Show the correct volume of medication to be provided on the measuring device.

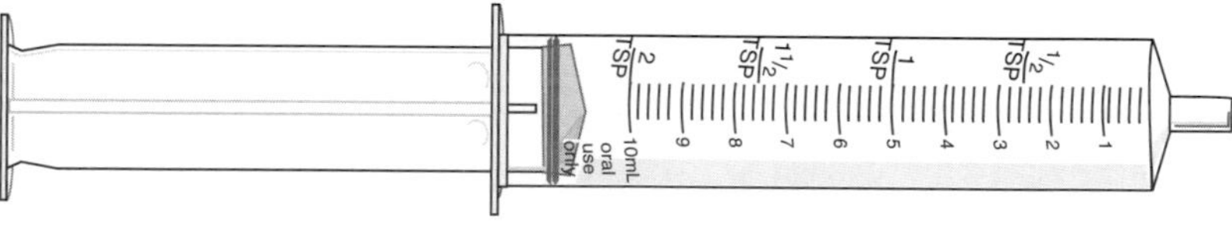

16. A physician orders an initial dose of vancomycin of 15 mg/kg for a 187-pound male. *How many mg are needed?*

Pretest, cont.

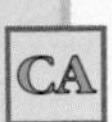
17. A female with breast cancer is prescribed paclitaxel 175 mg/m^2 IV over 3 hours every 3 weeks for 4 doses. Her BSA is 1.6 m^2. Paclitaxel is supplied in 6 mg/mL strength.

How many mg should she receive?

How many mL are required for this dose?

This amount is to be further diluted to 500 mL with 5% dextrose.

What is the final strength in mg per mL?

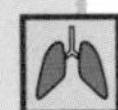
18. Medication order: aminophylline 20 mg/kg per day for a 72-lb child in *divided doses* q6h

Stock strength: aminophylline oral solution 105 mg/5 mL

How many mL are needed per dose?

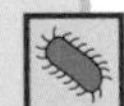
19. Prescription: nitrofurantoin 7 mg/kg/day given in four *divided doses* for a 39-lb child

Stock strength: nitrofurantoin oral suspension 25 mg/5 mL

What is the total strength of the medication the child should receive in a day?

What is the strength of one dose for the child?

How many milliliters are needed per dose?

Continued

Pretest, cont.

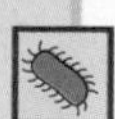

20. Prescription: griseofulvin 10 mg/kg per day for a 45-lb child for nail fungus

    Stock strength: griseofulvin oral suspension 125 mg/5 mL

    What is the strength of one dose for the child?

    How many milliliters are needed per dose?

INTRODUCTION

Patients other than average adults may require special medication dosing. Children are not small adults but rather a distinct population of individuals that exhibits different **pharmacokinetics** (medication absorption, distribution, metabolism, and excretion rates) than adults. The growth and development of the child, or the focus of the field of pediatrics, significantly affects medication dosing. According to the FDA, pediatric stages include **neonate**, **infant**, **child**, and **adolescent**.

Geriatric persons and persons with organ malfunctions also have differences in pharmacokinetics requiring the special calculation of many drug dosages. Most individuals with renal or liver dysfunction require dose adjustments of medications. With toxic medications such as chemotherapeutics, even nonelderly adults with normal organ function may require the use of **body surface area (BSA)** dosing based on height and weight for drug calculations. Emaciated patients, those who have excessively low body weight or muscle mass, and obese patients may also require dose adjustments for some medications. All of these groups are considered special populations because of the need for special dosing calculations. Since many dosing recommendations are standardized average adult doses, doses for special populations must be altered to meet the patients' needs according to age, body weight, BSA, and overall physical condition.

TECH ALERT

Any manufacturer-provided pediatric dose or dosage recommendation should be followed! When these are available, *never use rules that provide estimates.* If a physician's prescription does not agree with the manufacturer's recommendation, the pharmacist should contact the physician.

CALCULATING MEDICATION DOSES BY BODY WEIGHT

Pediatric doses of medications may be ordered according to body weight or body mass. The most common method of calculation uses grams, milligrams, or micrograms of drug per kilogram of body weight. The order therefore appears as g, mg, or mcg/kg. The child must be weighed with each visit to the hospital or physician's office to ensure the correct amount of medication is ordered. If weight is measured in pounds, it must be converted to kilograms. The conversion factor 2.2 lb = 1 kg is the basis for the conversion, which can be completed using ratio and proportion (R&P) or dimensional analysis (DA) (Example 12.1).

EXAMPLE 12.1

What is the weight of a 22-lb infant in kilograms?

R&P

$$\frac{1\text{ kg}}{2.2\text{ lb}} = \frac{x}{22\text{ lb}} \quad 2.2x = 22\text{ kg} \quad x = 10\text{ kg}$$

DA

$$\text{kg} = \frac{1\text{ kg}}{2.2\text{ lb}} \times \frac{22\text{ lb}}{1} = 10\text{ kg}$$

TECH NOTE

Because the calculations in Example 12.1 are normally going to be included in multistep conversions to obtain the weight or volume of a dose, it is advisable to practice them using DA.

EXAMPLE 12.2

An infant weighs 18 lb 4 oz. *What is the infant's weight in kilograms?*

If a person is weighed in pounds and ounces, the ounces must be converted to pounds first.

Convert ounces to pounds using 16 oz = 1 lb.

$$\text{lb} = \frac{1\text{ lb}}{16\text{ oz}} \times \frac{4\text{ oz}}{1} = \frac{1}{4}\text{ lb} \quad \text{so: } 18\text{ lb} + \tfrac{1}{4}\text{ lb} = 18\tfrac{1}{4}\text{ lb}$$

Fractions are *not* used in the metric system: $18\tfrac{1}{4}$ can be converted to 18.25 for the next step.

$$\text{kg} = \frac{1\text{ kg}}{2.2\text{ lb}} \times \frac{18.25\text{ lb}}{1} = 8.3\text{ kg}$$

! TECH ALERT

Conversions including a mixture of ounces and pounds need to be converted to pounds before using pounds in a DA or R&P equation because they involve addition.

Practice Problems A

Convert the following weights and round to the nearest hundredth of a kilogram. Show all of your calculations.

1. A child weighs 65 lb; what is the weight in kilograms? ______________

2. An infant weighs 8 lb 12 oz; what is the weight in kilograms? ______________

3. A child weighs 75 lb; what is the weight in kilograms? ______________

4. A child weighs 112 lb; what is the weight in kilograms? ______________

5. A child weighs 48 lb; what is the weight in kilograms? ______________

Although body weight calculations can be performed with a series of R&P calculations, DA is the preferred method because one equation can be used to obtain the final answer. This is the best way to keep track of units throughout multistep problems.

TECH NOTE

ORDER FOR DIMENSIONAL ANALYSIS

1. Set up a DA equation so that the units needed in the numerator of the *final* answer are in the numerator of the first fraction of the DA equation—this unit will *never* be canceled.
2. Set up the next fraction in the equation so that the units of its numerator are the same as the units of the denominator of the first fraction (so these units will cancel when the fractions are multiplied).
3. If necessary, set up the next fraction in the equation so that the units of its numerator are the same as the units of the denominator of the second fraction (so these units cancel when the fractions are multiplied).
4. Repeat with additional terms as many times as needed to solve the problem.
5. Multiply the fractions, and cancel units.

EXAMPLE 12.3

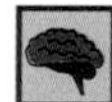

A 53-lb child has been diagnosed with epilepsy. The physician orders Dilantin (phenytoin) 30 mg Kapseals to be given at 2.5 mg/kg per dose.

How many Kapseals should be given per dose?

As with any DA calculation, identify your intended answer and work from there. In this case the answer will be the number of Kapseals per dose.

$$\frac{\#\text{Kapseals}}{\text{dose}} = \frac{1\text{ Kapseal}}{30\text{ mg}} \times \frac{2.5\text{ mg}}{\text{kg/dose}} \times \frac{1\text{ kg}}{2.2\text{ lb}} \times \frac{53\text{ lb}}{1} = 2.01\text{ Kapseals/dose}$$

Therefore the child should be administered two Kapseals with each dose of medication because this is the measurable dose, given that capsules (Kapseals) cannot be divided.

EXAMPLE 12.4

A physician orders amoxicillin 20 mg/kg per day to be given q8h to a 42-lb child. The concentration of amoxicillin is 125 mg/5 mL.

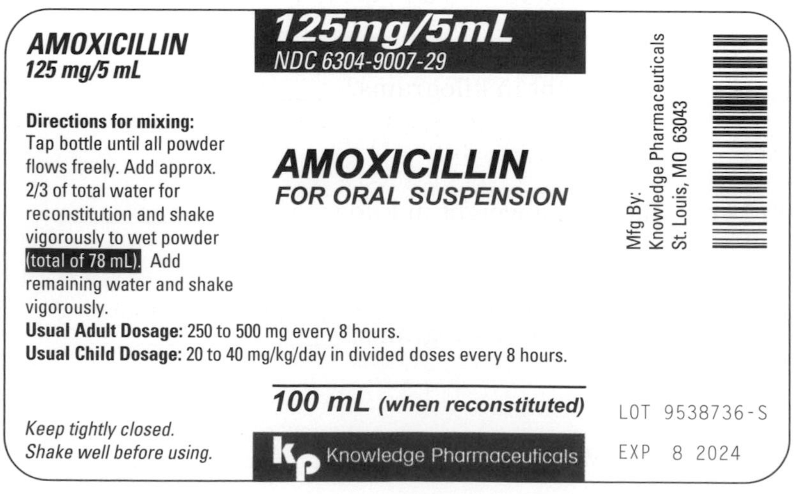

How many mg are needed **per dose***?*

$$\frac{\text{mg}}{\text{dose}} = \frac{20\text{ mg}}{\text{kg/day}} \times \frac{1\text{ day}}{3\text{ doses}} \times \frac{1\text{ kg}}{2.2\text{ lb}} \times \frac{42\text{ lbs}}{1} = 127.27\text{ mg/dose}$$

The more relevant question is, what amount or **volume** should be given per dose?

$$\frac{\text{mL}}{\text{dose}} = \frac{5\text{ mL}}{125\text{ mg}} \times \frac{20\text{ mg}}{\text{kg/day}} \times \frac{1\text{ day}}{3\text{ dose}} \times \frac{1\text{ kg}}{2.2\text{ lb}} \times \frac{42\text{ lbs}}{1} = 5.09\text{ mL/dose}$$

The amoxicillin dose can be rounded to 5 mL rather than 5.1 mL for a measurable quantity. As a shorter method, because you already calculated the dose in mg, the volume can be determined as follows:

$$\text{mL/dose} = 5\text{ mL}/125\text{ mg} \times 127.27\text{ mg/dose} = 5.1\text{ mL/dose}$$

If the question had been what volume of medication would be given per dose in household measurements, the DA sequence would be as follows:

$$\text{tsp} = \frac{1\text{ tsp}}{5\text{ mL}} \times \frac{5\text{ mL}}{125\text{ mg}} \times \frac{20\text{ mg}}{\text{kg/day}} \times \frac{1\text{ day}}{3\text{ doses}} \times \frac{1\text{ kg}}{2.2\text{ lb}} \times \frac{42\text{ lb}}{1} = 1.02\text{ tsp}$$

The measurable dose is 1 tsp.

EXAMPLE 12.5

A physician orders vancomycin 10 mg/kg IV (further diluted in 100 mL NS) for a 46-lb child, to run over 60 minutes q6h. After reconstitution, the vancomycin strength is 500 mg/10 mL.

The full 10 mg/kg is to be given 4 times a day, q6h, so use 10 mg/kg per dose in the calculation.

How many milliliters of reconstituted vancomycin for injection should be added to 100 mL of normal saline for injection to provide one dose?

$$\frac{\text{mL}}{\text{dose}} = \frac{10\text{ mL}}{500\text{ mg}} \times \frac{10\text{ mg}}{\text{kg/dose}} \times \frac{1\text{ kg}}{2.2\text{ \#}} = \frac{46\text{ \#}}{1} \times 4.18\text{ mL/dose}$$

The measurable amount of 4.2 mL should be added to a 100-mL IV bag of normal saline.

TECH NOTE

Not all medications can be rounded to a whole number. Typically, the smaller the dose and the more potent the medication, the less rounding is recommended.

! TECH ALERT

Read orders carefully to distinguish whether medication is being ordered per *dose* or per *day*!

Practice Problems B

*Use **body weight** calculations with DA to answer the following dosing questions.*

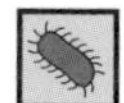

1. A physician orders Veetids 10 mg/kg q8h for a child who weighs 55 lb.

   Note: This dose is to be given every 8 hours for a total of three times per day.

   The medication strength is 250 mg/5 mL.

   What volume of medication (mL) should be given per dose?

   How many milligrams will the child receive per dose?

   How many milligrams will the child receive in 1 day?

   Indicate the amount of medication to be administered per dose on each of the following measuring devices.

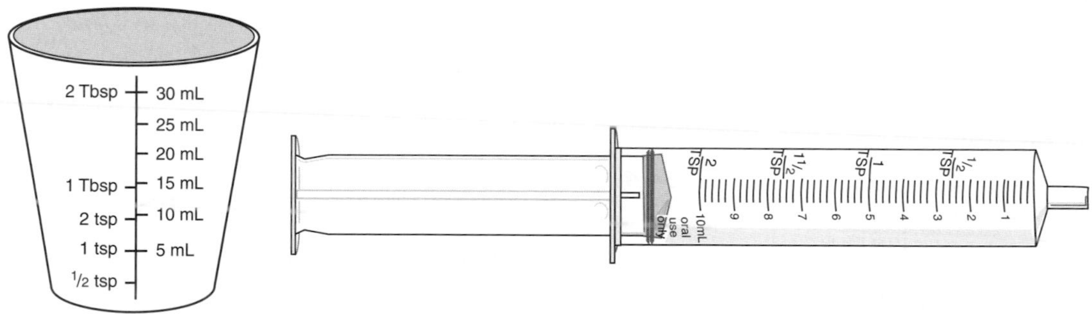

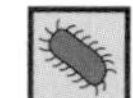

2. A physician orders Zithromax suspension 10 mg/kg daily for a 44-lb child with acute bronchitis. The medication available is 200 mg/5 mL.

   What is the dose in milligrams for the child?

What is the volume of medication to be given to the child for this dose?

Indicate the amount of medication to be administered on each of the following measuring devices.

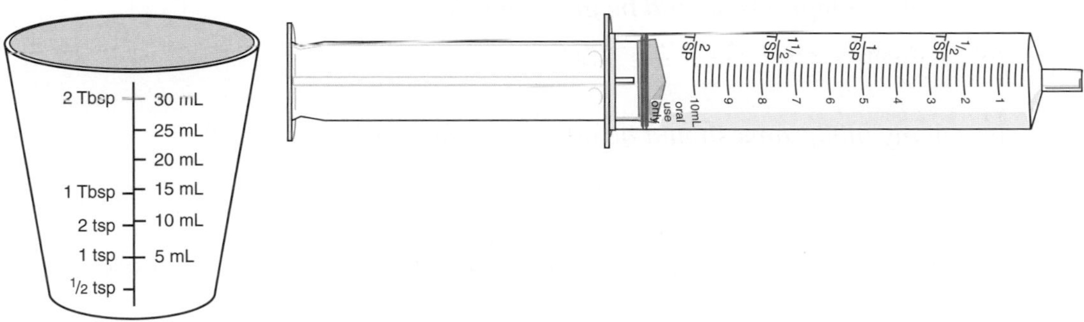

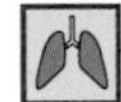

3. A physician orders Zyrtec syrup 0.1 mg/kg daily for a 55-lb child with allergies. The medication is available in 5 mg/5 mL.

What volume of medication in milliliters should be given to the child per dose?

What is this dose in the household measurement system?

Indicate the amount of medication to be administered on each of the following measuring devices.

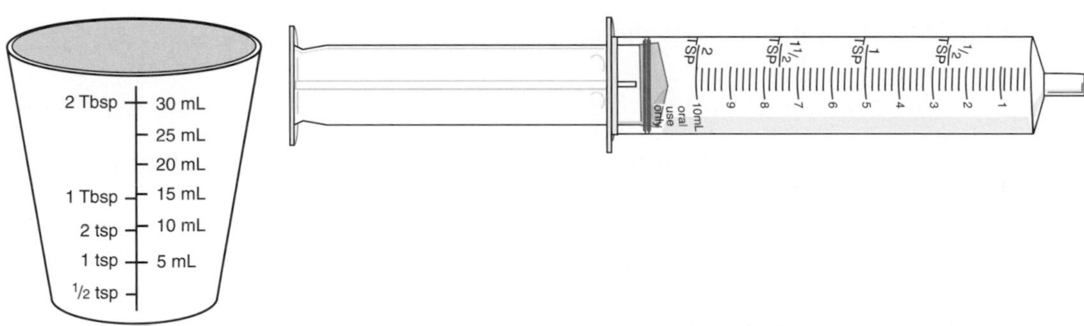

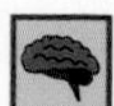

4. A physician orders Zarontin (*ethosuximide*) syrup 20 mg/kg per day in *divided* doses bid for a 54-lb child who has been diagnosed with seizures.

   Note: 20 mg/kg/day is the total daily dose.

   The medication available is Zarontin syrup 250 mg/5 mL.

   How many milligrams should be given in a day?

   How many milligrams should be administered for a single dose?

   What is the volume (mL) of medication to be given to the child per dose?

5. A physician orders Lanoxin (digoxin) elixir 8 mcg/kg for a 55-lb child. The available medication is 50 mcg/mL.

   What is the dose in micrograms for the child?

   What volume of medication should be given for one dose?

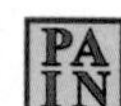

6. An 88-lb child has an order for Demerol (meperidine) syrup po 1 mg/kg per dose for postoperative pain.

   The medication available is meperidine 50 mg/5 mL.

   What volume of medication should be administered per dose?

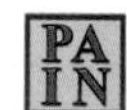

7. A physician wants a 53-lb child to have Tylenol (acetaminophen) elixir gr $\overline{\text{ss}}$/kg q8h prn high fever.

   The medication available is acetaminophen 325 mg/5 mL.

   Use the conversion gr i = 65 mg.

   What volume of medication should be given per dose?

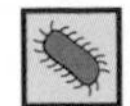

8. A physician orders erythromycin 10 mg/kg q6h for an 88-lb child. The available medications are erythromycin suspension 400 mg/5 mL and erythromycin 200 mg chewable tablets.

   What strength of erythromycin should be given to the child q6h?

   What volume of the suspension would be given for one dose?

   How many chewable tablets would be administered for one dose?

9. A physician orders Tofranil (imipramine) 0.3 mg/kg hs for a child with enuresis. The child weighs 72 lb. The available medication is 10-mg tabs.

   What dose strength of medication should be administered to the child each bedtime?

   How many tablets should be administered to the child for each dose?

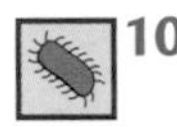

10. A physician orders Ceclor (cefaclor) 50 mg/kg per day to be administered in divided doses qid to a 38-lb child. The available medications are 250 mg/5 mL and 125 mg/5 mL.

    What weight of medication should be administered to the child for a single dose?

    Which concentration should be chosen for this child and why?

    What volume of medication should be administered to the child per dose using the chosen concentration of the medication?

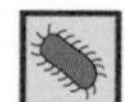

11. A physician orders ampicillin 100 mg/kg per day in 4 divided doses for a 12-pound infant. The available medication is 125 mg/5 mL.

What volume of medication should be given per dose?

What would be the measurable dose in household measurements?

What would be the measurable dose in household measurements if the concentration used was 250 mg/5 mL?

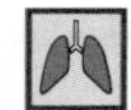

12. A physician orders aminophylline 2.5 mg/kg per dose q8h for a 40-lb child.

The available medication is aminophylline oral liquid 90 mg/5 mL.

What is the strength of one dose (mg)?

What volume of medication should be administered per dose?

How many teaspoons of medication should be administered to the child per dose?

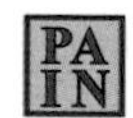

13. A physician orders acetaminophen elixir 6 mg/kg for a 45-lb child.

The available elixir contains 160 mg/5 mL.

What volume of medication should be administered to the child?

*What type of measuring device should be provided for the parent to administer this medication at home?*____

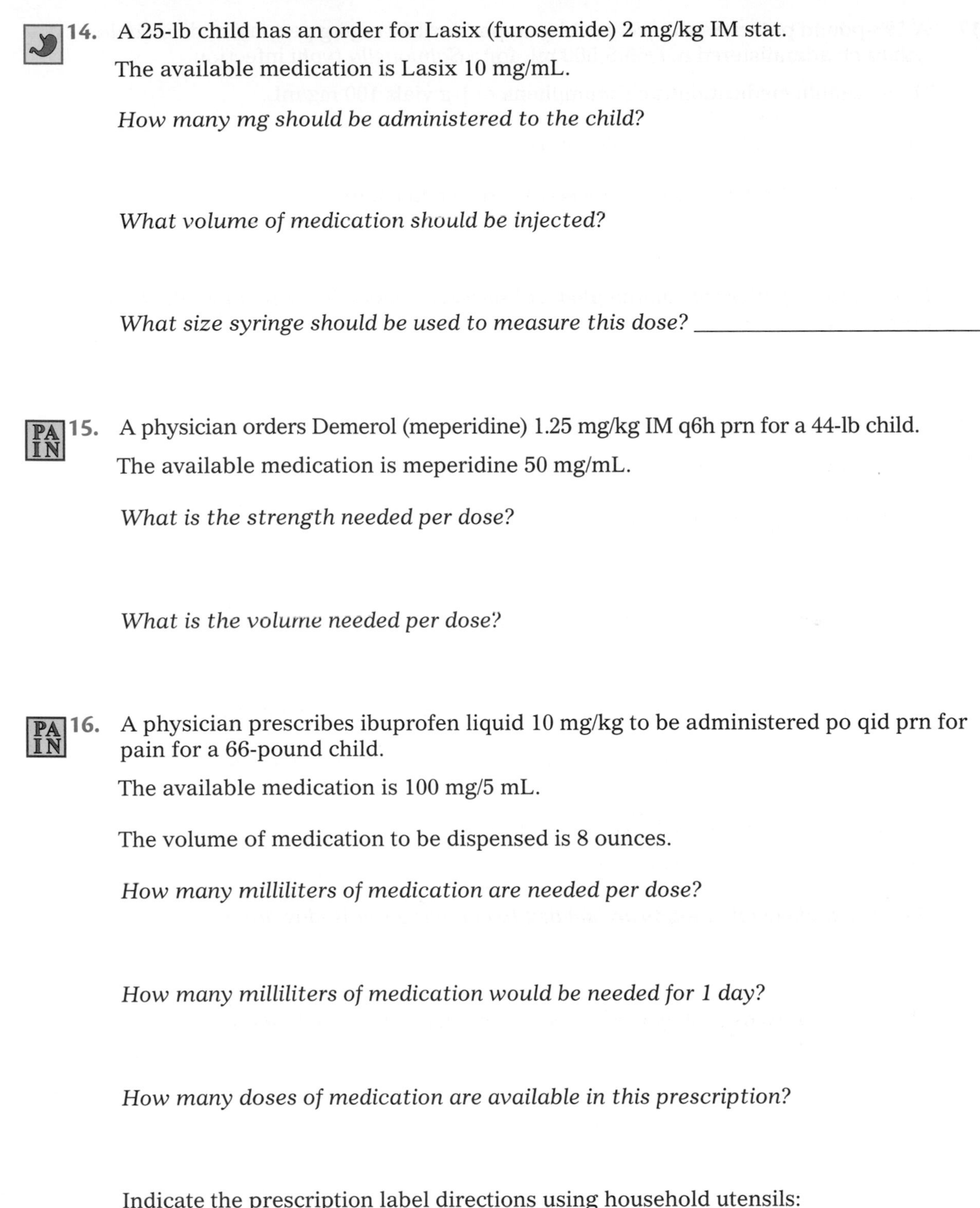

14. A 25-lb child has an order for Lasix (furosemide) 2 mg/kg IM stat.

The available medication is Lasix 10 mg/mL.

How many mg should be administered to the child?

What volume of medication should be injected?

What size syringe should be used to measure this dose? ______________________

15. A physician orders Demerol (meperidine) 1.25 mg/kg IM q6h prn for a 44-lb child.

The available medication is meperidine 50 mg/mL.

What is the strength needed per dose?

What is the volume needed per dose?

16. A physician prescribes ibuprofen liquid 10 mg/kg to be administered po qid prn for pain for a 66-pound child.

The available medication is 100 mg/5 mL.

The volume of medication to be dispensed is 8 ounces.

How many milliliters of medication are needed per dose?

How many milliliters of medication would be needed for 1 day?

How many doses of medication are available in this prescription?

Indicate the prescription label directions using household utensils:

____

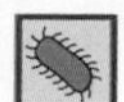

17. A 198-pound patient is to receive chloramphenicol 50 mg/kg per day in *divided doses* q4h to be administered in D5NS 500 mL for a *Salmonella typhi* infection.

The available medication is chloramphenicol 1-g vials 100 mg/mL.

Hint: Only full vials are available for use.

How many milliliters of chloramphenicol are in a full vial?

How many milliliters of chloramphenicol should be added to each bag of fluids per dose?

How many vials of chloramphenicol are needed for 1 day?

Explain your answer.

____

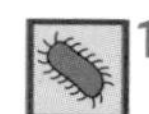

18. A 66-pound child has a streptococcal infection of the throat.

Sig: erythromycin 40 mg/kg per day in *divided doses* q6h for 10 days.

The medication is available as erythromycin 200 mg chewable tablets.

How many mg are needed per dose?

How many chewable tablets are needed to complete the 10-day order?

Write the directions as they would appear on the prescription label:

____

The parent states that the child will not chew the tablet but will take oral liquids. Erythromycin is also available as 400 mg/5 mL.

After obtaining the physician's permission for the change, how many milliliters should be dispensed?

How many milliliters would be needed per dose? (Round to the nearest tenth.)

19. A 36-kg child is prescribed an initial dose of Narcan (naloxone) 0.01 mg/kg subcut to counteract an opioid overdose.

    Stock available: naloxone 0.4 mg/mL (1-mL vials) for IM, IV, or SC use

    How many milliliters should be administered?

    How many micrograms is this?

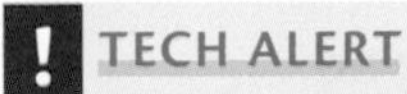

20. A 68-kg patient is prescribed heparin 250 units/kg subcut q12h.

    Stock strength to be used: heparin 20,000 units/mL

    How many milliliters should be administered every 12 hours?

Use of Clark's Rule for Pediatric Dosing

Clark's rule is a method for *approximating* pediatric doses based on the manufacturer's recommended average adult dose, by relating the child's body weight to an average adult body weight of 150 lb. Studies have shown that the average adult now weighs more than 150 lb. Clark's rule is being phased out as a means for calculating pediatric doses, but technicians should still be aware of the method.

! TECH ALERT

The *manufacturer-recommended* pediatric dose should always be used when available!

Clark's rule

$$\text{Child's dose} = \frac{\text{child's weight in pounds}}{150} \times \text{Adult dose}$$

TECH NOTE

An answer obtained with Clark's rule is an *approximation*; 150 pounds is an estimate of an average adult weight.

! TECH ALERT

Clark's rule would never be used to determine the dose of medication with a narrow therapeutic range—that is, one where there is little difference between therapeutic and toxic levels!

EXAMPLE 12.6

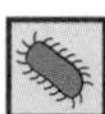

A physician orders Cefzil (cefprozil) for a 38-lb child with an upper respiratory infection. The adult dose for Cefzil is 500 mg q24h.

The physician did not order an amount per kilogram, so calculating this medication by the "mg/kg" body weight method is not possible.

Using Clark's Rule, how many milligrams should be given for one dose?

$$\text{Child's dose} = \frac{38}{150} \times 500 \text{ mg} = 126.7 \text{ mg}$$

If the prescription is filled with Cefzil 125 mg/5 mL, how many milliliters are needed per dose?

$$\text{mL} = \frac{5 \text{ mL}}{125 \text{ mg}} \times \frac{126.7 \text{ mg}}{\text{dose}} = 5.07 \text{ mL}$$

This dose should be rounded to 5 mL, which is a measurable amount. This is already an approximation due to the use of Clark's rule!

Practice Problems C

Round all calculations to a measurable dose for the device to be used in the final step. Show your calculations.

1. A 64-pound child is ordered a medication with an adult dose of 60 mg tid.

   What is the approximate dose for the child?

2. A 68-pound child is to receive a medication tid. The normal adult dose is 90 mg/day.

What is the strength of one ***dose*** *for the child?*

What is the total strength of the medication the child should receive in a ***day****?*

The medication is available as 10 mg/5 mL. *What volume of medication should the child receive per* ***dose****?*

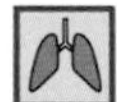

3. A physician orders Benylin (dextromethorphan) syrup for a 30-lb child. The normal adult dose is 20 mg q6h. The medication on hand is Benylin syrup 15 mg/5 mL.

How many milligrams should the child receive per dose?

What is the volume of one dose of medication in the metric system?

What is the approximate volume of one dose in household measurements?

Mark the amount of medication in milliliters on one side of the oral syringe and teaspoons on the other side. Observe that they are very close but not exactly the same.

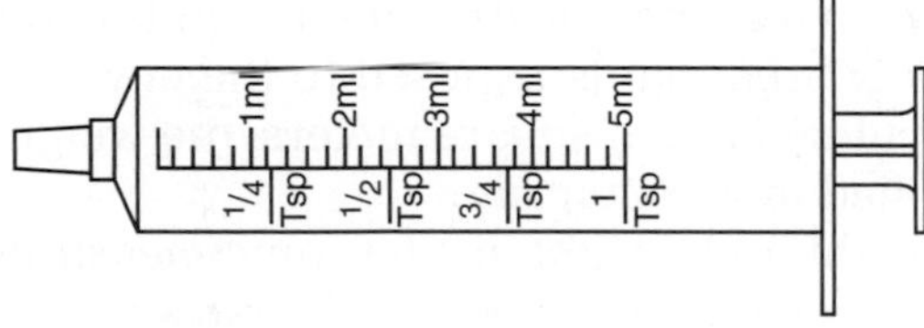

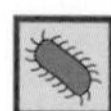

4. A 60-lb child is prescribed Biaxin (clarithromycin) suspension for sinusitis.

The adult dose is 500 mg bid.

The medication available is 125 mg/5 mL.

How many milligrams should the child receive per dose?

What is the volume of medication per dose?

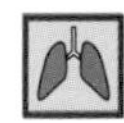

5. A physician orders Benadryl (diphenhydramine) elixir q4h for a 60-lb child.

The usual adult dose is 25 mg q4h.

The available medication is diphenhydramine elixir 12.5 mg/5 mL.

How many milligrams should the child receive per dose?

What is the volume of medication per dose?

CALCULATING MEDICATION DOSES BY BODY SURFACE AREA

Dosing based on body surface area is the most accurate method because it is based on *both* body weight and height. This form of calculation is often used for pediatric and geriatric patients and when dosing medications with a narrow therapeutic index, such as chemotherapeutics. BSA refers to the total body area that is exposed to the environment and is expressed in square meters (m^2). To calculate BSA in square meters, the weight and height of a person must be measured and applied to a **nomogram**.

To use a nomogram, locate the patient's height and weight, *in the same measurement system,* on the correct lines of the chart. Fig. 12.1 depicts the use of the child's nomogram for a child who is 41″ tall and weighs 36 lb. The intersection of the straight line on the BSA line is 0.68, so the BSA for this patient is 0.68 m^2. For a child of normal height and weight

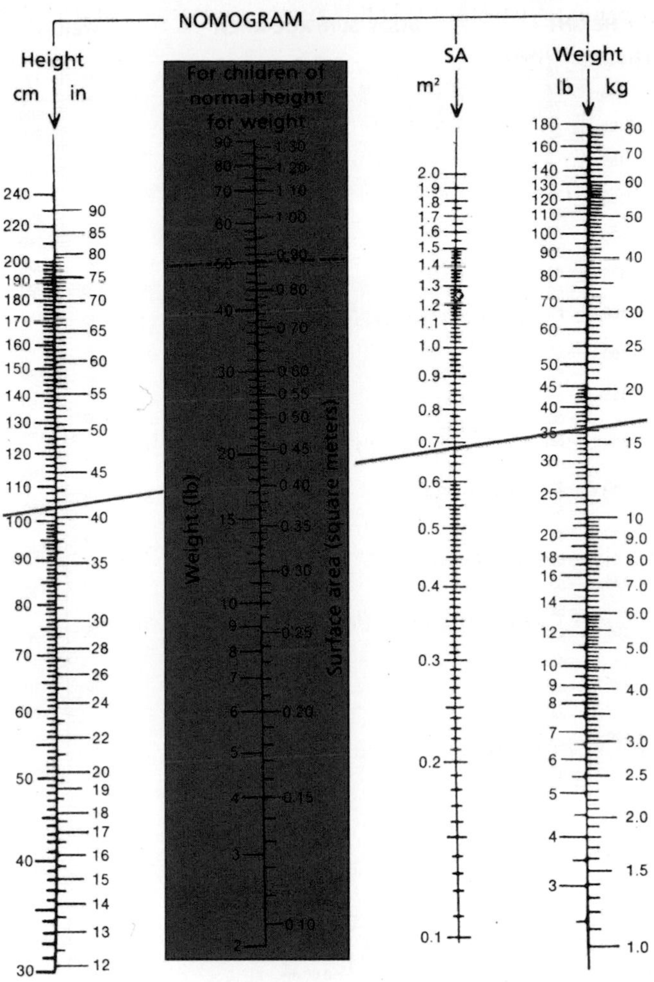

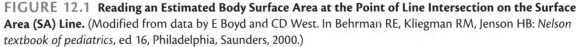

FIGURE 12.1 Reading an Estimated Body Surface Area at the Point of Line Intersection on the Surface Area (SA) Line. (Modified from data by E Boyd and CD West. In Behrman RE, Kliegman RM, Jenson HB: *Nelson textbook of pediatrics*, ed 16, Philadelphia, Saunders, 2000.)

for their age, BSA may be determined by weight alone using the additional column within the center box.

An adult nomogram (Fig. 12.2) is used for adults who fall outside of what is considered normal weight for height or those being administered medications with a narrow therapeutic index. The metric system is on the left side of *both* the height and weight columns. In comparison, the metric system is on the left side of the height measurement column and on the right side of the weight measurement column on the child's nomogram.

Pharmacy technicians rarely use a nomogram since they are typically used by a pharmacist or physician in a clinical hospital setting. It is still good to be familiar with the concept.

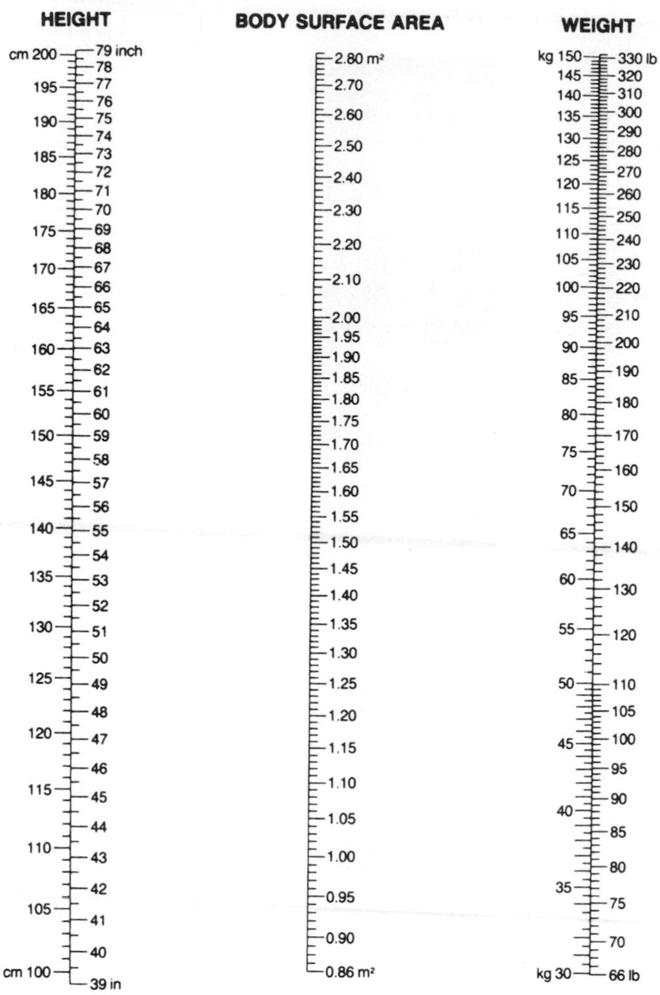

FIGURE 12.2 Nomogram for Calculating Body Surface Area for an Adult. (Lentner C: *Geigy Scientific Tables*, ed 8, vol 1, Basel, Switzerland, Ciba-Geigy, 1981.)

Practice Problems D

Use the proper nomogram to calculate the BSAs. Round to the nearest hundredth.

1. A 15-lb, 24″ child.

2. A 50-lb, 48″ child.

3. A 5-kg, 60-cm child.

4. A 40-lb child of normal height for weight.

5. A 20-kg, 100-cm child.

The most accurate method of determining a dose using BSA is when the medication is ordered in micrograms, milligrams, or grams per square meter. For calculating doses in milligrams, the BSA in square meters is multiplied by the dose ordered using DA.

$$\text{mg} = \text{mg/m}^2 \times \text{m}^2$$

EXAMPLE 12.7

A medication dose is ordered for a patient with a BSA of 1.6 at 1.5 mg/m^2

What is the dose?

$$\text{mg} = \frac{1.5\text{ mg}}{\text{m}^2} \bullet \frac{1.6\text{ m}^2}{1} = 2.4\text{ mg}$$

EXAMPLE 12.8

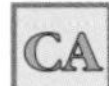

A physician orders the chemotherapeutic agent Cytoxan 50 mg/m^2/dose IV for a 160-lb adult who is 55″ tall.

Determine the BSA by plotting 55″ and 160 lb on the nomogram. The BSA is 1.75 m^2.

If the vial of medication is 200 mg/10 mL, what is the volume of the dose?

mL = 10 mL/200 mg × 50 mg/m2/dose × 1.75 m2/1 = 4.375 mL/dose

The measurable dose of this chemotherapeutic medication is 4.4 mL.

If a medication for a child is not ordered in an amount per square meters, a formula similar to Clark's rule may be used to calculate the dose. The "normal" BSA of 1.7 m^2 for adults and the normal adult dose may be used to *estimate* the child's dose. After using the nomogram for a child, the following formula may be used for calculating the dose.

Child's dose = child's BSA/1.7 × Adult dose

EXAMPLE 12.9

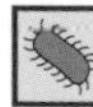

A physician orders amoxicillin tid for a 50-lb child who is 45″ tall.

Determine the BSA. BSA = 0.86 m^2

The normal adult dose is amoxicillin 500 mg tid.

Use formula above to obtain the desired strength of medication.

$$\text{Child's dose} = \frac{0.86}{1.7} \times 500\text{ mg} = 252.94\text{ mg}$$

What dose should be given to the child if the available medication is 250 mg/5 mL?

$$\text{mL} = \frac{5\text{ mL}}{250\text{ mg}} \times \frac{252.94\text{ mg}}{1} = 5.06\text{ mL}$$

The measurable dose to be given is 5 mL.

Practice Problems E

Calculate the following based on BSA. Determine the BSA if required, and insert it into the proper formula. Show your calculations. Round to the nearest hundredth for the dose in milligrams. Round to the nearest tenth for volume to be administered (measurable dose).

1. A 15-lb child is 25″ tall. *What is the child's BSA?* ____________

   The physician orders Lanoxin (digoxin) elixir daily. The adult dose of Lanoxin is 0.25 mg/day. The available medication is Lanoxin pediatric elixir 0.05 mg/mL.

   What is the daily dose of Lanoxin in milligrams for the child?

   What volume of medication would be administered per day?

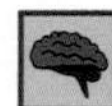

2. A child has a BSA of 0.88 m^2.

   The physician orders Tegretol (carbamazepine) for epilepsy. The adult dose of the medication is 200 mg qid. The medication is available in Tegretol suspension 100 mg/5 mL.

   What is the single-dose strength for the child?

   What is the volume of medication per dose?

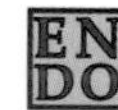

3. A physician orders prednisone for a 41-kg, 158-cm child with an allergic reaction.

   What is the child's BSA? ____________

   The usual adult dose is 5 mg tid.

   What strength of medication should be administered to the child per dose?

   The medication available is prednisone syrup 1 mg/1 mL.

   What volume of medication should be administered per dose?

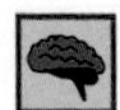

4. A 40-lb child is of normal height for weight. *What is the child's BSA?* ______________

The physician orders Dilantin (phenytoin) suspension for the child for seizures.

The normal adult dose is 100 mg tid.

What is the dose to be administered to the child?

The available medication is Dilantin suspension 125 mg/5 mL.

What is the volume of medication to be given to the child per dose?

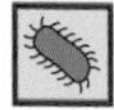

5. A physician orders erythromycin oral suspension for a child with acute bronchitis. BSA = 1.08 m^2.

The usual adult dose is erythromycin 250 mg qid.

What strength of medication should be given to the child per dose?

The medication available is an oral suspension 250 mg/5 mL.

What is the volume of medication to be given per dose?

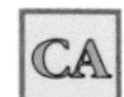

6. A 38-lb, 38-inch 5-year-old with leukemia is ordered vincristine 2 mg/m^2.
BSA = 0.7 m^2

The medication is supplied in 1 mg/mL concentration.

What volume of medication should be administered?

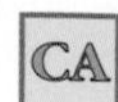

7. A 120-lb adult is 64″. What is her BSA? ______________

The physician ordered Vancocin (vancomycin) 600 mg/m^2 IV q12h.

The available medication is 1 g/10 mL after reconstitution.

Be sure to include the conversion factor between milligrams and grams in your DA setup.

What volume of medication should be prepared for administration of the infusion?

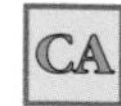

8. An adult with a BSA of 1.79 m^2 has been diagnosed with a malignant neoplasm.

The physician orders Oncovin (vincristine) 1.4 mg/m^2 IV, available in 1 mg/1 mL.

What volume of medication should be administered to this patient?

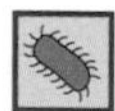

9. An adult with a BSA of 1.62 m^2 has severe herpes zoster.

The physician orders Zovirax (acyclovir) 500 mg/m^2 q8h in 400-mg tablets.

What exact dose of medication should be given to the patient q8h?

How many whole tablets should be given to come closest to this dose?

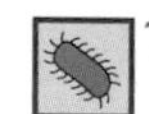

10. A physician orders Augmentin (amoxicillin/clavulanate) q8h for a 44-lb child of normal height for weight with streptococcal pneumonia.

What is her BSA? ______________

The usual adult dose is 500 mg q8h.

The medication is available in Augmentin pediatric chewable tablets 250 mg and Augmentin suspension 250 mg/5 mL.

What amount of medication in mg is needed per dose?

How many chewable tablets would be required per dose?

What volume of suspension would be required per dose?

Which form of medication is most accurate? ____________

CALCULATING MEDICATION DOSES FOR PEDIATRIC PATIENTS BASED ON AGE

Pediatric doses have also been estimated by age using Fried's or Young's rules, which are based on the normal adult dose. These formulas will yield approximate answers and *should not* be used with medications that have a narrow therapeutic index. Age is no longer considered a valid criterion for determining pediatric dosing, but a technician should still be aware of the following formulas.

Fried's rule is used for neonates and infants up to 24 months:

$$\text{dose} = \frac{\text{age in months}}{150} \times \text{Adult dose}$$

EXAMPLE 12.10

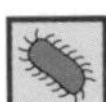

A physician orders amoxicillin for a 6-month-old infant. The usual adult dose is 500 mg. *How many milligrams should the infant receive per dose?*

$$\text{Infant's dose} = \frac{6}{150} \times 500\text{ mg} = 20\text{ mg}$$

The medication available is amoxicillin 50 mg/mL What dose would be given to the infant?

$$\text{mL} = 1\text{ mL}/50\text{ mg} \times 20\text{ mg}/1 = 0.4\text{ mL}$$

Young's rule is used to calculate medications for children 1 year of age to 12 years of age.

$$\text{Child's dose} = \frac{\text{child's age in years}}{\text{child's age in years} + 12} \times \text{Adult dose}$$

EXAMPLE 12.11

A physician orders amoxicillin for a 5-year-old child. The adult dose is 500 mg/dose. *What dose would be given to the child?*

$$\text{Child's dose} = \frac{5}{5 + 12} \times 500 \text{ mg} = 147.06 \text{ mg}$$

If the medication is available as amoxicillin suspension 400 mg/5 mL, what dose would be given to the child?

$$\text{mL} = \frac{5 \text{ mL}}{400 \text{ mg}} \times \frac{147.06 \text{ mg}}{1} = 1.84 \text{ mL}$$

The measurable dose is 1.8 mL.

TECH ALERT

If the manufacturer has a suggested amount for a pediatric dose, that dose should always be used. More and more physicians are using only medications that have suggested manufacturer's doses for children rather than using age or body weight as a basis for calculating doses.

Practice Problems F

Calculate the following doses. Show your calculations. Round to the nearest hundredth for weight calculations and the nearest tenth when providing volume calculations, unless otherwise noted.

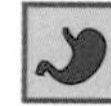

1. A physician orders Milk of Magnesia for a 3-year-old child. The adult dose is 30 mL.
   What volume of Milk of Magnesia should be given to the child?

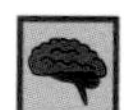

2. A physician wants a 6-month-old child to have phenobarbital.
   The usual adult dose is phenobarbital 30 mg.

   What dose of the medication should be given to the child?

   Phenobarbital is available as an elixir of 20 mg/5 mL.

   What volume of medication should be administered per dose?

3. A 12-year-old child is to take a medication bid. The normal adult dose is 200 mg/dose.

   What is the approximate strength of medication that the child should receive per ***dose****?*

   What is the total strength of medication the child should receive per ***day****?*

   If the stock liquid medication strength is 125 mg/5 mL, what volume of medication is required per ***dose****?*

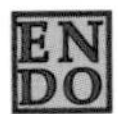

4. A physician prescribes prednisone for a 6-year-old child with a severe case of hives. The adult dose is 20 mg.

   What dose should be given to the child?

   The available medication is prednisone oral solution 5 mg/5 mL.

   What volume of medication should be given to the child?

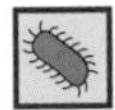

5. Prescription: Cefzil q12h for a 4-year-old child (Adult dose 500 mg q12h)

   Stock strength: Cefzil (cefprozil) 125 mg/5 mL oral suspension

   How many mL are needed per dose?

REVIEW

Whenever available, a manufacturer's recommendation should be the guideline for the amount of medication that is administered. Certain populations require special dosing considerations. Body weight and BSA calculations provide the most accurate doses. In the past, children's doses were estimated from adult doses based on weight or age using Clark's, Young's, or Fried's rules. These methods are not common now.

TECH ALERT

Remember that doses for a "normal" adult must be adjusted for certain characteristics of patients, such as body weight, organ function, and other parameters.

Posttest

Calculate the following problems using the correct formula for each situation provided. If measuring devices for administration are included, indicate the volume of medication on the appropriate measuring device(s). Show your calculations. If the volume of medication is less than 1 mL, the answer should be rounded to the hundredths position.

1. A child weighs 30 lb and the normal adult dose is 50 mg tid.

What method should be used? ______________

What is the approximate dose for the child?

2. A 22-lb child is to receive 0.05 mg/kg per day in two divided doses.

What method should be used? ______________

What is the total strength of medication that the child should receive per day?

What is the strength of medication that the child should receive per dose?

The medication is available as 1 mg/mL.

What volume of medication should the child receive per dose?

Posttest, cont.

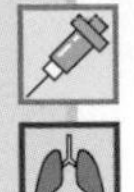

3. A 66-lb child is ordered Benadryl (diphenhydramine) elixir 0.4 mg/kg.

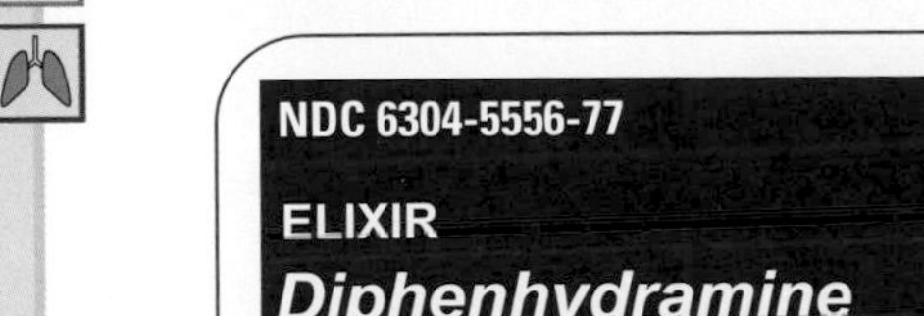

Elixir K-P 5556 for prescription dispensing only.
Contains-12.5 mg diphenhydramine hydrochloride in each 5 mL. Alcohol 14%.
Dose-Adults: 2-4 teaspoonfuls; children over 20 lb: 1-2 teaspoonfuls; 3-4 times daily

4 FLUIDOUNCES

Exp date and lot

KNOWLEDGE PHARMACEUTICALS
St. Louis, MO 63043 USA

5556A406 10 2024 P67419N

What method should be used? ______________

What is the strength of medication to be given in mg?

What dose should be given in mL using the diphenhydramine label?

What is the measurable dose in household measurements?

Continued

Posttest, cont.

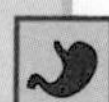

4. A 66-lb child is ordered Compazine (prochlorperazine) 0.5 mg/kg/day *in 3 divided doses.*

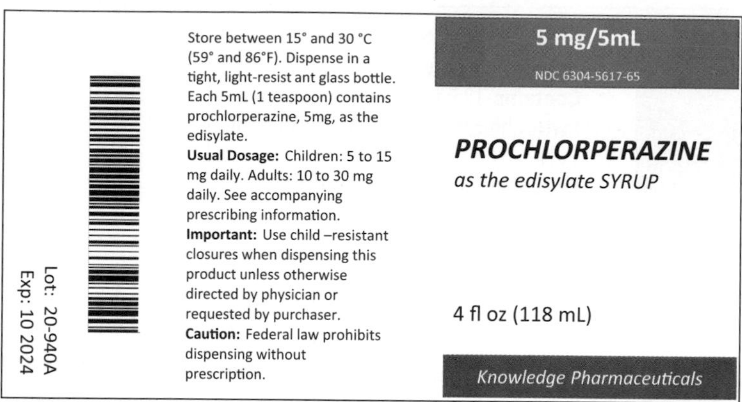

Store between 15° and 30 °C (59° and 86°F). Dispense in a tight, light-resist ant glass bottle. Each 5mL (1 teaspoon) contains prochlorperazine, 5mg, as the edisylate.
Usual Dosage: Children: 5 to 15 mg daily. Adults: 10 to 30 mg daily. See accompanying prescribing information.
Important: Use child –resistant closures when dispensing this product unless otherwise directed by physician or requested by purchaser.
Caution: Federal law prohibits dispensing without prescription.
Lot: 20-940A
Exp: 10 2024
5 mg/5mL
NDC 6304-5617-65
PROCHLORPERAZINE
as the edisylate SYRUP
4 fl oz (118 mL)
Knowledge Pharmaceuticals

What method should be used? ____________

What volume of medication should be administered per **dose**? ____________

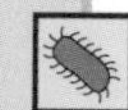

5. A 56-lb child of normal height for weight is prescribed amoxicillin.

The normal adult dose is amoxicillin 500 mg tid.

What method should be used? ____________

What is his BSA? ____________

How many milligrams should be administered per dose?

The medication is available as amoxicillin 125 mg/5 mL and 250 mg/5 mL.

Which strength is the most appropriate for this dose? ____________

What volume of the chosen medication should be given?

Posttest, cont.

6. A child has a BSA of 0.54 m^2. The physician orders Claritin (loratadine) for hay fever.

   The normal adult dose is 10 mg once a day.

   What method should be used? ____________

   The available medication is 1 mg/1 mL.

   What volume of medication should be given to the child daily?

7. A physician orders 6 mg/kg/day of Demerol (meperidine) q4h for a 66-lb child.

   What method should be used? ____________

   What is the total amount of medication that the child can receive in one day?

   How many mg should be given per dose?

   The medication available is 50 mg/5 mL.

   What is the volume of medication needed per dose?

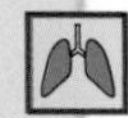

8. An emaciated 100-lb adult has a maintenance order for aminophylline 3 mg/kg per dose q8h.

   What method should be used? ____________

   What strength of medication should be given to this patient every 8 hours?

   The medication available is aminophylline oral liquid 105 mg/5 mL.

   What volume of medication should be taken per dose?

Continued

Posttest, cont.

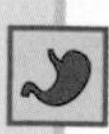

9. An 8-year-old child has an order for Tofranil (imipramine) one hour before bedtime to prevent bedwetting.

The usual adult dose is Tofranil 50 mg.

What method should be used? ______________

What strength of medication should be administered to the child?

The medication is available in 10 mg tablets.

How many tablets are needed for the dose? ______________

10. A 12-year-old child has an order for Motrin (ibuprofen) for elevated temperature.

The usual adult dose is 400 mg q6h.

What method should be used? ______________

What strength of medication should be given per dose?

Ibuprofen oral suspension is available in 100 mg/5 mL.

What volume of medication should be administered for each dose?

The medication is also available in 100 mg chewable tablets.

How many tablets should be given per dose? ______________

Posttest, cont.

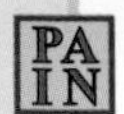

11. A 6-month-old infant is ordered acetaminophen q4h for a high fever.

The usual adult dose is 325 mg q4–6h.

What method should be used? ____________

What strength of medication should be given to the infant?

The medication available is acetaminophen 160 mg/5 mL.

What volume of medication should be given to the infant?

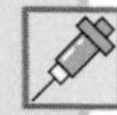

12. A 64-lb child with a severe allergic reaction to a bee sting is ordered Decadron (dexamethasone).

The normal adult dose is dexamethasone 4 mg.

What method should be used? ____________

What strength of medication should be given to the child?

The available medication is dexamethasone elixir 0.5 mg/5 mL.

What volume of medication should be given to the child?

13. A physician orders dexamethasone IM for a child with a BSA of 0.84 m^2.

The normal adult dose is Decadron 4 mg.

What method should be used? ____________

The available injection is Decadron 10 mg/mL.

What volume of medication is needed?

Show the dosage on the syringe.

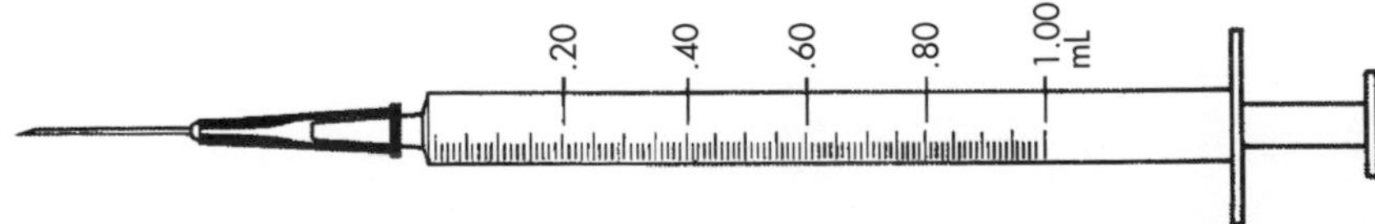

Continued

Posttest, cont.

14. A 48-lb child has an order for dexamethasone 0.08 mg/kg every 12 hours.

What method should be used? ____________

What strength of medication should be given to the child with each dose?

Dexamethasone is available as an *oral liquid* in 0.5 mg/5 mL and an *injection* in 4 mg/mL.

What volume of medication should be given to the child orally?

What volume of medication should be administered parenterally?

15. A 78-lb child is treated for status epilepticus with Valium (diazepam) 0.3 mg/kg.

Diazepam is available in 5 mg and 10 mg tablets, 5 mg/5 mL oral solution, and 5 mg/mL injectable solution.

What method should be used? ____________

What strength in milligrams should be administered to the child?

How many tablets would be given orally for this dose? ____________

What volume of oral solution would be given?

What volume of medication would be administered parenterally?

Posttest, cont.

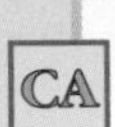

16. A 185-lb, 5′11″ male patient is being treated with cisplatin IV for testicular cancer at a dosage of 20 mg/m^2 IV over 60 minutes daily for 5 days.

What is the patient's BSA? ____________

What strength of medication should be administered per dose?

Cisplatin is available as a powder in 10-mg and 50-mg vials reconstituted to 1 mg/mL.

Which vial of medication should be reconstituted to provide the ordered dose? ____________

Show the amount of medication to be administered on the following syringe:

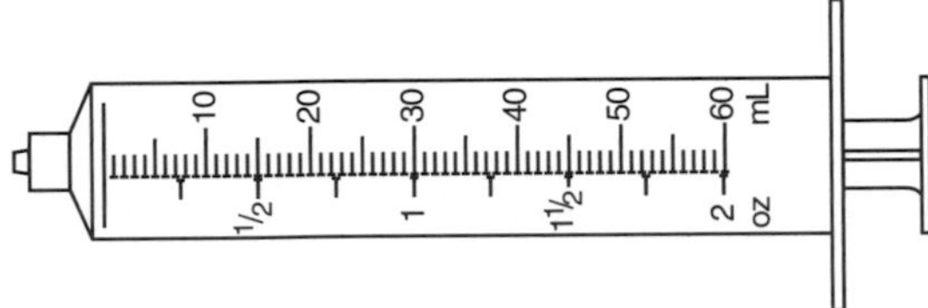

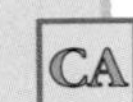

17. A patient with a BSA of 1.75 m^2 is being treated for Hodgkin disease with doxorubicin 65 mg/m^2 every 21 days.

How many milligrams of medication should this patient receive per dose?

Doxorubicin is available in 5-, 10-, 25-, 75-, and 100-mL vials in 2 mg/mL strength.

What volume of medication would be used to provide the patient's dose?

Which vial of medication is most appropriate to use? ____________

Continued

Posttest, cont.

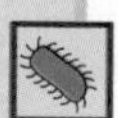

18. A 56-lb child has an order for Zithromax (azithromycin) oral suspension 10 mg/kg perday for the first day and 5 mg/kg per day for the next 4 days.

Use the label shown for the calculations of doses to be given.

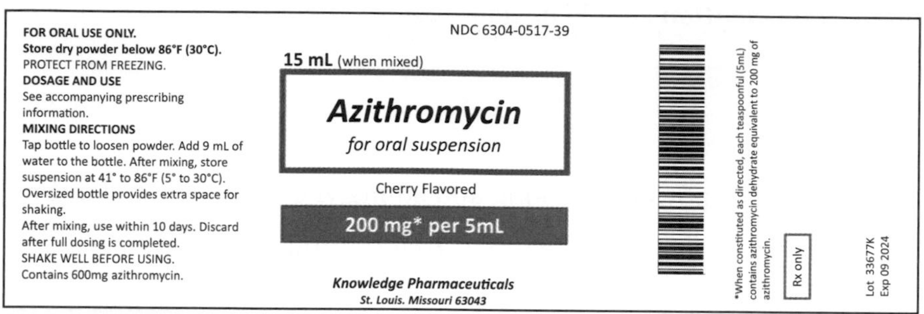

FOR ORAL USE ONLY.
Store dry powder below 86°F (30°C).
PROTECT FROM FREEZING.
DOSAGE AND USE
See accompanying prescribing information.
MIXING DIRECTIONS
Tap bottle to loosen powder. Add 9 mL of water to the bottle. After mixing, store suspension at 41° to 86°F (5° to 30°C). Oversized bottle provides extra space for shaking.
After mixing, use within 10 days. Discard after full dosing is completed.
SHAKE WELL BEFORE USING.
Contains 600mg azithromycin.
NDC 6304-0517-39
15 mL (when mixed)
Azithromycin
for oral suspension
Cherry Flavored
200 mg* per 5mL
Knowledge Pharmaceuticals
St. Louis. Missouri 63043
*When constituted as directed, each teaspoonful (5mL) contains azithromycin dehydrate equivalent to 200 mg of azithromycin.
Rx only
Lot 33677K
Exp 09 2024

What strength of medication should be given to the child on the first day?

What is the measurable amount of suspension that should be given the first day?

Show this amount on the following oral syringe:

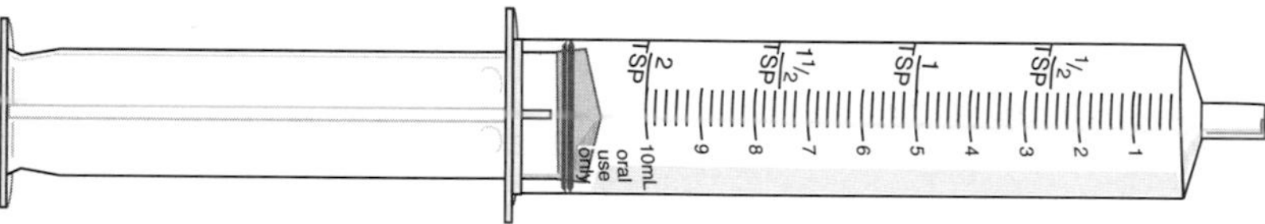

What strength of medication should be given to the child on subsequent days?

What volume of medication should be given to the child on subsequent days?

Show this amount on the following oral syringe:

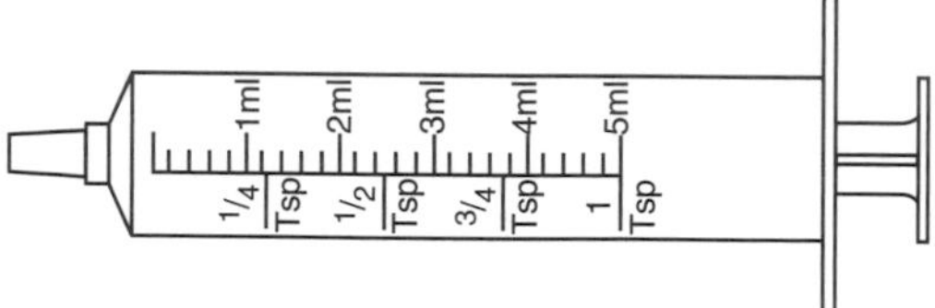

Posttest, cont.

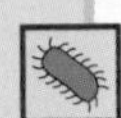

19. A 4-month-old child is being treated with ampicillin for a strep infection. The normal adult dose is ampicillin 500 mg/dose.

What rule is needed for this calculation? ______________

What strength of medication should be administered to this child?

Ampicillin is available as an oral suspension 125 mg/5 mL.

What volume of medication should be ordered for the child?

Show the amount on the following oral syringe:

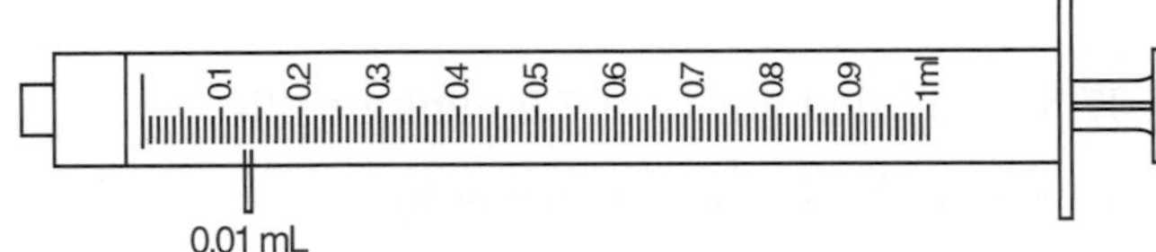

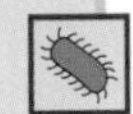

20. A 55-lb child has a prescription for penicillin V potassium q8h. The normal adult dose is penicillin V potassium 500 mg q8h. Use the following label for calculations.

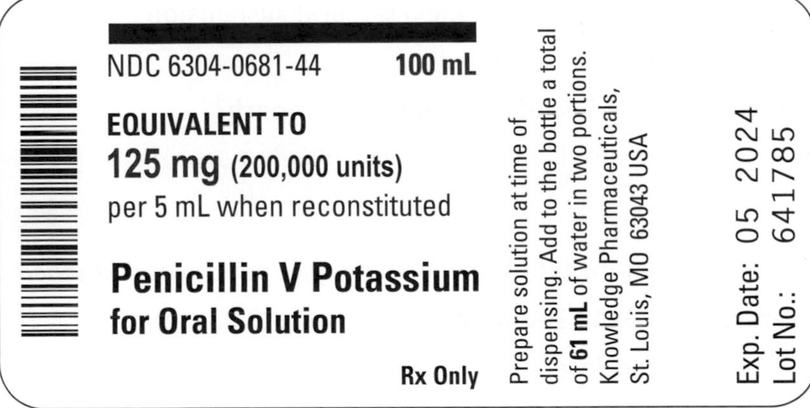
NDC 6304-0681-44 **100 mL**

EQUIVALENT TO
125 mg (200,000 units)
per 5 mL when reconstituted

Penicillin V Potassium
for Oral Solution

Rx Only

Prepare solution at time of dispensing. Add to the bottle a total of **61 mL** of water in two portions.
Knowledge Pharmaceuticals, St. Louis, MO 63043 USA

Exp. Date: 05 2024
Lot No.: 641785

What rule is needed for this calculation? ______________

What strength of medication should be given per dose?

What is the volume of medication to be given per dose?

Continued

Posttest, cont.

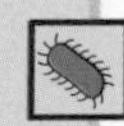
21. A child with a BSA of 0.9 m^2 is ordered codeine 15 mg/m^2 q6h prn for a severe aching related to influenza, not to exceed 60 mg/day.

What strength of medication should be administered per dose?

The strength available is 15 mg/5 mL.

What volume of the oral liquid should be administered per dose?

Is the dosage within acceptable range if the child receives the medication q6h? ____________

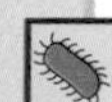
22. Prescription: Cefzil q24h for a 37.5-lb child at a rate of 7.5 mg/kg q12h

Stock strength: Cefzil (cefprozil) 125 mg/5 mL oral suspension

How many mL are needed per dose?

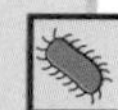
23. Prescription: amoxicillin for a 6-month-old infant / usual adult dose 500 mg qid

Stock strengths available: amoxicillin 125 mg/5 mL oral suspension

What method should be used? ____________

How many milliliters are needed per dose using this strength?

24. Prescription: Lanoxin for a 40-lb child based on 6 mcg/kg per *day* in **2 *divided doses***

Stock strength: Lanoxin (digoxin) Pediatric Elixir 50 mcg (0.05 mg)/mL

How many mL are needed ***per dose****?*

Posttest, cont.

25. A physician orders medication A 100 mg tid for a 60-lb child with a BSA of 0.85 m^2. Medication A can be dosed at 118 mg/m^2 tid or 10–12 mg/kg/day **in 3 divided doses**. *What is the* ***dose*** *calculated using BSA?*

Is the ordered dose adequate for the child? ____________

What is the range for one dose using body weight?

Is the ordered dose within this range? ____________

CHAPTER 13

Calculations With Ratio and Percentage Strengths

OBJECTIVES

1. Discuss the types of percentage strength.
2. Calculate the amount of solute in premade intravenous preparations.
3. Calculate the amount of active ingredient expressed in percentage strength.
4. Discuss the types of ratio strengths.
5. Convert from ratio to percentage strength, and from percentage strength to ratio.

KEY WORDS

Medication strength Concentration of active ingredient in a medication

Percentage strength An amount of active ingredient per 100 parts total ($x/100 = x\%$)

qs Quantity sufficient or required

qs ad Quantity sufficient to make

Ratio strength Expression of strength of weak solutions or liquid preparations; one part active ingredient in *x* parts total (1:*x*)

Solute The smaller portion of a solution; the component to be dissolved in the solvent

Solvent The larger portion of a solution; the component doing the dissolving; aka diluent

Pretest

If you are already comfortable with the subject matter, perform the following calculations to test your knowledge. If not, work your way through the chapter and return to them for extra practice. Show your calculations.

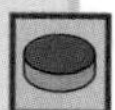

1. *How many grams of sodium chloride are in 1,000 mL of ½ NS?*
2. *How many grams of amino acids are in 300 mL of 5.5% Travasol (amino acids)?*
3. *If 12 g of medication are dissolved in 100 mL of solution, what is the percentage strength?*
4. *How many milliliters of a 25% solution will provide 5 g of active ingredient?*

Pretest, cont.

5. *If a 1 g vial of powdered medication is diluted to 10 mL, what is the strength in mg/mL?*

6. *What is the percentage strength of a 50 mg/mL solution?*

7. *How many grams of zinc oxide are needed to prepare 30 g of a 1.5% zinc oxide ointment?*

8. *What is the concentration in mg/mL of a 1:2,000 solution?*

9. *How many grams of sodium chloride are in 1,000 mL NS?*

10. *How many grams of dextrose are in 500 mL of D5W?*

11. A physician orders 250 mL D5W.

    How many grams of dextrose will the patient receive?

12. A physician orders 500 mL D5 ½ NS q8h as a continuous infusion.

    How many grams of dextrose will the patient receive in 8 hours?

    How many grams of sodium chloride will the patient receive in 8 hours?

Continued

Pretest, cont.

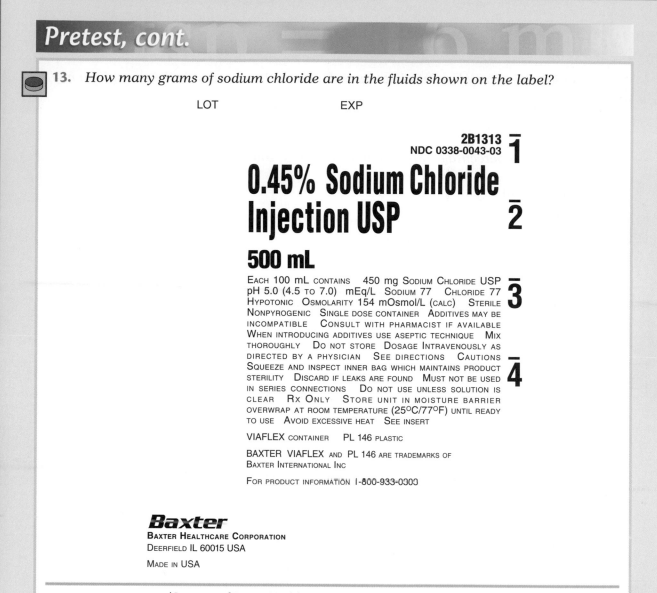
13. *How many grams of sodium chloride are in the fluids shown on the label?*

LOT EXP

2B1313
NDC 0338-0043-03

0.45% Sodium Chloride Injection USP

1 2

500 mL

EACH 100 mL CONTAINS 450 mg SODIUM CHLORIDE USP pH 5.0 (4.5 TO 7.0) mEq/L SODIUM 77 CHLORIDE 77 HYPOTONIC OSMOLARITY 154 mOsmol/L (CALC) STERILE NONPYROGENIC SINGLE DOSE CONTAINER ADDITIVES MAY BE INCOMPATIBLE CONSULT WITH PHARMACIST IF AVAILABLE WHEN INTRODUCING ADDITIVES USE ASEPTIC TECHNIQUE MIX THOROUGHLY DO NOT STORE DOSAGE INTRAVENOUSLY AS DIRECTED BY A PHYSICIAN SEE DIRECTIONS CAUTIONS SQUEEZE AND INSPECT INNER BAG WHICH MAINTAINS PRODUCT STERILITY DISCARD IF LEAKS ARE FOUND MUST NOT BE USED IN SERIES CONNECTIONS DO NOT USE UNLESS SOLUTION IS CLEAR RX ONLY STORE UNIT IN MOISTURE BARRIER OVERWRAP AT ROOM TEMPERATURE (25°C/77°F) UNTIL READY TO USE AVOID EXCESSIVE HEAT SEE INSERT

3 4

VIAFLEX CONTAINER PL 146 PLASTIC

BAXTER VIAFLEX AND PL 146 ARE TRADEMARKS OF BAXTER INTERNATIONAL INC

FOR PRODUCT INFORMATION 1-800-933-0303

Baxter
BAXTER HEALTHCARE CORPORATION
DEERFIELD IL 60015 USA
MADE IN USA

Pretest, cont.

14. A label reads Zephiran chloride 0.2%.

Interpret (w/v): ______________________________

How many grams are in 500 mL?

15. A label reads sodium hypochlorite 10%.

Interpret (w/v): ______________________________

How many grams are in 240 mL?

16. *How many grams of silver nitrate are in 250 mL of a 1:500 silver nitrate solution?*

How many milligrams of silver nitrate are necessary to prepare 250 mL of this solution?

What is the percentage strength of this solution?

17. A physician orders 5 mL of epinephrine 1% added to 45 mL of sterile water.

What is the weight in milligrams of the epinephrine that has been added?

18. A physician orders Prostigmin 0.4 mg IM stat.

How many milliliters of Prostigmin 1:2,000 are needed for this dose?

19. A dentist orders an antiseptic mouthwash of sodium bicarbonate 1:40.

How many grams of sodium bicarbonate are needed to make 6 oz of mouthwash?

20. *How many mL of boric acid solution are needed to prepare 500 mL of a 1:20 v/v solution?*

Continued

INTRODUCTION

Percentage and ratio strengths are two additional methods for indicating **medication strength**, the amount or concentration of active ingredient present in medications. When the **solute** or active ingredient is described as part of the total amount of preparation, the product may be labeled as **percentage strength** or **ratio strength**. Both express an amount of medication per unit of volume or weight of a total liquid or solid preparation. The labels indicate percentage strength, such as Lidocaine 1%, or ratio strength, such as epinephrine 1:1,000. Many medications expressed in ratio or percentage strengths also list the active ingredient amount, usually in the metric system, on the label. As with all medications, consider the total volume or weight of medication in the container to determine the total amount of active ingredient.

Ratio strengths are usually used for liquid medications with a *very low* concentration of active ingredients. Percentage strengths frequently express the amount of active ingredients in medications, the amount of solutes in premade intravenous (IV) solutions, and the strengths of various wound dressings and soaks.

Types of Percentage Strength

Percentage strength is always interpreted as an amount out of 100. It is used to describe various solutions and topically applied drugs. There are three basic types:

1. weight in volume (w/v) $= \dfrac{x \text{ g}}{100 \text{ mL}}$

This is read as *x* grams of active ingredient in 100 milliliters of total solution.

For example, 10% calcium gluconate injection has 10 g of calcium gluconate in 100 mL of total solution and 5% dextrose in water (D5W) has 5 g of dextrose in 100 mL of total solution. Normal saline (NS; 0.9% sodium chloride) has 0.9 g of sodium chloride in 100 mL of total solution.

2. volume in volume (v/v) $= \dfrac{x \text{ mL}}{100 \text{ mL}}$

This is read as *x* milliliters of active ingredient in 100 milliliters of total solution.

For example, 5% hydrogen peroxide solution has 5 mL of hydrogen peroxide in 100 mL of total solution.

3. weight in weight (w/w) $= \dfrac{x \text{ g}}{100 \text{ g}}$

This is read as *x* grams active ingredient in 100 grams of total preparation.

For example, 1% hydrocortisone cream has 1 g hydrocortisone in 100 g of total cream.

Working with the last two types may get confusing because *both* the active ingredient and total preparation have the same unit. Label them with an *a* or a *t* to help identify the active ingredient measurement and the total preparation measurement. The total preparation value will *always* be 100 when interpreting percentage strengths.

$$\frac{x \text{ mL}_{(a)}}{100 \text{ mL}_{(t)}} \text{ or } \frac{x \text{ g}_{(a)}}{100 \text{ g}_{(t)}}$$

TECH NOTE

Percentage strength is always *x*/100.

TABLE 13.1 Abbreviations for Common Intravenous Solutions

ABBREVIATION	SOLUTION
NS	0.9% Sodium chloride or normal saline
½ NS	0.45% Sodium chloride or half-normal saline
D5W	Dextrose 5% in water
D10W	Dextrose 10% in water
D5LR	Dextrose 5% in lactated Ringer's
RL or LR	Ringer's lactate or lactated Ringer's
D5NS	Dextrose 5% in 0.9% sodium chloride
D5 ½ NS	Dextrose 5% in 0.45% sodium chloride

TECH NOTE

All w/v percentage or ratio strength preparations are g/mL, so any question involving milligrams requires the conversion factor of 1,000 mg = 1 g and any question involving liters requires the conversion factor of 1,000 mL = 1 L. These are multistep problems that are more easily solved using dimensional analysis (DA).

Calculating Amounts of Solutes in Intravenous Fluids

The ingredients found in prepared IV fluids, such as dextrose or sodium chloride, are expressed in percentage strengths. These fluids are labeled with the percentage of solute found in the total solution. D5W, or 5% dextrose in water, indicates that 5% dextrose is present in the total solution, with water as the solvent. Remember that percentage is always based on 100, so the percentage is shown per 100 mL of solution, indicating that 5 g of dextrose is found in 100 mL of fluid. However, if the solution is larger than 100 mL, the total weight of the solute must be calculated. The easiest method for calculating the weight of solute in this case is by ratio and proportion (R&P).

In most cases the physician will use common abbreviations for ordering IV fluids. These are shown in Table 13.1. Dextrose solutions are always ordered as a percentage. However, the two most commonly prescribed sodium chloride solutions are sometimes referred to as normal saline, which is 0.9% sodium chloride (0.9% NaCl), and ½ NS, which is 0.45% sodium chloride (0.45% NaCl). These solutions have 0.9 g of NaCl and 0.45 g of NaCl per 100 mL, respectively.

Always begin percentage strength calculations by identifying the known value. Whatever the percentage strength is, place that number over 100. Then set up your unknown equivalent. The easiest method for calculating the amount of solute is by using R&P.

EXAMPLE 13.1

A physician orders 500 mL D5W for a patient.

What is the weight in grams of dextrose in this bag of fluids?

$$\frac{5\text{ g dextrose}}{100\text{ mL total solution}} = \frac{x}{500\text{ mL total solution}}$$

$$100x = 2{,}500\text{ g dextrose}$$

$$x = 25\text{ g dextrose}$$

There are 25 g of dextrose in 500 mL of the above fluids.

EXAMPLE 13.2

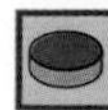

*How many **milligrams** of sodium chloride are in 250 mL of NS (0.9% sodium chloride)?*

The known information is 0.9 g NaCl/100 mL total solution.

This is a multistep problem requiring the conversion from grams to milligrams, so use DA.

$$\text{mg} = \frac{1{,}000\text{ mg}}{1\text{ g}} \bullet \frac{0.9\text{ g}}{100\text{ mL}} \bullet \frac{250\text{ mL}}{1} = 2{,}250\text{ mg}$$

There are 2,250 mg of NaCl in 250 mL of NS.

At this point in working with pharmaceutical calculations, some find it easy to convert between grams and milligrams mentally so that the calculation can be done with R&P as follows and then converted mentally to milligrams.

$$\frac{0.9\text{ g}}{100\text{ mL}} = \frac{x}{250\text{ mL}}$$

$$100x = 225\text{ g}$$

$$x = 2.25\text{ g, which is then converted to } 2{,}250\text{ mg}$$

TECH NOTE

Percentage is based on 100, so *x*% indicates that *x* (g or mL) is found in 100 (g or mL) of total product. When calculating combination products such as D5NS, there are 5 g of dextrose **and** 0.9 g of NaCl per 100 mL.

EXAMPLE 13.3

A physician orders 500 mL of 5.5% Travasol (amino acids) to be used in a total parenteral nutrition bag. How many grams of amino acids will be provided?

$$\frac{5.5\text{ g amino acids}}{100\text{ mL total solution}} = \frac{x}{500\text{ mL}}$$

$$100x = 2{,}750\text{ g}$$

$$x = 27.5\text{ g}$$

Practice Problems A

Calculate the amount of solute found in the IV fluids. Show your work.

1. *How many grams of dextrose are in 250 mL of D10W?*

2. *What is the weight in grams of dextrose in the IV?*

LOT EXP

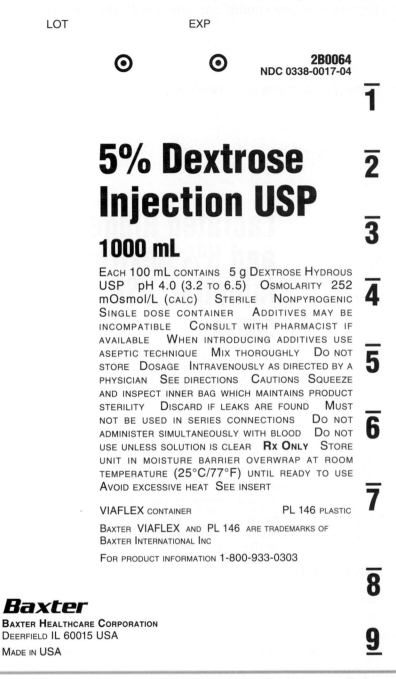

2B0064
NDC 0338-0017-04

1

5% Dextrose Injection USP

2

3

1000 mL

EACH 100 mL CONTAINS 5 g DEXTROSE HYDROUS USP pH 4.0 (3.2 TO 6.5) OSMOLARITY 252 mOsmol/L (CALC) STERILE NONPYROGENIC SINGLE DOSE CONTAINER ADDITIVES MAY BE INCOMPATIBLE CONSULT WITH PHARMACIST IF AVAILABLE WHEN INTRODUCING ADDITIVES USE ASEPTIC TECHNIQUE MIX THOROUGHLY DO NOT STORE DOSAGE INTRAVENOUSLY AS DIRECTED BY A PHYSICIAN SEE DIRECTIONS CAUTIONS SQUEEZE AND INSPECT INNER BAG WHICH MAINTAINS PRODUCT STERILITY DISCARD IF LEAKS ARE FOUND MUST NOT BE USED IN SERIES CONNECTIONS DO NOT ADMINISTER SIMULTANEOUSLY WITH BLOOD DO NOT USE UNLESS SOLUTION IS CLEAR **RX ONLY** STORE UNIT IN MOISTURE BARRIER OVERWRAP AT ROOM TEMPERATURE (25°C/77°F) UNTIL READY TO USE AVOID EXCESSIVE HEAT SEE INSERT

4

5

6

7

VIAFLEX CONTAINER PL 146 PLASTIC

BAXTER VIAFLEX AND PL 146 ARE TRADEMARKS OF BAXTER INTERNATIONAL INC

FOR PRODUCT INFORMATION 1-800-933-0303

8

Baxter

BAXTER HEALTHCARE CORPORATION
DEERFIELD IL 60015 USA
MADE IN USA

9

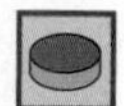

3. *What is the weight in grams of sodium chloride in 500 mL of D5LR?*
Note: Since the weight of sodium chloride in this IV is provided in milligrams/100 mL, change the weight of sodium chloride to g before using it in an R&P or use DA starting with "grams equals" and follow with the conversion factor.

What is the weight in grams of dextrose?

LOT EXP

2B2073
NDC 0338-0125-03

Lactated Ringer's and 5% Dextrose Injection USP

500 mL

1 2 3 4

EACH 100 mL CONTAINS 5 g DEXTROSE HYDROUS USP 600 mg SODIUM CHLORIDE USP 310 mg SODIUM LACTATE 30 mg POTASSIUM CHLORIDE USP 20 mg CALCIUM CHLORIDE USP pH 5.0 (4.0 TO 6.5) mEq/L SODIUM 130 POTASSIUM 4 CALCIUM 2.7 CHLORIDE 109 LACTATE 28 HYPERTONIC OSMOLARITY 525 mOsmol/L (CALC) STERILE NONPYROGENIC SINGLE DOSE CONTAINER **NOT FOR USE IN THE TREATMENT OF LACTIC ACIDOSIS** ADDITIVES MAY BE INCOMPATIBLE CONSULT WITH PHARMACIST IF AVAILABLE WHEN INTRODUCING ADDITIVES USE ASEPTIC TECHNIQUE MIX THOROUGHLY DO NOT STORE DOSAGE INTRAVENOUSLY AS DIRECTED BY A PHYSICIAN SEE DIRECTIONS CAUTIONS SQUEEZE AND INSPECT INNER BAG WHICH MAINTAINS PRODUCT STERILITY DISCARD IF LEAKS ARE FOUND MUST NOT BE USED IN SERIES CONNECTIONS DO NOT ADMINISTER SIMULTANEOUSLY WITH BLOOD DO NOT USE UNLESS SOLUTION IS CLEAR RX ONLY STORE UNIT IN MOISTURE BARRIER OVERWRAP AT ROOM TEMPERATURE (25°C/77°F) UNTIL READY TO USE AVOID EXCESSIVE HEAT SEE INSERT

VIAFLEX CONTAINER PL 146 PLASTIC

BAXTER VIAFLEX AND PL 146 ARE TRADEMARKS OF BAXTER INTERNATIONAL INC

FOR PRODUCT INFORMATION 1-800-933-0303

Baxter

BAXTER HEALTHCARE CORPORATION
DEERFIELD IL 60015 USA
MADE IN USA

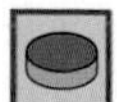 4. *What is the weight of sodium chloride in grams in the fluids shown below?*

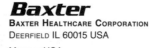

LOT EXP

2B1313
NDC 0338-0043-03 1

0.45% Sodium Chloride
Injection USP 2

500 mL

Each 100 mL contains 450 mg Sodium Chloride USP
pH 5.0 (4.5 to 7.0) mEq/L Sodium 77 Chloride 77 3
Hypotonic Osmolarity 154 mOsmol/L (calc) Sterile
Nonpyrogenic Single dose container Additives may be
incompatible Consult with pharmacist if available
When introducing additives use aseptic technique Mix
thoroughly Do not store Dosage Intravenously as
directed by a physician See directions Cautions
Squeeze and inspect inner bag which maintains product 4
sterility Discard if leaks are found Must not be used
in series connections Do not use unless solution is
clear Rx Only Store unit in moisture barrier
overwrap at room temperature (25°C/77°F) until ready
to use Avoid excessive heat See insert

VIAFLEX container PL 146 plastic

BAXTER VIAFLEX and PL 146 are trademarks of
Baxter International Inc

For product information 1-800-933-0303

Baxter
Baxter Healthcare Corporation
Deerfield IL 60015 USA
Made in USA

5. *How many grams of dextrose are in 1 L of 3% dextrose?*

If only 400 mL of the IV are administered, how many grams did the patient receive?

6. *How many grams of dextrose are in 50 mL of D5W?*

7. A physician orders 1 L of D10 ½ NS.

   How many grams of dextrose will the patient receive?

   How many grams of sodium chloride will the patient receive?

8. *How many grams of dextrose are in 500 mL of D50W (50% dextrose solution)?*

9. A physician orders 300 mL of 5.5% Travasol (amino acids) in a total parenteral nutrition bag.

   How many grams of amino acids will be provided?

10. A physician orders 250 mL of 8.5% Travasol (amino acids) in a total parenteral nutrition bag.

    How many grams of amino acids will be provided?

Calculations With Percentage Strength

Percentages are also used for some liquid and semisolid medications to show different strengths, such as 1% lidocaine. When interpreting percentage labels, the amount of medication is expressed as either weight per volume (solid in liquid) such as 0.9% sodium chloride solution, weight per weight (solid in solid) such as 1% hydrocortisone cream, or volume per volume (liquid in liquid) such as 70% isopropyl alcohol, which is 70 mL of alcohol with enough sterile water to make 100 mL of total solution.

EXAMPLE 13.4

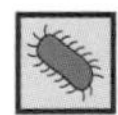

Interpret the following medication: 15% neomycin solution (w/v)

15 g of neomycin in 100 mL of total solution

What is the strength in mg/mL? Use DA because the answer has two units.

$$\frac{\text{mg}}{\text{mL}} = \frac{1{,}000\ \text{mg}}{1\ \text{g}} \bullet \frac{15\ \text{g}}{100\ \text{mL}} = 150\ \text{mg/mL}$$

EXAMPLE 13.5

How many grams of neomycin are in 200 mL of 15% neomycin solution (w/v)?

$$\frac{15\text{ g}}{100\text{ mL}} = \frac{x}{200\text{ mL}} \quad x = 30\text{ g}$$

How many milligrams of neomycin are in 4 oz of 15% solution?

Use DA because this involves two conversion factors.

$$\text{mg} = \frac{1{,}000\text{ mg}}{1\text{ g}} \bullet \frac{15\text{ g}}{100\text{ mL}} \bullet \frac{30\text{ mL}}{1\text{ oz}} \bullet \frac{4\text{ oz}}{1} = 18{,}000\text{ mg}$$

How much neomycin powder is needed to make 50 mL of 15% neomycin solution?

$$\frac{15\text{ g}}{100\text{ mL}} = \frac{x}{50\text{ mL}}$$

$$x = 7.5\text{ g}$$

EXAMPLE 13.6

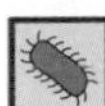

A physician orders 3,000 mL of 15% neomycin solution to use for irrigation of a wound.

The available neomycin is 0.5 g tablets.

How many grams of neomycin are needed to fulfill the order?

$$\frac{15\text{ g}}{100\text{ mL}} = \frac{x}{3{,}000\text{ mL}} \quad x = 450\text{ g}$$

How many tablets of neomycin are needed?

$$\frac{0.5\text{ g}}{1\text{ tab}} = \frac{450\text{ g}}{x} \quad x = 900\text{ tabs}$$

The answer to how many tablets are needed can be obtained in one step with DA.

$$\text{tabs} = \frac{1\text{ tab}}{0.5\text{ g}} \bullet \frac{15\text{ g}}{100\text{ mL}} \bullet \frac{3{,}000\text{ mL}}{1} = 900\text{ tabs}$$

Percentage strength can be determined when given the amount of active ingredient in a total amount of product.

EXAMPLE 13.7

What is the percentage strength of a solution containing 25 g of active ingredient in 500 mL of total solution?

$$\frac{x\text{ g}}{100\text{ mL}} = \frac{25\text{ g}}{500\text{ mL}} \quad x = 5\text{, therefore } 5\text{ g}/100\text{ mL} = 5\%$$

Percentage strength can also be used to determine how many milliliters contain a specific amount of medication, which is necessary when calculating a specific dosage that is needed.

EXAMPLE 13.8

How many mL of a 25% solution will provide 5 g of active ingredient?

$$\frac{25\text{ g}}{100\text{ mL}} = \frac{5\text{ g}}{x\text{ mL}}$$

$x = 20$ mL

EXAMPLE 13.9

How many milliliters of D50W (50% dextrose) should be administered to a hypoglycemic patient to provide 150 mg of dextrose?

Think of this as, "How much 50% dextrose contains 150 mg?"

In situations when the dose is ordered in milligrams, use DA and invert the percentage:

$$\text{mL} = \frac{100\text{ mL}}{50\text{ g}} \bullet \frac{1\text{ g}}{1{,}000\text{ mg}} \bullet \frac{150\text{ mg}}{1} = 0.3\text{ mL}$$

TECH NOTE

Fractional values may be inverted as necessary as long as the units of the numerators and denominators of both fractions are in the same position with R&P and as long as the units are in the correct position to cancel with DA.

When making a specific quantity of a *solution*, there is no way to know exactly how much solvent is needed. The abbreviations **qs** or **qs ad** will be seen with many formulation instructions. These mean *quantity sufficient* and *quantity sufficient to make*, respectively. Once the amount of solute is calculated, the solvent is added in a quantity sufficient to make the total solution. For instance, in Example 13.6, the instructions would be as follows:

900 Neomycin 0.5 g tablets; qs ad 3,000 mL with sterile water

Even v/v solutions do not always add as expected. For example, making 100 mL of 70% alcohol requires 70 mL of 100% alcohol in 100 mL total solution. Adding 30 mL of water in this instance does not make 100 mL of total solution because the alcohol molecules fit in between the water molecules, resulting in a smaller total volume. Thus the instructions would read as follows:

70 mL 100% alcohol, qs ad 100 mL with water

EXAMPLE 13.10

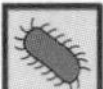

How many milliliters of 15% neomycin solution can be made from 150 g neomycin?

$$\frac{15\text{ g}}{100\text{ mL}} = \frac{150\text{ g}}{x}$$

$x = 1{,}000$ mL

How would the formulation instructions read for this preparation?

neomycin 150 g

qs ad sterile water 1,000 mL

Practice Problems B

Interpret the strengths of the medications as g/100 mL, mL/100 mL, or g/100 g.

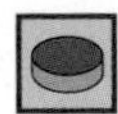

1. 7.5% magnesium sulfate solution (w/v)

____

What is the strength in mg/mL?

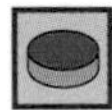

2. 5% sodium chloride solution (w/v)

____

What is the strength in mg/mL?

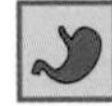

3. 0.5% glycerol solution (w/v)

____

What is the strength in mg/mL?

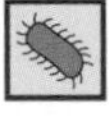

4. 5% formaldehyde solution (w/v)

____

What is the strength in mg/mL?

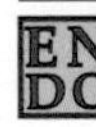

5. 1% hydrocortisone cream (w/w)

____

What is the strength in $mg_{(a)}/g_{(t)}$?

6. ciprofloxacin ophthalmic solution 0.3%

Interpret (w/v): ______________________________

____

How many milligrams of active ingredient are in a 2.5-mL bottle?

7. Betadine solution (10% povidone-iodine)

Interpret (w/v): ______________________________

____

How many grams of povidone-iodine are present in a 3.78-L bottle?

8. Mucomyst-20 (20% acetylcysteine solution)

Interpret (w/v): ______________________________

____

How many grams are in one 10-mL vial?

9. A physician orders 1 L of a 10% boric acid solution to be used for compresses.

How many grams of boric acid are needed for this order?

10. *How many grams of sucrose are needed to make 500 mL of a 75% solution?*

How many grams are needed to make 1,000 mL?

How many grams are needed to make 250 mL?

11. *How many milliliters of 10% solution can be made from 750 g of active ingredient?*

How many liters is this?

12. A 20-mL vial contains 50 mg/mL.

What is the total weight of the medication in the vial in grams?

What is the percentage strength of the medication?

13. *How many grams of boric acid are needed to make 60 mL of a 5% solution?*

14. *What total volume of 2.5% solution can be prepared from 75 g of sucrose?*

How would the formula instructions for this solution be written?

15. How many milliliters of D50W (50% dextrose) should be administered to a hypoglycemic patient to provide 300 mg of dextrose? Hint: How much 50% dextrose contains 300 mg?

16. *How many grams of dextrose are needed to prepare 3 L of a 10% solution?*

17. How many 650 mg tablets of sodium bicarbonate are needed to prepare 325 mL of a 1% sodium bicarbonate solution? Hint: Use DA starting with tabs = 1 tab/650 mg.

How much solvent is needed?

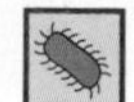
18. *How many milliliters of 10% silver nitrate solution are needed to provide 150 mg of silver nitrate?*

19. *What is the percentage strength of a solution containing 10 g in 200 mL?*

20. *What is the percentage strength of a 6 mg/mL w/v solution?*

Types of Ratio Strengths

The numerical amount of active ingredient in ratio strengths is *always* 1. Ratio strength is expressed as 1:*x*, with *x* representing the total amount of product. It is frequently used to describe solutions with a very small amount of active ingredient. The three types are as follows:

1. weight : volume 1 g : *x* mL

   This is read as 1 gram of active ingredient in *x* milliliters of total solution.
   For example, epinephrine 1:1,000 is 1 g of epinephrine in 1,000 mL of total solution.

2. volume : volume 1 mL : *x* mL

   This is read as 1 milliliter of active ingredient in *x* milliliters of total solution.
   For example, 1:15 sodium hypochlorite solution is 1 mL sodium hypochlorite in 15 mL of total solution.

3. weight : weight 1 g : *x* g

   This is read as 1 gram of active ingredient in *x* grams of total preparation.
   For example, a 1:500 hydrocortisone cream contains 1 g of hydrocortisone in 500 g of total product.

   Performing calculations with the last two types may be confusing because *both* the active ingredient and total preparations have the same unit. Label them as follows to help identify the active ingredient measurement and the total preparation measurement:

   $1\ mL_{(a)} : x\ mL_{(t)}$ or $1\ g_{(a)} : x\ g_{(t)}$

TECH NOTE

Ratio strength is always in the form of 1:*x*.

TECH NOTE

Ratio strength is typically used to describe liquid medications with very low concentrations.

Calculations with Ratio Strength

EXAMPLE 13.11

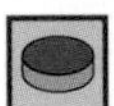

Interpret the following: 1:1,000 sodium bicarbonate solution

1 g of sodium bicarbonate in each 1,000 mL of total solution

How many grams of sodium bicarbonate are in 300 mL of 1:1,000 sodium bicarbonate solution?

$$\frac{1\text{ g sodium bicarbonate}}{1{,}000\text{ mL total solution}} = \frac{x}{300\text{ mL}} \quad x = 0.3\text{ g}$$

What is the strength in mg/mL?

$$\frac{\text{mg}}{\text{mL}} = \frac{1{,}000\text{ mg}}{1\text{ g}} \bullet \frac{1\text{ g}}{1{,}000\text{ mL}} = 1\text{ mg/mL}$$

EXAMPLE 13.12

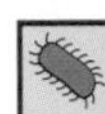

A physician orders 75 mL of a 1:15 sodium hypochlorite solution to be used in the office.

How many grams of sodium hypochlorite are needed to prepare the solution?

$$\frac{1\text{ g}}{15\text{ mL}} = \frac{x}{75\text{ mL}} \quad x = 5\text{ g}$$

How many milliliters of solvent are needed? qs to 75 mL

When ratio strength questions involve the use of milligrams, a conversion factor is needed since weight-to-volume and weight-to-weight ratio strengths are expressed as 1 g : x mL and 1 g/ x g.

EXAMPLE 13.13

How many milliliters of epinephrine 1:1,000 solution are needed to provide a 0.5 mg IM dose?

$$\text{mL} = \frac{1{,}000\text{ mL}}{1\text{ g}} \bullet \frac{1\text{ g}}{1{,}000\text{ mg}} \bullet \frac{0.5\text{ mg}}{1} = 0.5\text{ mL}$$

EXAMPLE 13.14

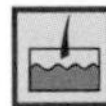

What ratio strength solution is made by dissolving Benadryl (diphenhydramine) 50 mg in a lotion to make 150 mL?

Begin by changing 50 mg to 0.05 g:

$$\frac{0.05\text{ g}}{150\text{ mL}} = \frac{1\text{ g}}{x} \quad 0.05x = 150\text{ mL} \quad x = 3{,}000\text{ mL}$$

Ratio strength = 1 : 3,000

Practice Problems C

Interpret the strengths of the medications as 1 g/ x mL, 1 mL/ x mL, or 1 g/ x g.

1. epinephrine solution 1:10,000 (w/v)

   ____

   How many grams are in 100 mL of solution?

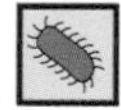

2. 1:100 potassium permanganate solution (w/v)

   ____

   How many grams are in 200 mL of solution?

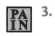

3. 1:50,000 lidocaine solution (w/v)

   ____

   How many grams are in 20 mL of solution?

   How many micrograms are in 20 mL of solution?

   What is the strength in milligrams per milliliter?

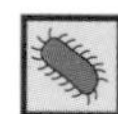

4. 1:1,000 Zephiran chloride solution

   ____

   How many grams are in 100 mL of solution?

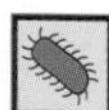

5. *How many grams of sodium perborate are in 200 mL of 1:50 solution?*

   How many grams are in 100 mL of solution?

6. *How many grams of epinephrine are in 1 mL of epinephrine 1:1,000?*

   What is the strength in milligrams per milliliter?

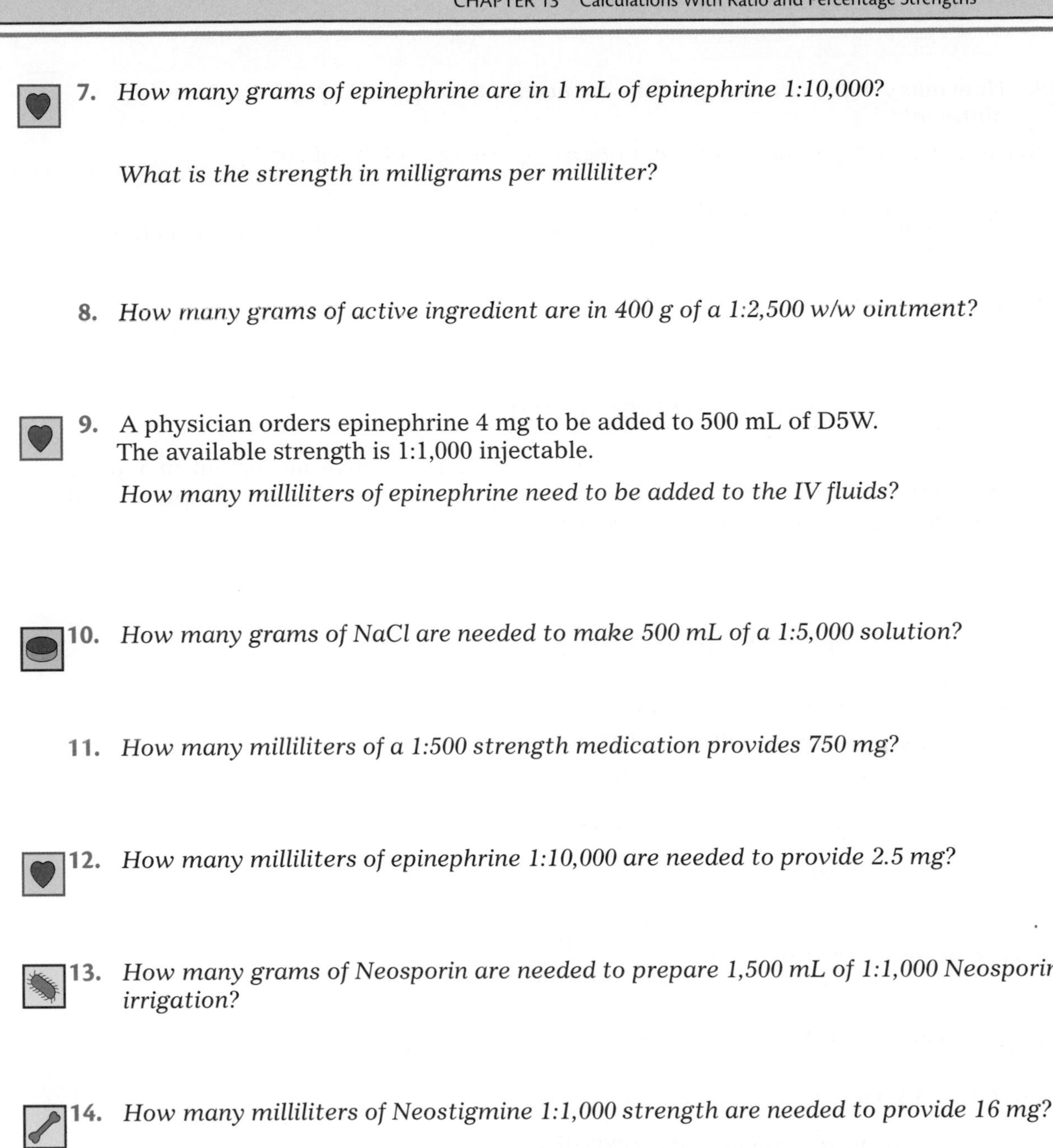

7. *How many grams of epinephrine are in 1 mL of epinephrine 1:10,000?*

   What is the strength in milligrams per milliliter?

8. *How many grams of active ingredient are in 400 g of a 1:2,500 w/w ointment?*

9. A physician orders epinephrine 4 mg to be added to 500 mL of D5W. The available strength is 1:1,000 injectable.

   How many milliliters of epinephrine need to be added to the IV fluids?

10. *How many grams of NaCl are needed to make 500 mL of a 1:5,000 solution?*

11. *How many milliliters of a 1:500 strength medication provides 750 mg?*

12. *How many milliliters of epinephrine 1:10,000 are needed to provide 2.5 mg?*

13. *How many grams of Neosporin are needed to prepare 1,500 mL of 1:1,000 Neosporin irrigation?*

14. *How many milliliters of Neostigmine 1:1,000 strength are needed to provide 16 mg?*

15. *A medication contains 5 mg/mL. What is the ratio strength of the solution?*

16. *What is the concentration in mg/mL of a 1:2,000 solution?*

17. *What is the ratio strength of a 4 mg/mL w/v solution?*

18. *How many grams of Neosporin powder are needed to prepare 2 L of a 1:1,000 w/v bladder irrigation?*

19. *How many mg of active ingredient are needed to prepare 60 g of a 1:2,500 w/w ointment?*

20. *How many milligrams are in one 10-mL pre-filled syringe of epinephrine injection 1:10,000?*

Changing From Ratio to Percentage Strength

Set up an R&P that asks the question, "If there is 1 part active ingredient in x parts total preparation, how many parts of active ingredient would be in 100 parts total preparation?"

$$\frac{1}{x} = \frac{x}{100}$$

EXAMPLE 13.15

What is the percentage strength of a 1:10,000 w/v solution?

If there is 1 g active ingredient in 10,000 mL, how many grams would be in 100 mL?

$$\frac{1\text{ g}}{10{,}000\text{ mL}} = \frac{x}{100\text{ mL}}$$ 1 times 100 equals 100, divided by 10,000 equals 0.01

This means there are 0.01 g in 100 mL: $\frac{0.01\text{ g}}{100\text{ mL}}$

Answer: 0.01%

EXAMPLE 13.16

What is the percentage strength of a 1:200 w/w ointment?

If there is 1 g active ingredient in 200 g total, how many $g_{(a)}$ would be in $100g_{(t)}$?

$$\frac{1\text{ g}_{(a)}}{200\text{ g}_{(t)}} = \frac{x}{100\text{ g}_{(t)}}$$ 1 times 100 equals 100, divided by 200 equals 0.5

This means that there are 0.5 g in 100 g: $\frac{0.5\text{ g}_{(a)}}{100\text{ g}_{(t)}}$

Answer: 0.5%

A shortcut for changing ratio strength to percentage strength is to express the ratio as a fraction and multiply it by 100. That is essentially what is being done with the R&P method.

EXAMPLE 13.17

What is the percentage strength of a 1:5,000 preparation?

$$\frac{1}{5,000} \bullet 100 = 0.02\%$$

Practice Problems D

Change the following ratio strengths to percentage strengths.

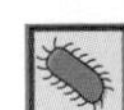

1. 1:100 potassium permanganate solution (w/v)

2. 1:50 Chloraseptic solution (w/v)

3. 1:1,000 Zephiran chloride solution (w/v)

4. 1:2,000 (w/v)

5. 1:100,000 (w/v)

6. *What is the percentage strength of 1:500 silver nitrate solution?*

   How many milligrams of silver nitrate are in 250 mL?

Changing From Percentage to Ratio Strength

Set up an R&P that asks the question, "If there are x parts active ingredient in 100 parts total preparation, 1 part active ingredient would be in how much total preparation?"

$$\frac{x}{100} = \frac{1}{x}$$

EXAMPLE 13.18

What is the ratio strength of a 0.04% w/v solution?

$$\frac{0.04 \text{ g}}{100 \text{ mL}} = \frac{1 \text{ g}}{x} \quad \text{1 times 100 divided by } 0.04 = 2{,}500$$

This means that there is 1 g in 2,500 mL, so the answer is 1:2,500.

EXAMPLE 13.19

What is the ratio strength of a 0.01% w/v solution?

$$\frac{0.01 \text{ g}}{100 \text{ mL}} = \frac{1 \text{ g}}{x} \quad \text{1 times 100 divided by } 0.01 = 10{,}000\text{, so the answer is 1:10,000.}$$

Practice Problems E

Change the following percentage strengths to ratio strengths.

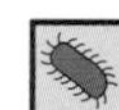

1. 5% formaldehyde solution

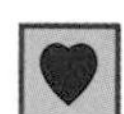

2. 0.01% epinephrine solution

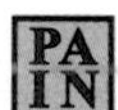

3. 1% lidocaine solution

4. 0.025% solution

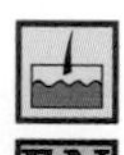

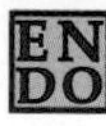

5. 0.5% hydrocortisone cream

6. 0.25% cream

REVIEW

Percentage and ratio strengths represent the amount of solute in a total amount of product. Percentage strength depicts the amount of active ingredient (solute) in 100 parts of total product. Ratio strength depicts one part of active ingredient (solute) in a total amount of product. Ratio strength is most commonly used for weak solutions. Percentage is expressed using % as an indication of the amount of active ingredient in a medication. The ratio is divided by a colon (:) to separate the solute and the solution.

Posttest

Show all calculations.

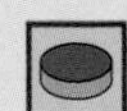

1. A.

LOT EXP

2B1064
NDC 0338-0089-04

5% Dextrose and 0.9% Sodium Chloride Injection USP

1000 mL

EACH 100 mL CONTAINS 5 g DEXTROSE HYDROUS USP 900 mg SODIUM CHLORIDE USP pH 4.0 (3.2 TO 6.5) mEq/L SODIUM 154 CHLORIDE 154 HYPERTONIC OSMOLARITY 560 mOsmol/L (CALC) STERILE NONPYROGENIC SINGLE DOSE CONTAINER ADDITIVES MAY BE INCOMPATIBLE CONSULT WITH PHARMACIST IF AVAILABLE WHEN INTRODUCING ADDITIVES USE ASEPTIC TECHNIQUE MIX THOROUGHLY DO NOT STORE DOSAGE INTRAVENOUSLY AS DIRECTED BY A PHYSICIAN SEE DIRECTIONS CAUTIONS SQUEEZE AND INSPECT INNER BAG WHICH MAINTAINS PRODUCT STERILITY DISCARD IF LEAKS ARE FOUND MUST NOT BE USED IN SERIES CONNECTIONS DO NOT USE UNLESS SOLUTION IS CLEAR RX ONLY STORE UNIT IN MOISTURE BARRIER OVERWRAP AT ROOM TEMPERATURE (25°C/77°F) UNTIL READY TO USE AVOID EXCESSIVE HEAT SEE INSERT

VIAFLEX CONTAINER PL 146 PLASTIC

BAXTER VIAFLEX AND PL 146 ARE TRADEMARKS OF BAXTER INTERNATIONAL INC

Baxter
BAXTER HEALTHCARE CORPORATION
DEERFIELD IL 60015 USA
MADE IN USA

FOR PRODUCT INFORMATION 1-800-933-0303

1 2 3 4 5 6 7 8 9

B.

LOT EXP

2B0064
NDC 0338-0017-04

5% Dextrose Injection USP

1000 mL

EACH 100 mL CONTAINS 5 g DEXTROSE HYDROUS USP pH 4.0 (3.2 TO 6.5) OSMOLARITY 252 mOsmol/L (CALC) STERILE NONPYROGENIC SINGLE DOSE CONTAINER ADDITIVES MAY BE INCOMPATIBLE CONSULT WITH PHARMACIST IF AVAILABLE WHEN INTRODUCING ADDITIVES USE ASEPTIC TECHNIQUE MIX THOROUGHLY DO NOT STORE DOSAGE INTRAVENOUSLY AS DIRECTED BY A PHYSICIAN SEE DIRECTIONS CAUTIONS SQUEEZE AND INSPECT INNER BAG WHICH MAINTAINS PRODUCT STERILITY DISCARD IF LEAKS ARE FOUND MUST NOT BE USED IN SERIES CONNECTIONS DO NOT ADMINISTER SIMULTANEOUSLY WITH BLOOD DO NOT USE UNLESS SOLUTION IS CLEAR RX ONLY STORE UNIT IN MOISTURE BARRIER OVERWRAP AT ROOM TEMPERATURE (25°C/77°F) UNTIL READY TO USE AVOID EXCESSIVE HEAT SEE INSERT

VIAFLEX CONTAINER PL 146 PLASTIC

BAXTER VIAFLEX AND PL 146 ARE TRADEMARKS OF BAXTER INTERNATIONAL INC

FOR PRODUCT INFORMATION 1-800-933-0303

Baxter
BAXTER HEALTHCARE CORPORATION
DEERFIELD IL 60015 USA
MADE IN USA

1 2 3 4 5 6 7 8 9

How many grams of NaCl are in the IV labeled A?

How many grams of dextrose are in the IV labeled A?

If a patient receives 400 mL of IV B, how much dextrose has been administered?

Continued

Posttest, cont.

2. A label for isopropyl alcohol reads "70% isopropyl alcohol in water."

   Interpret (v/v): ______________________________

   How many milliliters of alcohol are in a pint of 70% alcohol?

3. *How many g of dextrose are in 250 mL of D5W?*

4. *How many g of sodium chloride are in 1,000 mL of ½ NS?*

5. *How many grams of amino acids are in 300 mL of 5.5% Travasol (amino acids)?*

6. *If 12 g of medication are dissolved in 100 mL of solution, what is the percentage strength?*

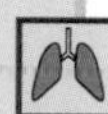

7. A label reads "epinephrine 2.25% nebulizer."

   Interpret (w/v): ______________________________

   ____

   How many milligrams are in a 0.5-mL vial?

   What is the strength in milligrams per milliliter?

8. 2% Xylocaine (lidocaine) Viscous Solution is used for oral anesthesia

   How many milligrams of lidocaine are in each milliliter of fluids?

9. *If 15 mg of amoxicillin is added to 100 mL of sterile water, what is the percentage strength of the total volume of prepared medication? (Do not round.)*

10. *How many grams of NaCl are in a 25-mL vial of 1:25 solution?*

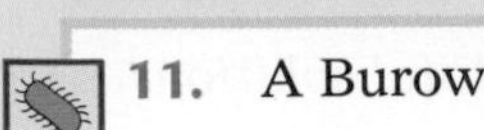

Posttest, cont.

11. A Burow's solution 100 mL label reads 1:7.5 v/v.

    What is the volume of Burow's solution in the total volume? (Round to tenths.)

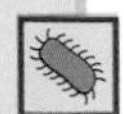

12. *How many milliliters of vinegar are in 500 mL of a 1:200 (v/v) vinegar solution?*

    What is the percentage strength of this solution?

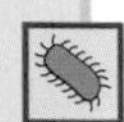

13. *How many grams of silver nitrate are in 1 L of 1:25,000 silver nitrate solution to be used by a urologist?*

    What is the percentage strength of silver nitrate?

14. *How many milligrams of a drug are in 1.5 mL of a 1:5,000 solution?*

15. *How many milligrams of a drug are found in 1,500 mL of a 1:750 solution?*

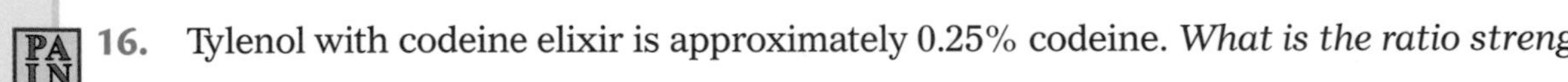

16. Tylenol with codeine elixir is approximately 0.25% codeine. *What is the ratio strength?*

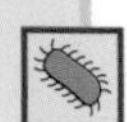

17. A physician asks for 0.4 g of potassium permanganate qs ad 480 mL of solution. *(Round to hundredths.)*

    What is the percentage strength of the solution?

    What is the ratio strength of the solution?

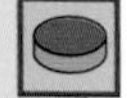

18. A physician orders a 1-L solution of sodium chloride 1:200.

    How many grams of sodium chloride would be necessary to complete this order?

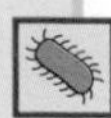

19. *How many milliliters of a 10% solution of boric acid can be prepared from 20 g of boric acid?*

Continued

Posttest, cont.

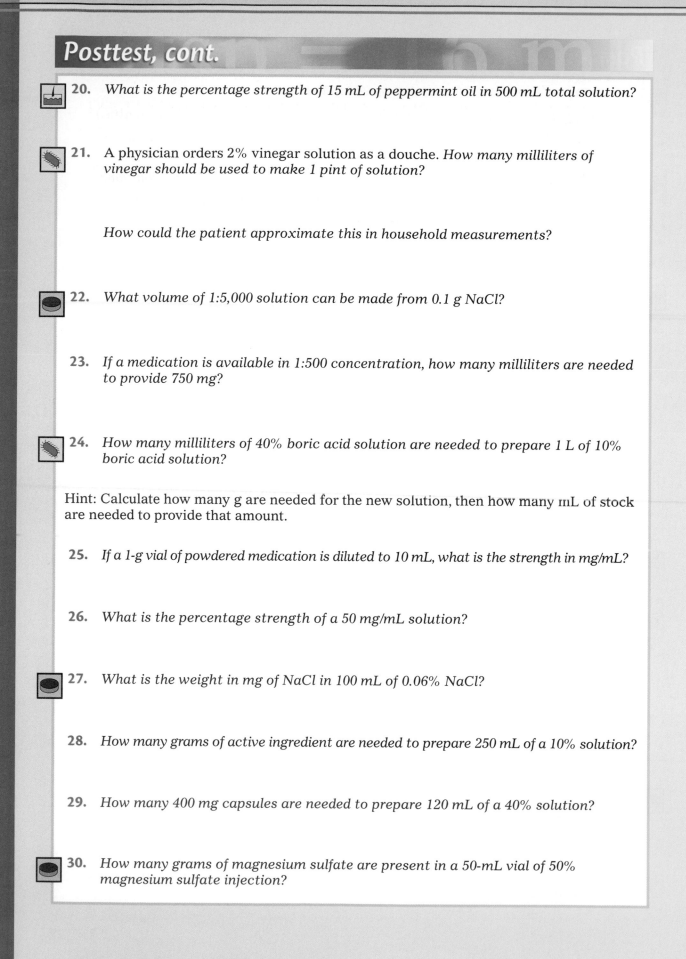

20. *What is the percentage strength of 15 mL of peppermint oil in 500 mL total solution?*

21. A physician orders 2% vinegar solution as a douche. *How many milliliters of vinegar should be used to make 1 pint of solution?*

How could the patient approximate this in household measurements?

22. *What volume of 1:5,000 solution can be made from 0.1 g NaCl?*

23. *If a medication is available in 1:500 concentration, how many milliliters are needed to provide 750 mg?*

24. *How many milliliters of 40% boric acid solution are needed to prepare 1 L of 10% boric acid solution?*

Hint: Calculate how many g are needed for the new solution, then how many mL of stock are needed to provide that amount.

25. *If a 1-g vial of powdered medication is diluted to 10 mL, what is the strength in mg/mL?*

26. *What is the percentage strength of a 50 mg/mL solution?*

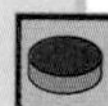
27. *What is the weight in mg of NaCl in 100 mL of 0.06% NaCl?*

28. *How many grams of active ingredient are needed to prepare 250 mL of a 10% solution?*

29. *How many 400 mg capsules are needed to prepare 120 mL of a 40% solution?*

30. *How many grams of magnesium sulfate are present in a 50-mL vial of 50% magnesium sulfate injection?*

REVIEW OF RULES

- To calculate the amount of drug in a specific amount of preparation using R&P, write the percentage or ratio strength as a fraction to show the amount of medication found in the total amount (known value) and set up an equivalent fraction to solve for the unknown value.
- To change from ratio strength to percentage strength, write the ratio as a fraction and set it equal to $x/100$.
- To change from percentage to ratio strength, write the percentage as a fraction and set it equal to $1/x$.
- To calculate milligrams per milliliter, use the known strength with the conversion factor 1,000 mg = 1 g in a DA equation, cancel units, and solve.

Calculations for Simple Dilutions, Mixtures, and Compounding

OBJECTIVES

1. Dilute stock medications to the required strength.
2. Use alligation to calculate the weight/volume of stock medications needed to prepare a desired strength.
3. Interpret formulations for compounded preparations.
4. Enlarge and decrease compounding formulations as necessary.

KEY WORDS

Alligation alternate Mathematical method for determining the amount of *two* preparations of different strengths needed to prepare a required strength in between the two; aka **tic-tac-toe**

Alligation medial Calculation method by which the weighted average strength of a mixture of *two or more* preparations of known quantity and concentration may be determined

Compounding Preparing a product in the pharmacy that is *not* commercially available in the ordered dose or dosage form

Compounding formulation Similar to a recipe; list of all components needed for a particular compound

Diluent An inert component in which other components (such as the active ingredient) are mixed or dissolved (e.g., water, elixir, cream, or ointment bases); aka **base or solvent**

Dilution Process of making a more concentrated preparation less concentrated by adding a diluent containing no active ingredient, such as water or white petrolatum

Nonsterile compounding The mixing of two or more components that does not require a sterile environment

Stock medication Medication provided by a manufacturer and kept on hand for use in preparing medication orders or prescriptions

Pretest

If you are already comfortable with the subject matter, perform the following calculations to test your knowledge. If not, work your way through the chapter and return to them for extra practice. Round answers to tenths if needed. Show calculations.

1. Order: 30 g of 0.5% ointment. The available stock is 10% ointment.

   How many grams of 10% ointment are needed to prepare 30 g?

   How many grams of petrolatum are needed to prepare 30 g?

Pretest, cont.

2. Prepare 400 mL of 6% solution from a stock solution of 7.5% and water.

   How many milliliters of the stock solution are needed?

   How many milliliters of the solvent (water) are needed?

3. Prepare 15 g of 0.5% ointment from a stock ointment of 2.5% and petrolatum.

   How many grams of 2.5% ointment are needed?

   How many grams of petrolatum are needed?

4. An order is to supply 10 mL of a drug at 50 mg/mL. The stock supply is 2.5 g/10 mL.

   How many milliliters of stock solution (solute) are needed?

   How many milliliters of solvent (diluent) are needed?

5. A physician asks that 500 mL of 10% solution of a medication be prepared. The stock supply of the solution is 75%.

   How many milliliters of stock solution (solute) are needed?

   How many milliliters of solvent (diluent) are needed?

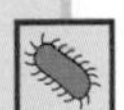

6. A physician asks the pharmacy to prepare 1 L of 1:2,000 silver nitrate solution to be used as an irrigation. The stock solution is 1% silver nitrate solution.

   How many milliliters of silver nitrate stock solution are needed?

   How many milliliters of solvent are needed?

Continued

Pretest, cont.

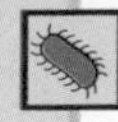

7. Prepare 250 mL of 0.02% benzalkonium chloride solution for cleansing skin before surgery. Stock strength of the solute is 1%.

   How many milliliters of stock solution (solute) are needed?

   How many milliliters of solvent (diluent) are needed?

   *How many mL of solute would be needed to prepare 500 mL of solution?*__________

   *How many mL of solvent would be needed to prepare 500 mL of solution?*__________

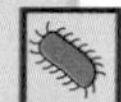

8. A medical office needs 0.25 L of 10% Lysol solution for disinfecting the office.

   How many milliliters of 25% Lysol are needed to prepare the solution?

   How many milliliters of water (solvent) are needed?

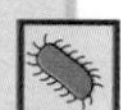

9. A physician orders 100 mL of 50% creosol solution.

   How many milliliters of 1:2 creosol solution are needed to prepare this order?

   How many milliliters of solvent should be added?

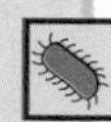

10. *How many mL of 10% methyl salicylate are needed to prepare 3 pints of 4% lotion?*

    Hint: Remember that the units must be in the same measurement.

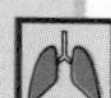

11. Epinephrine is available as a 5% solution.

    How many milliliters are needed to prepare 10 mL of 2.5% solution of epinephrine?

Pretest, cont.

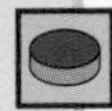

12. Use a 15% solution of sodium hypochlorite to prepare 1 L of 0.15% solution.

    How many milliliters of sodium hypochlorite are needed?

    How many milliliters of solvent should be added?

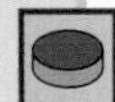

13. A stock L contains 50% sodium bicarbonate. A physician desires 2 L of 6% solution.

    How many milliliters of 50% sodium bicarbonate are needed to fill this order?

    How many milliliters of solvent are needed?

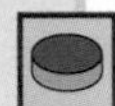

14. A physician orders 20% KCl solution. There are 10% and 50% solutions in stock.

    How much of each are needed to prepare 100 mL of 20% solution?

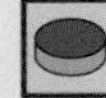

15. Prepare 750 mL of 0.75% sodium chloride solution from 0.9% NaCl and 0.45% NaCl.

    How many mL of each solution need to be combined to fill this order?

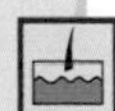

16. A physician orders 50 g of 1.5% hydrocortisone ointment.

    100 g of 5% ointment and 100 g of petrolatum ointment base are in stock.

    Hint: Just because 100 g of 5% hydrocortisone ointment and 100 g of petrolatum are available does not mean that the entire amount will be used.

    How many grams of each are needed?

Continued

Pretest, cont.

17. A physician orders 30 g of ointment containing 3% of Drug A and 7% of Drug B. Both are available as pure powders (100% strength).
How many grams of each are needed?

Drug A

Drug B

Ointment base

18. *How much water should be added to 300 mL of a 25% solution to make a 10% solution?*

19. 500 mL of a 1:1,000 solution is diluted to 1,000 mL.
What is the ratio strength of the new solution?

20. *How much of a 4% solution is needed to make 120 mL of a 1:200 solution?*

INTRODUCTION

This chapter covers simple **dilution**, mixtures, and basic compounding calculations. Dilution may be necessary to compound a lower strength ordered by a physician. **Stock medications** may be ordered from manufacturers in concentrated strengths for storage and economic reasons and diluted later with a specific volume or weight of **diluent**. By using stock solutions that are purer and stronger forms of a drug, larger amounts of medication may be prepared from small quantities. The solute and solvent (aka diluent) may be in solid form, as well as liquid. A solid diluent is frequently referred to as a base. The pharmacy staff is responsible for diluting to fill prescriptions and medication orders.

A solution is made of a solute (the drug dissolved) and a solvent or diluent (the substance in which the solute is dissolved). Various methods may be used to determine the amount of concentrated medication and diluent needed to compound an ordered strength. Simple dilution is used when *one* product concentration is combined with a diluent that has zero concentration of active ingredient, thus making a more concentrated product less concentrated. Alligation alternate is a mathematical calculation that determines the necessary amount of *two* different concentrations required to compound a concentration in between the two. Alligation medial can be used to calculate the concentration of a mixture of *two or more* different concentrations of medications.

The following procedures will make these calculations easier:

1. *Convert all strengths to percents before performing calculations.*
2. *Convert all amounts to metric measurements before performing calculations.*

Compounding is preparing medications according to prescription orders for medications that are *not* commercially available in the desired strength or dosage form. Whereas many solutions are prepared for use in an inpatient setting, other compounded prescriptions are intended for dispensing to a consumer. Compounding medications in specially ordered doses has become very popular, giving rise to compounding pharmacies. Special populations such as geriatric or pediatric patients often require different medication strengths than those found in stock medications from the manufacturer. Individualized hormone replacement therapy, as well as other medication, requires specialty compounding. Specific requirements governing the process of **nonsterile compounding** are found in USP <795>. Pharmacy technicians can earn special certification in compounding.

TECH NOTE

All compounding calculations should be performed using the metric system.

Simple Dilution of Stock Medications

With simple dilution, the amount of active ingredient or solute remains the same and the solvent amount is increased, thus reducing the strength of the **stock medication**. Simple dilution is the process of making a more concentrated product less concentrated by adding a diluent with no active ingredient. Common diluents with no active ingredient (0% medication strength) include sterile water (SW) for liquid solutions and petrolatum (ointment base) for solid solutions. Various cream bases are also used.

The following method can be used to solve dilution problems as long as they involve only *one* stock strength solution to be diluted with a diluent containing no active ingredient—for example, a 50% solution diluted with water to a 40% solution or a 1% ointment diluted to a 0.25% ointment with petrolatum. The most important thing to remember with this method is that the volume units of the stock and desired product should be milliliters, the weight units must be the same, and the strength units of the stock and desired product must be the same; usually both are changed to percentages.

Equation for Diluting Stock Liquids

Volume units must be the same! Strength units must be the same!

$$SV \bullet SS = DV \bullet DS$$

SV = stock volume SS = stock strength

DV = desired volume DS = desired strength

Equation for Diluting Stock Solids

Weight units must be the same! Strength units must be the same!

$SW \bullet SS = DW \bullet DS$

SW = stock weight   SS = stock strength

DW = desired weight   DS = desired strength

Solute—substance being dissolved; the stock strength that is being diluted
Solvent—substance doing the dissolving; diluent or base with 0% active ingredient
To determine the amount of solvent needed, use one of the following:

Solvent volume = DV – SV

Solvent weight = DW – SW

Follow these steps to solve simple dilution problems:

1. Identify the *three known variables,* and use a question mark to identify the unknown variable.
2. Make certain that the units of volume or weight are the same and the units of strength are the same.
   a. Calculations for compounding and diluting are *always* performed in the metric system, so change all weight and volume measurements to the metric system before placing them in the formula.
   b. It is easiest to work with percentage strengths so convert all strengths to percentages. (The formula will work no matter what strength designation is used as long as both the SS and DS are the *exact* same unit. If using both in ratio strength, write them as fractions and solve. As long as both values are in mg/1 mL, that value can be used also.)
3. Write the equation.
4. Fill in the variables, and solve for the unknown value.
5. Round to the nearest whole number if dealing with large quantities, tenths if dealing with small quantities, and hundredths if dealing with answers less than zero.

EXAMPLE 14.1

A physician orders 250 mL of 15% solution to be prepared from a stock supply of 80% solution.

How many milliliters of stock solution and solvent are needed?

SV = ?   SS = 80%   DV = 250 mL   DS = 15%

$SV \bullet SS = DV \bullet DS$

$SV \bullet 80\% = 250 \text{ mL} \bullet 15\%$

$SV \bullet 80 = 3{,}750 \text{ mL}$ (Divide both sides by 80.)

$SV = 46.9 \text{ mL} = 47 \text{ mL}$

How many milliliters of the solvent/diluent (sterile water) are needed?

Solvent volume = DV − SV

Solvent volume = 250 mL − 47 mL = 203 mL

Directions: Combine 47 mL of 80% solution and 203 mL of sterile water to make 250 mL of 15% solution.

EXAMPLE 14.2

An order is received for 10 g of petrolatum to be combined with 25 g of 0.2% hydrocortisone ointment.

This example, where the unknown value is the desired strength, is for instructional purposes only since one would not mix ingredients without having a specific desired strength.

What is the strength of the final product?

$SW = 25\text{ g} \quad SS = 0.2\% \quad DW = 35\text{ g } (10\text{ g} + 25\text{ g}) \quad DS = ?$

$SW \bullet SS = DW \bullet DS$

$25\text{ g} \bullet 0.2\% = 35\text{ g} \bullet DS$

$5\% = 35 \bullet DS$

$5\% = 35 \bullet DS$ (Divide both sides by 35.)

$0.14\% = DS$

TECH NOTE

It is always important to identify your variables in order to identify the unknown value. Any time a question states, "A physician orders" or "prepare," what follows will be the desired value.

EXAMPLE 14.3

Prepare 500 mL 5% creosol solution from a stock solution of creosol 1:10.

How many milliliters of stock solution and solvent are needed?

$SV = ? \quad SS = 1:10 \quad DV = 500\text{ mL} \quad DS = 5\%$

The first step is to convert the 1:10 strength to a percent so that it can be used in the formula.

$\frac{1\text{ g}}{10\text{ mL}} = \frac{x}{100\text{ mL}} \quad x = 10\text{ g} \quad 1:10 = 10\%$

$SV = ? \quad SS = 10\% \quad DV = 500\text{ mL} \quad DS = 5\%$

$SV \bullet SS = DV \bullet DS$

$SV \bullet 10\% = 500\text{ mL} \bullet 5\%$

$SV \bullet 10 = 2{,}500\text{ mL}$ (Divide both sides by 10.)

$SV = 250\text{ mL}$

Solvent volume = DV − SV

Solvent volume = 500 mL − 250 mL = 250 mL

Directions: Combine 250 mL of 1:10 creosol solution with 250 mL of sterile water to make 500 mL of 5% solution.

TECH NOTE

When diluting a product to exactly half the original strength, equal parts of solute and solvent will be used.

EXAMPLE 14.4

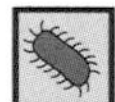

Prepare 1 oz of a 0.002% solution of merthiolate from a 1% stock solution.

How many milliliters of stock solution and solvent are needed?

SV = ? SS = 1% DV = 1 oz DS = 0.002%

First, convert oz to mL so that the calculations can be performed in the metric system.

1 oz = 30 mL is a common conversion factor.

SV = ? SS = 1% DV = 30 mL DS = 0.002%

SV • SS = DV • DS

SV • 1% = 30 mL • 0.002%

SV = 0.06 mL Such a small volume of stock should not be rounded.

Solvent volume = DV − SV

Solvent volume = 30 mL − 0.06 mL = 29.94 mL

Directions: Combine 0.06 mL of 1% solution and 29.94 mL of sterile water to make 30 mL of 0.002% solution.

EXAMPLE 14.5

A physician orders 15 mL of a 10 mcg/mL dilution of a drug for a child.

The stock medication is 40 mcg/mL.

How many milliliters of stock solution and solvent are needed?

SV = ? SS = 40 mcg/mL DV = 15 mL DS = 10 mcg/mL

Because both strengths are in the *exact* same unit (mcg/1 mL), they can be used in this formula:

SV • SS = DV • DS

SV • 40 mcg/mL = 15 mL • 10 mcg/mL

SV • 40 = 150 mL (Divide both sides by 40.)

SV = 3.75 mL = 3.8 mL

Solvent volume = DV − SV

Solvent volume = 15 mL − 3.8 mL = 11.2 mL

Directions: Combine 3.8 mL of 40 mcg/mL solution and 11.2 mL of sterile water to make 15 mL of 10 mcg/mL strength solution.

Other variables are sometimes used to represent this equation such as IV or IW and IS, for initial volume or weight and initial strength, and FV or FW and FS, for final volume or weight and final strength. The concept is the same no matter what variables are used to represent the equation.

Practice Problems A

Calculate the following problems. Show your work.

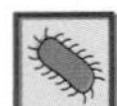

1. Prepare 1 L of Lysol 3% from a stock solution of Lysol 10%.

   How many milliliters of stock solution (solute) are needed?

   How many milliliters of solvent are needed?

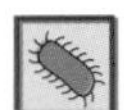

2. Prepare 8 oz of 40% solution of isopropyl alcohol from a 70% stock solution.

   How many milliliters of stock solution (solute) are needed?

   How many milliliters of solvent are needed?

   (Remember, from Ch 13 page 359, what happens when alcohol and water are combined.)

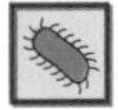

3. Prepare 1.5 L of creosol 1:200 from a 2% stock solution.

   How many milliliters of stock solution (solute) are needed?

   How many milliliters of solvent are needed?

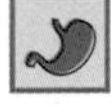

4. A physician orders 250 mL of 15% glycerin solution as an enema. The available stock solution is glycerin 25%.

   How many milliliters of stock solution (solute) are needed?

   How many milliliters of solvent are needed?

5. A physician orders 1 pint of 7.5% dextrose in water. The stock solution is 50%.

   How many milliliters of stock solution (solute) are needed?

   How many milliliters of solvent are needed?

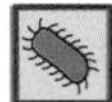

6. *How many milliliters of 20% Zephiran chloride are needed to prepare 8 oz of 7.5% solution?*

   How many milliliters of solvent are needed?

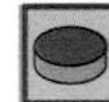

7. 1.5 L of potassium chloride 15% is to be prepared from a 20% stock solution.

   How many milliliters of stock solution (solute) are needed?

   How many milliliters of solvent are needed?

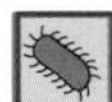

8. A medical office needs 3 L of a 1:10 solution of hypochlorous acid. The stock solution is 25% hypochlorous acid.

   How many milliliters of stock solution (solute) are needed?

   How many milliliters of solvent are needed?

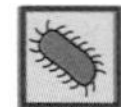

9. A physician orders 8 oz of 2% Betadine solution. The stock solution is 10% Betadine.

   How many milliliters of stock solution (solute) are needed?

   How many milliliters of solvent are needed?

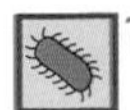

10. Prepare 3 L of hydrogen peroxide 1:40. The stock solution is hydrogen peroxide 5%.

    How many milliliters of stock solution (solute) are needed?

    How many milliliters of solvent are needed?

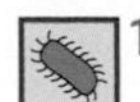

11. Prepare 600 mL of a 2.5% solution from a 10% hydrogen peroxide solution.

    How many milliliters of stock solution (solute) are needed?

    How many milliliters of solvent are needed?

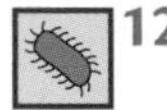

12. Prepare 4 L of a 1:50 solution of potassium permanganate from a 5% potassium permanganate stock solution.

    How many milliliters of stock solution (solute) are needed?

    How many milliliters of solvent are needed?

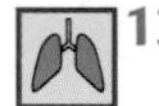

13. Prepare 10 mL of 0.01% adrenaline solution for injection from a 2% adrenaline ampule. *Do not round answer!*

    How many milliliters of stock solution (solute) are needed?

    How many milliliters of solvent are needed?

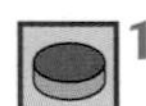

14. A physician orders 500 mL of 2% calcium chloride solution. The stock solution is calcium chloride 10%.

    How many milliliters of stock solution (solute) are needed?

    How many milliliters of solvent are needed?

    If calcium chloride is available in 5-mL ampules, how many ampules are needed?

15. *How many milliliters of a 6% solution can be made from 30 mL of a 36% solution?*

    Hint: Take care when identifying the three known variables.

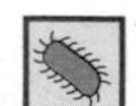

16. A stock solution of 1:50 mercuric chloride is used to prepare 250 mL of 0.02% solution.

    How many milliliters of stock solution (solute) are needed?

    How many milliliters of solvent are needed?

17. *If 300 mL of a 20% stock solution is added to 2.7 L of sterile water, what is the percentage strength of the final solution?* Hint: See Example 14.2.

18. A physician orders 80 mL of a 1:1,000 solution. In stock is a 1:250 solution.

    How many milliliters of stock solution (solute) are needed?

    How many milliliters of solvent are needed?

19. Prepare 1 L of 15% dextrose from a 50% dextrose solution.

    How many mL of 50% dextrose (stock solution) are needed?

    How many mL of solvent (water) are needed?

20. *What is the percentage strength of the resultant solution if 250 mL of a 10% solution is combined with 750 mL of water?*

    Hint: Start with determining the "desired" volume.

CALCULATIONS USING ALLIGATION

Alligation is a mathematical method of solving questions involving the mixing of solutions or compounds possessing different percentage strengths. The process is the same whether dealing with weight or volume solutions.

Alligation Alternate

Alligation alternate, also known as *tic-tac-toe,* is a method that is used to calculate the number of parts of two different percentage strengths of medication that can be mixed together to prepare a third strength that is not available. If a physician orders 20% KCl solution and only 10% and 50% KCl solutions are in stock, the amount of each solution needed to prepare the prescribed amount of the 20% solution can be calculated. This can *only* be achieved when the strength desired is *in between* the two strengths being mixed. Mixing a 5% and a 10% solution cannot result in a 15% solution, but mixing a 5% and a 15% solution can result in a 10% solution.

All strengths should be converted to percentages before performing alligation alternate. As mentioned, the final strength of the mixture must lie somewhere between the strengths of the component parts. This means that the prepared mixture must be stronger than its weakest component and weaker than its strongest component. If the mixture contains more of the weaker component, the prepared mixture will be closer to the strength of the weaker component. If the mixture contains more of the stronger component, the mixture will be closer to the strength of the stronger component.

Alligation alternate:

Step 1—Prepare a graph, similar to a box for tic-tac-toe.

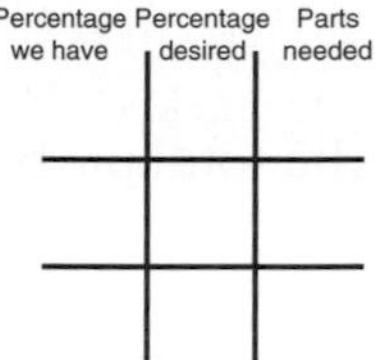

Step 2—Place the strength to be calculated in the center box.

Percentage we have	Percentage desired	Parts needed
	70%	

Step 3—Place the highest percentage concentration in the upper left corner.

Percentage we have	Percentage desired	Parts needed
95%		
	70%	

Step 4—Place the lowest percentage concentration in the lower left corner.

Percentage we have	Percentage desired	Parts needed
95%		
	70%	
50%		

Step 5—Subtract the center square amount from the upper left corner amount, and place the answer in the lower right corner to determine the number of parts of the lowest percentage concentration to be used in the mixture.

Percentage we have	Percentage desired	Parts needed
95%		
	70%	
50%		25 parts

Step 6—Subtract the lower left corner amount from the center square amount, and place the answer in the upper right corner to reveal the number of parts of the highest percentage concentration to be used in the mixture.

Percentage we have	Percentage desired	Parts needed
95%		20 parts
	70%	
50%		25 parts

Step 7—Add the two calculated parts in the far-right column to find the total parts of the two ingredients in the compound.

Percentage we have	Percentage desired	Parts needed
95%		20 parts
	70%	
50%		25 parts 45 parts

Step 8—When a specific quantity is included in the order, the two parts of the mixture are written as fractions of the whole, and each is multiplied by the total amount needed to calculate the exact amount of each ingredient needed.

EXAMPLE 14.6

Prepare 1,000 mL of 70% w/v solution from a 50% solution and a 95% solution.

Step 1—Draw a graph.
Step 2—Place the desired strength in the center box.
Step 3—Place the highest percentage concentration in the upper left corner.
Step 4—Place the lowest percentage concentration in the lower left corner.
Step 5—Subtract the center square amount from the upper left corner amount, and place the answer in the lower right corner to determine the parts of the lowest percentage concentration needed.
Step 6—Subtract the lower left corner amount from the center box amount, and place the answer in the upper right corner to reveal the parts of the highest percentage concentration needed.
Step 7—Add both parts to obtain the total parts in the compound.

To prepare this solution: Use 20 parts of 95% and 25 parts of 50%

$\frac{20}{45}$ will be 95% solution, which can be written to the right of the top row of the graph

$\frac{25}{45}$ will be 50% solution, which can be written to the right of the bottom row of the graph

These are the fractional parts that are used to find the exact amounts to be mixed when the total weight or volume of the compound is indicated.

! TECH ALERT

Notice that the answers are in parts, not unit values.

Step 8—The total desired amount of the 70% solution is 1,000 mL.

$$\frac{20 \text{ parts}}{45 \text{ parts}} \times 1,000 \text{ mL} = 444.4 \text{ mL} = 444 \text{ mL of } 95\% \text{ solution}$$

$$\frac{25 \text{ parts}}{45 \text{ parts}} \times 1,000 \text{ mL} = 555.6 \text{ mL} = 556 \text{ mL of } 50\% \text{ solution}$$

Adding the two amounts equals 1,000 mL:

$$444 \text{ mL of } 95\% \text{ solution} + 556 \text{ mL of } 50\% \text{ solution} = 1,000 \text{ mL of } 70\% \text{ solution}$$

TECH NOTE

Always check your calculations to be sure the total volume/weight of the calculated compound equals the desired prescription weight/volume.

Steps 1 to 7 determine the *parts* of each stock medication needed. Step 8 is to determine the volume/weight of each stock medication needed to prepare a *specific* amount.

If one component has a zero percent strength, such as water or petrolatum, the alligation method can still be used by placing a zero in the bottom left square and proceeding in the same manner. The other choice is to use the equation from the dilution section because it is a simple dilution.

Alligation Medial

Alligation medial is a method of calculation that may be used to determine the total percentage strength when *two or more* substances with known quantities and strengths are mixed. This method allows for the rapid calculation of final strengths. The quantities must be expressed in common measurements such as the same weight or volume.

Steps

Step 1—Add the number of milliliters or grams being mixed to obtain the total volume or weight that is being prepared.

Step 2—Multiply the percentage strength of each component, written in decimal form, by the total number of grams or milliliters being used in the preparation, to obtain the total number of g or mL of active ingredient that component will add to the total product as shown in the following equation:

$$\text{Decimal form of percentage strength times g or mL used}$$
$$= \text{g or mL provided by that component}$$

Step 3—Add the amounts of active ingredient provided by each component.

Step 4—Place the total amount of active ingredient over the total amount of milliliters or grams and multiply by 100 to determine the percentage strength of the new product.

EXAMPLE 14.7

What is the final percentage strength of a w/v solution when 300 mL of 95%, 1,000 mL of 70%, and 200 mL of 50% solutions are combined?

Step 1—Add the number of milliliters being mixed to obtain the total volume being prepared.

$$300 \text{ mL} + 1{,}000 \text{ mL} + 200 \text{ mL} = 1{,}500 \text{ mL}$$

Step 2—Determine how many grams of medication are in each quantity to be mixed.

How many grams of active ingredient are in 300 mL of 95% solution?

$$0.95 \times 300 = 285 \text{ g}$$

This calculation is actually a shortcut of the following calculation that was covered in Chapter 13. The shortcut from step 2 can be used in place of the following:

$$\frac{95 \text{ g}}{100 \text{ mL}} = \frac{x}{300 \text{ mL}} \quad 100x = 95 \text{ g} \bullet 300$$

$$x = 285 \text{ g}$$

300 mL of 95% solution contains 285 g of medication

How many grams of active ingredient are in 1,000 mL of 70% solution?

$$0.7 \times 1{,}000 = 700 \text{ g}$$

How many grams of active ingredient are in 200 mL of 50% solution?

$$0.5 \times 200 = 100 \text{ g}$$

Step 3—Add all three amounts.

$$285 \text{ g} + 700 \text{ g} + 100 \text{ g} = 1{,}085 \text{ g}$$

Step 4—Place total number of grams over the total milliliters and multiply by 100.

$$\text{Total number of } \frac{\text{grams}}{\text{milliliters}} \times 100$$

$$\frac{1{,}085 \text{ g}}{1{,}500 \text{ mL}} \times 100 = 72.3\%$$

This is a shortcut for solving a ratio and proportion between the fraction in step 4 and $\frac{x}{100}$ *to determine the percentage strength of the total mixture.*

$$\frac{1{,}085 \text{ g}}{1{,}500 \text{ mL}} = \frac{x}{100 \text{ mL}} \quad 1{,}500\,x = 108{,}500 \text{ g} \quad x = 72.3 \text{ g}$$

$$\text{By definition, } \frac{72.3 \text{ g}}{100 \text{ mL}} = 72.3\%.$$

What is the ratio strength of the final answer?

$$\frac{72.3 \text{ g}}{100 \text{ mL}} = \frac{1 \text{ g}}{x} \quad 72.3x = 100 \text{ mL} \quad x = 1.4$$

The ratio strength is 1:1.4.

TECH NOTE

If the original strengths are provided as ratios, step 1 will be to change the ratio strengths to percentages.

Alligation medial can also be used as a quick means of verifying alligation alternate results.

EXAMPLE 14.8

Use alligation medial to verify the results of Example 14.6.

What is the final percentage strength of a solution when 444 mL of 95% solution is mixed with 556 mL of 50% solution? (It should be 70%.)

Step 1 : $444\ \text{mL} + 556\ \text{mL} = 1{,}000\ \text{mL}$

Step 2: $444\ \text{mL} \times 0.95 = 421.8 = 422\ \text{g}$ of active ingredient

$556\ \text{mL} \times 0.5 = 278\ \text{g}$ of active ingredient

Step 3: $422\ \text{g} + 278\ \text{g} = 700\ \text{g}$ of active ingredient

Step 4 : $\dfrac{700\ \text{g}}{1{,}000\ \text{mL}} \times 100 = 70\%$

This verifies that the calculations in Example 14.6 using alligation alternate are correct.

When performing calculations with v/v or w/w solutions, it may help to label which portion is the active ingredient and which part is the total product because both the amount of active ingredient and the total amount of preparation will have the same unit.

Practice Problems B

Complete these problems using alligations. Round to tenths unless otherwise indicated. Label answers as g or mL and identify the appropriate percentage strength of each.

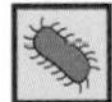

1. *How many milliliters of 6% and 15% sodium hypochlorite solution are needed to prepare 500 mL of a 10% solution?*

2. In stock are two ointment strengths containing 5% and 20% boric acid. *How many grams of each are needed to prepare 1 g of a 12.5% ointment?*

3. A physician orders 20 g of a 15% tannic acid ointment. *How many grams of 12% and 25% tannic acids are needed?* Use alligation medial to verify your answers.

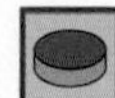

4. Prepare 500 mL of 15% potassium chloride solution using 20% potassium chloride and 5% potassium chloride solution.

   How many milliliters of each solution need to be combined to fill this order?

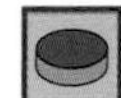

5. Prepare 500 mL of 0.9% sodium chloride solution from a 10% sodium chloride solution.

   How many milliliters of each solution need to be combined to fill this order?

   Hint: The diluent of sterile water necessary for this calculation has 0% sodium chloride. Use alligation alternate and SV • SS = DV • DS and compare your answers.

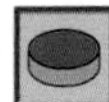

6. Prepare 750 mL of 3% sodium bicarbonate solution from a 15% solution and 1% solution. *How many milliliters of each solution need to be combined to fill this order?*

7. Prepare 200 mL of 10% dextrose solution using 5% dextrose and 50% dextrose solutions. *How many milliliters of each solution need to be combined to fill this order?*

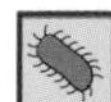

8. Prepare 3 L of 3% Lysol solution using 1.5% Lysol and 5% Lysol solutions. *How many milliliters of each need to be combined to fill this order?* (Round to whole numbers.)

9. A physician orders 50 g of a 7.5% ointment. The available ointments are 2.5% and 15%.

   How many grams of each need to be combined to fill this order?

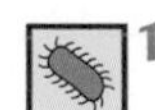

10. Prepare 1,800 mL of 40% alcohol from 10% alcohol and 55% alcohol.

How many milliliters of each solution need to be combined to fill this order?

11. Prepare 500 mL of 4% potassium permanganate solution using 1:10 potassium permanganate solution and 1:50 potassium permanganate solution.

How many milliliters of each solution need to be combined to fill this order?

Hint: Change ratio strengths to percentage strengths first.

12. Prepare 250 mL of 8% dextrose solution from D5W and D10W.

How many milliliters of each solution need to be combined to fill this order?

13. A physician orders 50 mL dextrose 7.5% to be administered IV stat. The available strengths are D5W and D50W. *How many milliliters of each solution are needed?*

14. Prepare 200 mL of 5% potassium chloride. The available potassium chloride is 20%.

How many milliliters of 20% KCl and sterile water need to be combined to fill this order?

15. Prepare 50 mL of 1.8% sodium chloride solution from 0.9% and 5% NaCl. *How many milliliters of each solution are needed?*

16. Prepare 2.5 g of 7.6% ointment from stock strengths of 2.5% and 10%.

How many grams of each need to be combined to fill this order?

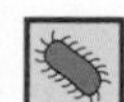

17. A physician orders 1.5 L of 12% Burow's solution to be made from 5% and 25%. *How many milliliters of each solution need to be combined to fill this order?*

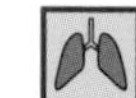

18. A patient is ordered 100 mL of epinephrine 4% for an acute asthma attack. The available epinephrine is 1:10 and 1:100.

    How many milliliters of each solution need to be combined to fill this order?

19. Prepare 30 g of 1% ointment from 0.5% ointment and 5% ointment.

    How many g of 5% and 0.5% ointment are needed?

20. Prepare 400 mL of 6% Travasol solution from 5.5% Travasol and 8.8% Travasol.

    How many mL of each strength are needed?

COMPOUNDING

Developing a Medication Formula From a Prescription

Sometimes physicians order a particular strength of medication that is not manufactured commercially. In these cases, pharmacy personnel need to calculate the correct formula. The compounding pharmacy may maintain a book, similar to a recipe book, containing frequently prescribed formulations of medications. Calculations to determine formulas can be performed using the following methods.

EXAMPLE 14.9

How much hydrocortisone (solute) and how much Eucerin cream (commercially prepared base/solvent with no active ingredient) should be combined to prepare this prescription?

hydrocortisone 2.5% cream 30 g

Amount of hydrocortisone needed:

$$\frac{2.5\ g_{(a)}}{100\ g_{(t)}} = \frac{x}{30\ g_{(t)}}\quad x = 0.75\ g$$

Amount of Eucerin cream needed:

$$30\ g_{(t)} - 0.75\ g_{(a)} = 29.25\ g$$

This question can also be thought of as follows: *How much hydrocortisone (100% powder) and how much Eucerin cream are needed to prepare 30 g of hydrocortisone 2.5% cream?*

Amount of hydrocortisone needed:

$$SW = ?\quad SS = 100\%\quad DW = 30\ g\quad DS = 2.5\%$$

$$SW \bullet SS = DW \bullet DS$$

$$SW \bullet 100\% = 30\ g \bullet 2.5\%$$

$$SW \bullet 100 = 75\ g$$

$$SW = 0.75\ g$$

Amount of Eucerin cream needed: 30 g – 0.75 g = 29.25 g

If more than one active ingredient is to be added to a compound, the strength or amount of each is calculated according to the total amount to be prepared.

EXAMPLE 14.10

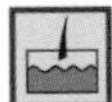

Prepare 1 g of 0.25% menthol and 0.5% phenol in petrolatum. Use DA because the answers are requested in mg, requiring a conversion factor.

How many milligrams of menthol are needed?

$$mg = \frac{1{,}000\ mg}{1\ g} \times \frac{0.25\ g_{(a)}}{100\ g_{(t)}} \times \frac{1\ g_{(t)}}{1} = 2.5\ mg$$

How many milligrams of phenol are needed?

$$mg = \frac{1{,}000\ mg}{1\ g} \times \frac{0.5\ g_{(a)}}{100\ g_{(t)}} \times \frac{1\ g_{(t)}}{1} = 5\ mg$$

How many milligrams of petrolatum are needed?

1 g total product is equal to 1,000 mg.

$$1{,}000\ mg - 2.5\ mg - 5\ mg = 992.5\ mg\ petrolatum$$

Sometimes a compound must be prepared using another strength of commercially prepared product. This can be calculated using strategies from Chapter 13 or simple dilution.

EXAMPLE 14.11

A physician orders 200 g of 2.5% cream. The commercially prepared cream is 10%.

How many grams of active ingredient are needed to prepare 200 g of 2.5% cream?

$$\frac{2.5\ g_{(a)}}{100\ g_{(t)}} = \frac{x}{200\ g_{(t)}}$$

$$x = 5\ g$$

How many grams of 10% cream contain 5 g of active ingredient?

$$\frac{10\ g_{(a)}}{100\ g_{(t)}} = \frac{5\ g_{(a)}}{x} \quad x = 50\ g \text{ of } 10\% \text{ cream provide } 5\ g$$

To compound 200 g of 2.5% cream from 10% cream and a base cream, measure 50 g of 10% cream and add 150 g base.

This question can also be approached as a simple dilution.

How many grams of 10% cream are needed to prepare 200 g of 2.5% cream?

$$SW = ? \quad SS = 10\% \quad DW = 200\ g \quad DS = 2.5\%$$

$$SW \bullet SS = DW \bullet DS$$

$$SW \bullet 10\% = 200\ g \bullet 2{:}5\%$$

$$SW \bullet 10 = 500\ g$$

$$SW = 50\ g \text{ of } 10\% \text{ cream}$$

How many grams of base cream are needed?

$$200\ g - 50\ g = 150\ g \text{ base}$$

Practice Problems C

Calculate the following problems. Show your calculations.

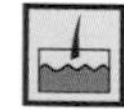

1. A prescription is written to prepare 30 g of 0.05% triamcinolone ointment using Aristocort A Ointment (0.1% triamcinolone) and white petrolatum. *How much of each is needed?*

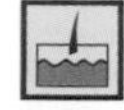
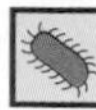

2. *How many grams of 100% zinc oxide and white petrolatum are needed to prepare 4 oz of a 10% ointment?* Hint: Convert ounces to grams first.

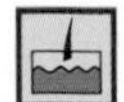

3. A dermatologist writes a prescription for 0.5% menthol and 0.6% phenol in petrolatum to make 30 g of ointment.

   How many grams of menthol are needed?

   How many grams of phenol are needed?

   How many grams of petrolatum are needed?

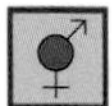

4. Prepare 30 mL of 5 mg/mL tadalafil suspension.

   How many milligrams of tadalafil are needed?

   How many tadalafil 20 mg tablets are needed?

   How much suspending agent is needed?

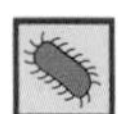

5. Prepare 5 mL of ceftazidime fortified eye drops 50 mg/mL in a hood for sterility.

   How many total milligrams of ceftazidime are needed?

   How many milliliters of ceftazidime 1 g/10 mL sterile injection are needed?

   How much sterile water is needed?

Preparing a Compounded Prescription From a Formula

If the **compounding formulation** is written, the instructions need to be followed exactly to prepare the prescription correctly. The abbreviations **qs**, meaning quantity required, and **qs ad**, meaning quantity sufficient to make, are frequently found in compounding formulations.

The following example illustrates some of the information that can be calculated from a formula.

EXAMPLE 14.12

Mouthwash

tetracycline	*1 g*
nystatin suspension	*60 mL*
diphenhydramine	*48 mL*
dexamethasone	*qs ad 240 mL*

What is the percentage of tetracycline (w/v) in the final compound?

The known information is that there is 1 g of tetracycline in 240 mL, so the question is, *How many grams would be in 100 mL?*

$$\frac{1\ \text{g}}{240\ \text{mL}} = \frac{x}{100\ \text{mL}} \quad x = 0.42\ \text{g (rounded to the hundredths place)}$$

Therefore the strength of tetracycline is 0.42%.

What is the percentage of nystatin (v/v) suspension in the final mixture?

$$\frac{60\ \text{mL}}{240\ \text{mL}} = \frac{x}{100\ \text{mL}} \quad x = 25\ \text{mL}$$

Therefore the strength of nystatin is 25%.

What is the percentage of diphenhydramine (v/v) in the final mixture?

$$\frac{48\ \text{mL}}{240\ \text{mL}} = \frac{x}{100\ \text{mL}} \quad 240x = 4{,}800\ \text{mL} \quad x = 20\ \text{mL}$$

Therefore the strength of diphenhydramine is 20%.

What volume of dexamethasone is needed to prepare the desired volume?

This cannot be determined exactly because it is not known how much volume 1 g of tetracycline will displace, so the answer is qs ad 240 mL.

TECH NOTE

When compounding, it can be helpful to know that 1 mL of water weighs 1 g.

In addition to the abbreviations qs and qs ad, the abbreviation $\overline{\text{aa}}$, meaning *of each,* is frequently found in compounding formulations. When used in a formulation, it means to use equal amounts of each component listed as follows.

EXAMPLE 14.13

A dentist sends a prescription for a mouthwash to swish and spit for pain.

Lidocaine 0.5%

Benadryl

Maalox

Sig: $\overline{\text{aa}}$ *qs 120 mL*

Determine the volume of each medication needed to prepare this prescription.

Because there are three parts to the formulation and there is to be an equal amount of each used, divide 120 mL by 3 to get 40 mL of each component.

Lidocaine	*40 mL*
Benadryl	*40 mL*
Maalox	*40 mL*
Total	*120 mL*

Determine the percentage (v/v) strength of each component.

Each one is one-third of the total, so each would be 33.3%.

Use ratio and proportion to prove this:

$$\frac{40 \text{ mL}}{120 \text{ mL}} = \frac{x}{100 \text{ mL}} \quad 120x = 4{,}000 \text{ mL} \quad x = 33.3 \text{ mL}$$

33.3 mL/100 mL is 33.3%.

A compounding prescription may also be written in parts.

EXAMPLE 14.14

Calculate the amounts required to make 2 oz (60 g) of the following formula:

coal tar	*1 part*
zinc oxide	*5 parts*
wool fat	*10 parts*
white paraffin	*20 parts*

Step 1—Find the total of all of the parts: 1 + 5 + 10 + 20 = 36.

Step 2—Determine how much of each ingredient is needed:

Coal tar:

$$\frac{1 \text{ part}}{36 \text{ parts}} = \frac{x}{60 \text{ g}} \quad 36x = 60 \text{ g} \quad x = 1.7 \text{ g}$$

Zinc oxide (g):

$$\frac{5 \text{ parts}}{36 \text{ parts}} = \frac{x}{60 \text{ g}} \quad 36x = 300 \text{ g} \quad x = 8.3 \text{ g}$$

Wool fat (g):

$$\frac{10 \text{ parts}}{36 \text{ parts}} = \frac{x}{60 \text{ g}} \quad 36x = 600 \text{ g} \quad x = 16.7 \text{ g}$$

White paraffin:

$$\frac{20 \text{ parts}}{36 \text{ parts}} = \frac{x}{60 \text{ g}} \quad 36x = 1{,}200 \text{ g} \quad x = 33.3 \text{ g}$$

Step 3—Check your calculations.

If the calculations are correct, adding all of the parts will equal 60 g.

$$1.7 \text{ g} + 8.3 \text{ g} + 16.7 \text{ g} + 33.3 \text{ g} = 60 \text{ g}$$

Practice Problems D

1. Calculate the amount of grams of each required to make 30 g of the following:

drug B	*1 part*
lanolin	*1 part*
petrolatum	*8 parts*

drug B

lanolin

petrolatum

2. Calculate the amounts needed to prepare 30 g of the following prescription:

salicylic acid	*0.9%*
menthol	*0.4%*
1% triamcinolone cream	*qs ad 30 g*

salicylic acid (mg)

menthol (mg)

1% triamcinolone cream (g)

3. Prepare a solution containing:

hydrochlorothiazide 50 mg tablets	*24*
purified water	*qs ad 120 mL*

What is the strength of the resulting solution in milligrams per milliliter?

4. Prepare a cream from the following formula:

hydrocortisone	*600 mg*
cream base	*29.4 g*

What is the percentage strength of the cream? (Round to a whole number.)

5. Calculate the amount needed to make 120 g of the following ointment:

coal tar	*1 part*
starch	*5 parts*
zinc oxide	*3 parts*
petrolatum	*7 parts*

coal tar

starch

zinc oxide

petrolatum

6. Calculate the amounts of the following ingredients needed to prepare 44 g of ointment.

All-Purpose Nipple Ointment[1]

STOCK[a]	FINAL CONCENTRATION
Bactroban (mupirocin) 2% Ointment	*1%*
betamethasone dipropionate	*0.05%*
miconazole	*2%*
Yellow color 2% solution	*1 drop*
Aquaphor Ointment	*qs 44 g*

[a]If the stock strength is not listed, it is 100% as with betamethasone and miconazole.

mupirocin

betamethasone dipropionate *(Do not round.)*

miconazole

7. Calculate how much of each ingredient is needed to prepare 45 mL of mouthwash.

lidocaine 0.5%	*1 part*
diphenhydramine	*1 part*
Maalox	*1 part*

lidocaine

diphenhydramine

Maalox

8. White Ointment, USP contains 5 parts white wax and 95 parts white petrolatum. *How many grams of each are needed to prepare 180 g?*

Reducing and Enlarging Compounded Prescriptions

When an amount of a compounding formulation requires reducing or enlarging to meet a physician's order, the original amounts in the formulation are used to calculate the new formulation by ratio and proportion.

EXAMPLE 14.15

Decreasing the amount of product

Formulation: 3% ibuprofen gel

ibuprofen	*3 g*
base	*97 g*

Prepare 30 g.

ibuprofen:

$$\frac{3\text{ g}}{100\text{ g}} = \frac{x}{30\text{ g}} \quad 100x = 90\text{ g} \quad x = 0.9\text{ g ibuprofen}$$

Base:

$$\frac{97 \text{ g}}{100 \text{ g}} = \frac{x}{30 \text{ g}} \quad 100x = 2{,}910 \text{ g} \quad x = 29.1 \text{ g base}$$

EXAMPLE 14.16

Increasing the amount of product

Formulation: 3% ibuprofen gel

ibuprofen	*3 g*
base	*97 g*

Prepare 120 g.

ibuprofen:

$$\frac{3 \text{ g}}{100 \text{ g}} = \frac{x}{120 \text{ g}} \quad 100x = 360 \text{ g} \quad x = 3.6 \text{ g ibuprofen}$$

Base:

$$\frac{97 \text{ g}}{100 \text{ g}} = \frac{x}{120 \text{ g}} \quad 100x = 11{,}640 \text{ g} \quad x = 116.4 \text{ g base}$$

TECH NOTE

The amounts calculated when reducing or increasing a formulation must add up to the new amount ordered.

EXAMPLE 14.17

The following recipe is for 10 mg/mL of drug A:

Drug A 100 mg	*#10*
Sterile water	*18 mL*
Cherry flavoring	*5 mL*
Simple syrup	*qs ad 100 mL*

Prepare 4 oz.

Change 4 oz to 120 mL because compounding is *always* calculated using the metric system.

Set up a ratio and proportion:

If 10 tablets are needed to make 100 mL, how many are needed to make 120 mL?

Drug A:

$$\frac{10 \text{ tabs}}{100 \text{ mL}} = \frac{x}{120 \text{ mL}} \quad 100x = 1{,}200 \text{ tabs} \quad x = 12 \text{ tabs}$$

Follow the same process with the other ingredients.

Sterile water: (This will be used to dissolve the crushed tablets.)

$$\frac{18 \text{ mL water}}{100 \text{ mL}} = \frac{x}{120 \text{ mL}} \quad 100x = 2{,}160 \text{ mL water} \quad x = 21.6 \text{ mL water}$$

Cherry flavoring:

$$\frac{5 \text{ mL flavoring}}{100 \text{ mL}} = \frac{x}{120 \text{ mL}} \quad 100x = 600 \text{ mL flavoring} \quad x = 6 \text{ mL flavoring}$$

Simple syrup qs ad 120 mL

Practice Problems E

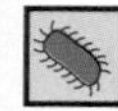

1. A prescription is written for a mouthwash:

tetracycline	*800 mg*
nystatin suspension	*40 mL*
diphenhydramine elixir	*60 mL*
qs ad dexamethasone elixir	*240 mL*

How much of each ingredient is needed to prepare 90 mL?

tetracycline (mg)

nystatin suspension

diphenhydramine elixir

dexamethasone elixir

2. A prescription for a hydrocortisone enema is to be prepared from the following formulation:

hydrocortisone	*4.5 g*
emulsifier	*5 mL*
methylcellulose 1%	*240 mL*
normal saline	*qs ad 500 mL*

How much of each ingredient is needed to prepare 30 mL?

hydrocortisone (mg)

emulsifier

methylcellulose 1%

normal saline

3. *How much of each of the following is needed to make 60 suppositories?*

Glycerin suppositories #20

glycerin	*36 g*
sodium stearate	*3.6 g*
purified water	*1.8 mL*

glycerin

sodium stearate

water

4. *How much of each ingredient is needed to make 4 oz?*

Meloxicam 3 mg/mL Gel[2]

meloxicam	*300 mg*
triethanolamine	*2 g*
carbomer (Carbopol 940)	*1.6 g*
purified water	*qs 100 mL*

meloxicam

triethanolamine

carbomer

purified water

5. *How much of each ingredient is needed to prepare 30 g of the following?* (Do not round.)

ingredient A	*500 mg*
ingredient B	*10 g*
cream base	*109.5 g*

ingredient A

ingredient B

cream base

What is the percentage strength of ingredient A? (Round to nearest tenth.)

6. *How much urea is needed to prepare 18 g of the following formulation?*

urea	*20 g*
propylene glycol	*20 mL*
cream base	*qs to 60 g*

7. *How much of each ingredient is needed to prepare 240 mL of the following syrup?*

sucrose	*85 g*
cherry flavoring	*2 mL*
purified water	*qs ad 100 mL*

sucrose

cherry flavoring

purified water

What is the percentage strength of the sucrose?

8. *How many **grams** of each ingredient are needed to make 90 suppositories?*

Glycerin Suppositories #20

glycerin	*36 g*
sodium stearate	*3.6 g*
purified water	*1.8 mL (same as 1.8 g since the specific gravity of water is 1)*

glycerin

sodium stearate

purified water

What is the percentage of glycerin in this preparation? (Round to nearest whole number.)

REVIEW

Stock supplies in concentrated strengths are often used to prepare compounds that are less concentrated. To prepare the correct strength of medication for a physician's order or to administer a more accurate dose of medication, the stock medication may need dilution. Simple dilution involves adding more solvent to prepare a weaker product. This can be calculated using the following formulas: SV • SS = DV • DS or SW • SS = DW • DS.

When two or more medications are combined, alligation is used. Alligation alternate can be used when combining *two* strengths of medications. However, if the "weighted average" percentage strength is necessary for mixture of *two or more* substances with a known quantity and concentration, alligation medial is used. As a pharmacy technician, you must know how to calculate the strength and must also know the correct method for calculation on the basis of the information given.

Although dilution and alligation calculations are frequently used in inpatient settings, compounding pharmacies may also use these calculations for filling outpatient prescription orders. The pharmacy personnel may need to formulate a prescription, interpret a compounding prescription, or increase or decrease the amount of a compounding prescription.

Posttest

Calculate the following problems using the appropriate method for each. Show your work. Round to tenths, unless otherwise indicated.

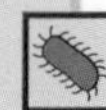

1. *How many milliliters of 1:10 boric acid solution are needed to prepare 100 mL of 5% solution?*

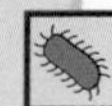

2. An order is written for 1,500 mL of a 1:10 antiseptic solution. Stock solution is 1:5.

   How many milliliters of stock solution (solute) are needed?

   How many milliliters of solvent (diluent) are needed?

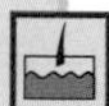

3. A lotion of 5% methyl salicylate is to be prepared for a patient with allergic dermatitis.

   What amount of a 10% methyl salicylate lotion is needed to prepare 240 mL?

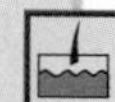

4. 250 mL of 3% calamine lotion is to be prepared from 7.5% calamine lotion.

   How many milliliters of stock solution (solute) are needed?

   How many milliliters of solvent are needed?

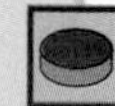

5. A stock pint of sodium bicarbonate contains 60% solution. The physician prescribes 1.5 L of 15% sodium bicarbonate solution.

   Hint: Just because the stock bottle is a pint, the whole pint does not have to be used.

   How many milliliters of stock solution (solute) are needed?

   How many milliliters of solvent are needed?

Posttest, cont.

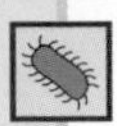

6. A stock boric acid solution of 1:5 is available. Prepare 300 mL of 15% solution.

   How many milliliters of 1:5 strength boric acid are needed?

   How many milliliters of solvent (sterile water) are needed?

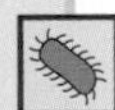

7. A stock boric acid solution of 1:5 is available. Prepare 300 mL of 2% solution.

   How many milliliters of 1:5 strength boric acid are needed?

   How many milliliters of solvent (sterile water) are needed?

8. A liquid is available in a 1:350 concentration. Prepare a pint of 1:500 solution.

   How many milliliters of stock solution (solute) are needed?

   How many milliliters of solvent are needed?

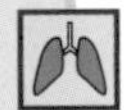

9. A physician orders 250 mL 0.05% epinephrine solution. The available epinephrine is 1:500 in 10-mL vials.

   How many milliliters of 1:500 epinephrine are needed?

   How many milliliters of sterile water are needed as a solvent?

   How many vials of medication are needed to complete the order?

10. A physician orders 250 mL of 15% dextrose in water. The stock solution is 50% dextrose in 10-mL ampules.

    How many milliliters of stock solution are needed?

    How many milliliters of sterile water are needed?

Continued

Posttest, cont.

How many ampules of dextrose are needed to complete the order?

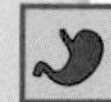

11. A physician orders 4 oz of glycerin solution 7.5% to be used as a retention enema. The available stock glycerin solution is 25%.

    How many milliliters of stock solution are needed?

    How many milliliters of solvent are needed?

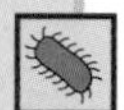

12. Prepare 250 mL of 3% hydrogen peroxide solution from 12% hydrogen peroxide solution.

    How many milliliters of stock solution (solute) are needed?

    How many milliliters of solvent are needed?

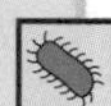

13. *How many milliliters of 2.5% hydrogen peroxide solution can be prepared from 1 pint of 15% hydrogen peroxide stock solution?* In this case use the entire pint.

14. In stock are 5% sodium hypochlorite solution and 20% sodium hypochlorite solutions.

    How many milliliters of each solution need to be combined to prepare 1 L of 12% sodium hypochlorite solution? (Round to whole numbers and label your answers.)

15. Prepare 500 mL of a 12.5% dextrose solution. Available are D5W and D50W.

    How many milliliters of each solution need to be combined to fill this order?

Posttest, cont.

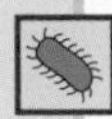

16. Prepare 1.5 L of 6% Lysol solution using 5% Lysol and 8% Lysol. *How many milliliters of each solution need to be combined to fill this order?* Check your answers using alligation medial.

17. Calculate the amount of the following ingredients needed to make 120 mL.

Bromhexine hydrochloride 0.8-mg/mL syrup[3]

bromhexine hydrochloride	*80 mg*
glycerin	*20 mL*
sodium benzoate	*240 mg*
fruit flavor	*qs*
tartaric acid	*340 mg*
sorbitol 70% solution	*45 mL*
sodium carboxymethylcellulose	*200 mg*
purified water	*qs 100 mL*

bromhexine HCl

glycerin

sodium benzoate

tartaric acid

70% sorbitol

sodium carboxymethylcellulose

purified water

What is the percentage of sorbitol in the final preparation?

Continued

Posttest, cont.

18. Calculate how much capsaicin (mg) is needed to prepare the following.

Capsaicin 0.05% clear Medication Stick[4]—#20 tubes

capsaicin	?
sodium stearate	7 g
alcohol	65 g
propylene glycol	25 g
cyclomethicone	3 g

19. Order: 10 mL of 25 mg/mL solution

Stock on hand: 60 mL of 100 mg/mL solution (Hint: not all of the stock will be needed.)

How many milliliters of the stock solution are needed?

How many milliliters of the solvent (water) are needed?

20. 60 mL of a 15% solution is diluted to 100 mL.

What is the percentage strength of the resultant solution?

21. Order: ophthalmic suspension to contain 100 mg/5 mL

Stock on hand: 5% ophthalmic suspension in normal saline

How much 5% suspension is needed?

How much sterile normal saline solution is needed?

22. Prepare 250 mL of a 4% solution from a 3% solution and an 8% solution.

How many milliliters of each solution are needed?

REVIEW OF RULES

- Simple dilution: diluting one strength

  SV • SS = DV • DS

  SW • SS = DW • DS

- Alligation alternate: diluting one strength or combining two strengths
- Alligation medial: combining two or more strengths

REFERENCES

1. Int J Pharm Compd. 14(6):485, 2010.
2. Int J Pharm Compd. 14(6):482, 2010.
3. Int J Pharm Compd. 14(6):516, 2010.
4. Int J Pharm Compd. 14(6):517, 2010.

CHAPTER 15

Calculations for Preparation of Intravenous Infusions

OBJECTIVES

1. Calculate amounts of additives for large- and small-volume parenterals.
2. Calculate intravenous infusion rates and the amount of medication a patient has received.
3. Calculate intravenous flow rates in drops per minute.
4. Calculate time needed to infuse an ordered volume of IV fluids.
5. Calculate parenteral nutrition formulations.

KEY WORDS

Additives Medications to be added to IV infusions including total parenteral nutrition (TPN) solutions and peripheral parenteral nutrition (PPN) solutions; electrolytes, multiple vitamins, trace elements, regular insulin, and other medications

Base solution Solution for a TPN or PPN that contains carbohydrates (dextrose), protein (amino acids), and sometimes lipids (fatty acids)

Continuous infusion Introduction of IV fluids without interruption of therapy

Dose time Amount of time needed to administer a medication dose

Dose volume Volume of medication administered per dose

Drip rate Specific type of flow rate calculated in drops per minute; gtt/min

Drop factor Size of drop from the drip chamber; found on IV tubing (gtt/mL)

Flow rate Speed at which IV medications are infused into the body; aka infusion rate

Infusion Slow administration of fluids, other than blood, into a vein

Large-Volume Parenteral (LVP) IV bag sized over 250 mL up to 3 L for infusion

Macrodrip infusion sets Infusion sets used for measuring rate of IV fluids; macrodrip sets provide large drops of fluid called *macrodrops*

Microdrip infusion sets Infusion sets used for measuring rate of IV fluids; microdrip sets supply small drops called *microdrops*

Parenteral nutrition IV solution used to provide nutrition to a patient; aka hyperalimentation

Peripheral parenteral nutrition (PPN) IV containing a low concentration of amino acids, dextrose, electrolytes, and sometimes lipids, which is administered through a peripheral vessel

Piggyback A small-volume parenteral; IV sized 50 to 250 mL with added medication that is administered through an established IV line

Small-Volume Parenteral (SVP) IV bag 250 mL or less

Total parenteral nutrition (TPN) IV containing a high concentration of amino acids, dextrose, and sometimes lipids with electrolytes and other medications, which is administered through a large central vessel

Pretest

If you are already comfortable with the subject matter, perform the following calculations to test your knowledge. If not, work your way through the chapter and return to them for extra practice. Round drip-rate answers to the nearest whole drop. When adding medication to fluids, the volume of medication(s) added should be included when calculating the total volume of fluids.

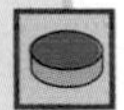

1. A physician orders KCl 20 mEq in 1 L IV fluids for a patient with electrolyte imbalance.

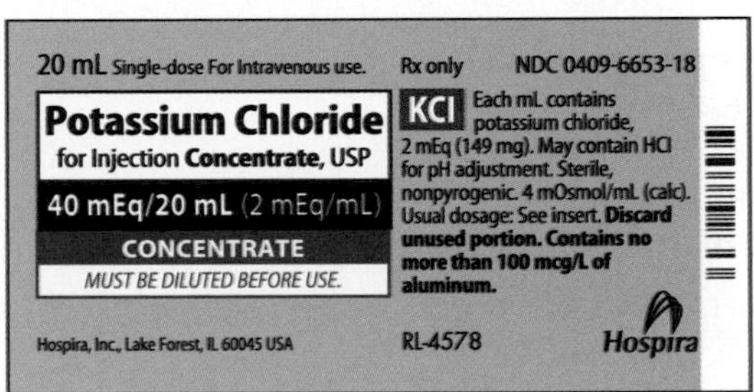

20 mL Single-dose For Intravenous use.
Rx only
NDC 0409-6653-18
Potassium Chloride
for Injection Concentrate, USP
40 mEq/20 mL (2 mEq/mL)
CONCENTRATE
MUST BE DILUTED BEFORE USE.
KCl
Each mL contains potassium chloride, 2 mEq (149 mg). May contain HCl for pH adjustment. Sterile, nonpyrogenic. 4 mOsmol/mL (calc). Usual dosage: See insert. Discard unused portion. Contains no more than 100 mcg/L of aluminum.
Hospira, Inc., Lake Forest, IL 60045 USA
RL-4578
Hospira

(© Pfizer. Used with permission.)

What is the strength of KCl in mEq/mL? ____________

What is the total volume of medication of the vial? ____________

What is the total amount (mEq) of medication in the vial? ____________

What volume of medication should be added to the liter of IV fluids for this order?

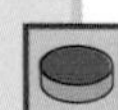

2. A physician orders a continuous infusion of 1,000 mL D5W with 20 mEq KCl q8h.

How many milliliters will the patient receive per hour?

How many milliequivalents of KCl will the patient receive each hour?

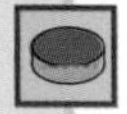

3. A physician orders 1 L of D5NS to be infused over 8 hours.

What is the flow rate in milliliters per hour?

How many milliliters per minute will the patient receive?

Continued

Pretest, cont.

Using a drop factor of 20 gtt/mL, how many drops per minute should be administered?

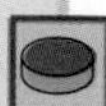

4. A physician orders 3,000 mL lactated Ringer's solution to infuse over 16 hours.
How many milliliters per hour should be administered?

How many milliliters per minute should be administered?

Using a drop factor of 10 gtt/mL, how many drops per minute should be administered?

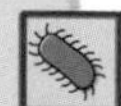

5. A physician orders Ancef (cefazolin) 1 g in 100 mL D5W IVPB. Infuse over 1 hour.
The tubing drop factor is 20 gtt/mL.
How many drops per minute should the patient receive?

6. A 250-mL IV is to be administered over 45 minutes using a 20gtt/mL infusion set.
How many drops per minute should be administered?

7. A physician orders 1,500 mL 0.45% NaCl IV over 24 hours.
The drop factor on the infusion set is 20 gtt/mL.
What is the weight in grams of sodium chloride in the total solution?

Pretest, cont.

How many milliliters of solution should be administered to the patient in 8 hours?

How many drops per minute should the patient receive?

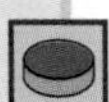

8. A physician orders Ringer's lactate solution to be administered with a 20-gtt/min set.
How much fluid is needed for 24 hours if administered at 2 mL/min?

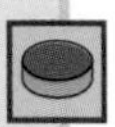

9. A physician orders D5NS q24h with a flow rate of 50 mL/h.
How many milliliters will the patient receive in 1 day?

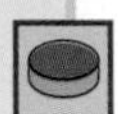

10. *What total amount of D5NS will be administered over 24 hours at 40 mL/h?*

How many liter bags of fluids are needed for 24 hours?

How many gtt/min should be administered using tubing with a drop factor of 20 gtt/mL?

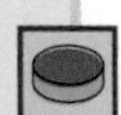

11. *How many grams of dextrose are in the fluid for the label shown below?*

How many minutes will it take to infuse at 2 mL/min?

How many drops per minute should be administered with a drop factor of 15 gtt/mL?

Continued

Pretest, cont.

LOT EXP

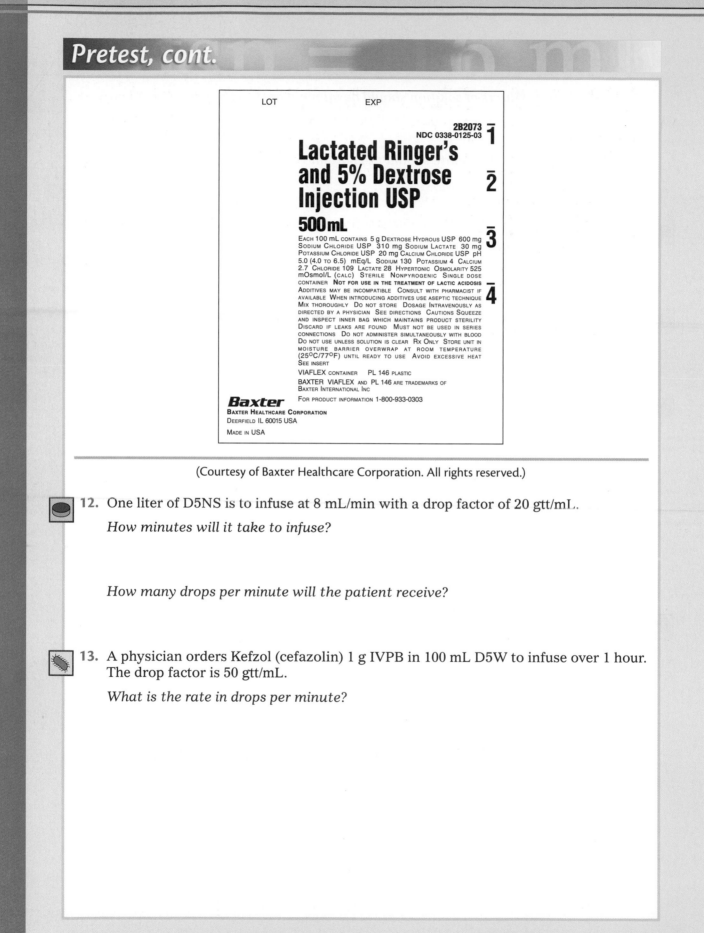

2B2073
NDC 0338-0125-03

Lactated Ringer's and 5% Dextrose Injection USP

500 mL

EACH 100 mL CONTAINS 5 g DEXTROSE HYDROUS USP 600 mg SODIUM CHLORIDE USP 310 mg SODIUM LACTATE 30 mg POTASSIUM CHLORIDE USP 20 mg CALCIUM CHLORIDE USP pH 5.0 (4.0 TO 6.5) mEq/L SODIUM 130 POTASSIUM 4 CALCIUM 2.7 CHLORIDE 109 LACTATE 28 HYPERTONIC OSMOLARITY 525 mOsmol/L (CALC) STERILE NONPYROGENIC SINGLE DOSE CONTAINER **NOT FOR USE IN THE TREATMENT OF LACTIC ACIDOSIS** ADDITIVES MAY BE INCOMPATIBLE CONSULT WITH PHARMACIST IF AVAILABLE WHEN INTRODUCING ADDITIVES USE ASEPTIC TECHNIQUE MIX THOROUGHLY DO NOT STORE DOSAGE INTRAVENOUSLY AS DIRECTED BY A PHYSICIAN SEE DIRECTIONS CAUTIONS SQUEEZE AND INSPECT INNER BAG WHICH MAINTAINS PRODUCT STERILITY DISCARD IF LEAKS ARE FOUND MUST NOT BE USED IN SERIES CONNECTIONS DO NOT ADMINISTER SIMULTANEOUSLY WITH BLOOD DO NOT USE UNLESS SOLUTION IS CLEAR Rx ONLY STORE UNIT IN MOISTURE BARRIER OVERWRAP AT ROOM TEMPERATURE (25°C/77°F) UNTIL READY TO USE AVOID EXCESSIVE HEAT SEE INSERT

VIAFLEX CONTAINER PL 146 PLASTIC

BAXTER VIAFLEX AND PL 146 ARE TRADEMARKS OF BAXTER INTERNATIONAL INC

FOR PRODUCT INFORMATION 1-800-933-0303

Baxter
BAXTER HEALTHCARE CORPORATION
DEERFIELD IL 60015 USA
MADE IN USA

1
2
3
4

12. One liter of D5NS is to infuse at 8 mL/min with a drop factor of 20 gtt/mL.

How minutes will it take to infuse?

How many drops per minute will the patient receive?

13. A physician orders Kefzol (cefazolin) 1 g IVPB in 100 mL D5W to infuse over 1 hour. The drop factor is 50 gtt/mL.

What is the rate in drops per minute?

Pretest, cont.

How many milliliters will be infused within 30 minutes?

How many milligrams of Kefzol will be administered in 15 minutes?

14. Three liters of D10W are to be infused over 24 hours.

What is the infusion rate in mL/h?

How many milliliters per minute will the patient receive?

If the drop factor is 10 gtt/mL, how many drops per minute will the patient receive?

15. One liter of D5NS is infusing at the rate of 45 gtt/min. The drop factor is 15 gtt/mL.

How many milliliters per hour will the patient receive?

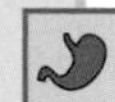

16. A physician orders Pepcid (famotidine) 20 mg in 100 mL lactated Ringer's solution IVPB to infuse over 30 minutes q12h.

Famotidine is available in 10-mg/mL vials.

How many milliliters of famotidine should be added to each 100 mL PB?

If the drop factor is 20 gtt/mL, how many drops per minute are infused?

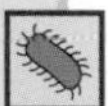

17. A physician orders amphotericin B 40 mg IV in 500 mL D5W infused over 12 hours. After reconstitution, the amphotericin strength is 50 mg/10 mL.

How many milliliters of amphotericin B would be added to 500 mL of fluids?

Continued

Pretest, cont.

How many milliliters should be administered per hour?

If the drop factor is 25 gtt/mL, how many drops per minute will be administered?

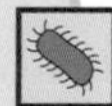

18. A physician orders ampicillin 2 g IV in 500 mL of D5 ½ NS, administered over 2 hours using a drop factor of 10 gtt/mL.

Ampicillin is available in 1-g vials to be reconstituted with 2.5 mL NS for a total of 3 mL.

How many milliliters need to be added to the 500-mL IV?

How many milliliters per hour will be given to the patient?

How many drops per minute will be administered?

19. Prepare a 3 L TPN solution containing 20% dextrose and 4.25% amino acids.

How many milliliters of 50% dextrose injection are needed?

How many milliliters of 8.5% amino acids injection are needed?

How many milliliters of sterile water for injection are needed?

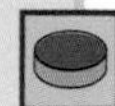

20. An order is received for the following to be added to a standard TPN solution containing 50% dextrose, 10% amino acids, and 20% lipids.

Calculate the amount of each additive needed (see below).

Pretest, cont.

TOTAL PARENTERAL NUTRITION ADDITIVE ORDERS	ADDITIVE STOCK STRENGTHS
sodium chloride 15 mEq	50 mEq/20 mL vial
magnesium sulfate 16 mEq	40.6 mEq/10 mL vial
potassium chloride 8 mEq	40 mEq/20 mL vial
MVI 10 mL	10 mL two-chambered single-dose vial

sodium chloride

magnesium sulfate

potassium chloride

MVI

INTRODUCTION

Intravenous (IV) medications require precise measurements and sterile preparation because the medication immediately enters the bloodstream with 100% bioavailability. Hospital pharmacy technicians usually prepare and deliver a 24-hour supply of IV solutions to nursing stations. **Large-volume parenterals (LVPs)** contain more than 250 mL of solution, whereas **small-volume parenterals (SVPs)** contain 250 mL or less.

LVPs for **continuous infusion**, with or without added medications, drip slowly into a vein either by gravity or through a pump. An IV infusion set includes tubing for carrying fluid from the container to the patient. Medication added to a small volume of fluids, called an IV **piggyback** (IVPB), is administered on an intermittent basis either through an injection port in the tubing or another line (Fig. 15.1). Most IVPBs are SVPs that are delivered over 30 to 60 minutes. The physician determines the type and volume of IV fluids, whether medications are added, and the amount of time over which they should be administered.

Parenteral nutrition (PN) is an IV that provides patient's nutritional needs via infusion. It is generally prescribed when a patient is unable to ingest and process nutrients orally. It can be used to maintain nutritional needs on a short- or long-term basis. Standardized PN solutions are available, but they can also be customized to meet individual nutritional requirements. Because of the regulations that surround the compounding of parenteral solutions, many pharmacies and hospitals contract out their PN orders to compounding companies that specialize in this area. Familiarization with the basic calculations necessary to fill such an order is still important.

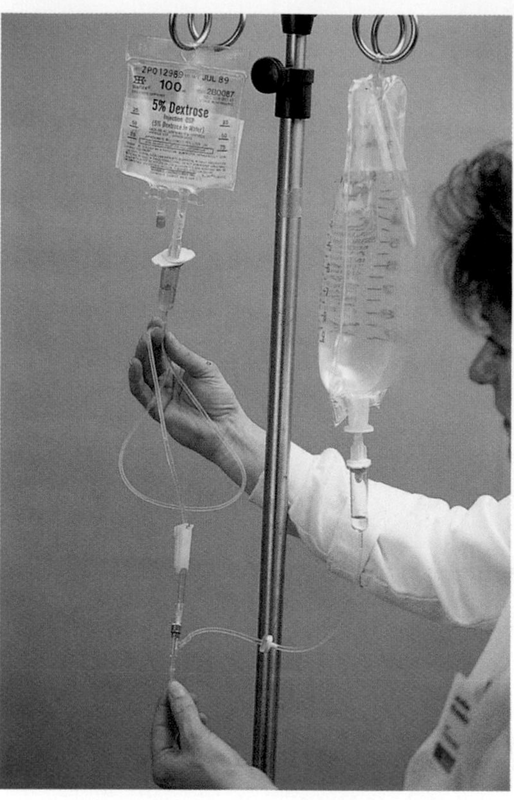

FIGURE 15.1 **Intravenous Piggyback Being Added to a Primary Line.** (From Potter P, Perry A: *Fundamentals of nursing*, ed 8, St. Louis, MO, Mosby, 2013.)

PREPARING LARGE- AND SMALL-VOLUME PARENTERALS

Physicians frequently order LVPs and SVPs with additives.

EXAMPLE 15.1

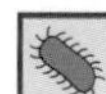

A physician orders ampicillin 0.2 g/kg/day IV to be delivered in *divided doses* q6h for a 110-lb patient. The physician wants each dose placed in 500 mL 5% Dextrose.

How many mg are needed per dose?

$$\frac{\text{mg}}{\text{dose}} = \frac{1{,}000\ \text{mg}}{1\ \text{g}} \bullet \frac{0.2\ \text{g}}{\text{kg/ day}} \bullet \frac{1\ \text{kg}}{2.2\ \text{lb}} \bullet \frac{110\ \text{lb}}{1} \bullet \frac{1\ \text{day}}{4\ \text{doses}} = 2{,}500\ \text{mg/dose}$$

2-g vials of ampicillin for injection are available to be reconstituted with 6.8 mL of sterile water resulting in 8 mL of fluid.

How many milliliters need to be added to each IV?

$$\text{mL} = \frac{8\ \text{mL}}{2\ \text{g}} \bullet \frac{1\ \text{g}}{1{,}000\ \text{mg}} \bullet \frac{2{,}500\ \text{mg}}{\text{dose}} = 10\ \text{mL}$$

Note that this will require the reconstitution of 2 vials per dose since 1 vial only contains 2 g or 2,000 mg.

How many total milliliters of fluids will the patient receive daily?

$$500 \text{ mL} + 10 \text{ mL} = 510 \text{ mL every 6 hours (4 doses), which equals 2,040 mL}$$

When preparing regular insulin drips or adding regular insulin to PN, the number of units ordered needs to be converted to milliliters to calculate the volume of regular insulin to be added. With U-100 insulin, this is a simple calculation. If any order is written to add regular insulin U-100 to an IV, remember the following: U-100 insulin contains 100 units/mL.

EXAMPLE 15.2

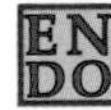

A physician orders an insulin infusion of Humulin R 50 Units in 1,000 mL NS.

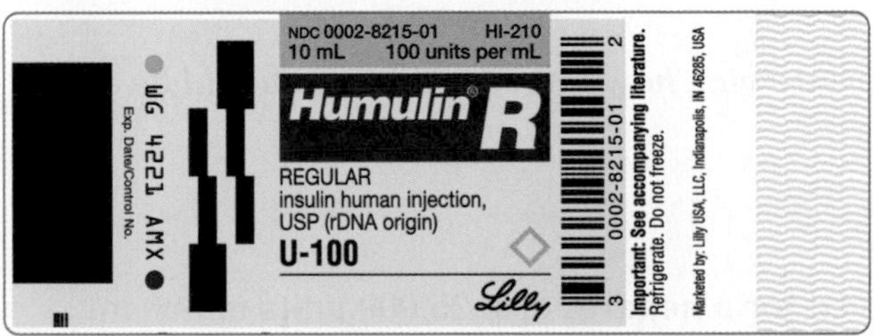

What volume of medication should be added to the fluid?

$$\frac{100 \text{ units}}{1 \text{ mL}} = \frac{50 \text{ units}}{x}$$

$$x = 0.5 \text{ mL}$$

After cross-multiplying, solving this equation for any amount of insulin involves dividing the number of units required by 100. Therefore, a 40-unit dose of U-100 measures 0.4 mL, 95 units measures 0.95 mL, 10 units measures 0.1 mL, and so on.

$$\frac{100 \text{ units}}{1 \text{ mL}} = \frac{x \text{ units}}{x \text{ mL}}$$

$$\frac{100 \text{ units}}{1 \text{ mL}} = \frac{80 \text{ units}}{x} \quad 80 \text{ mL} = 100x \quad x = 0.8 \text{ mL}$$

Practice Problems A

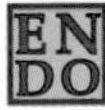

1. An order reads to add 80 units of regular insulin U-100 to an IV bag.

   How many milliliters are equivalent to 80 units?

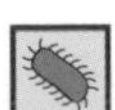

2. A 44-lb child is prescribed cefazolin 25 mg/kg per day in 4 divided doses.

   Each dose is to be added to a 50-mL IVPG of NS.

   Cefazolin IV is supplied in 500-mg and 1-g vials for reconstitution.

How many milligrams should be administered per dose?

If you are preparing 4 doses for a 24-hour supply, which size vial should you reconstitute?

Reconstitution instructions are as follows:

500 mg vial	Add 2 mL of sterile water for injection	Final volume 2.2 mL
1 g vial	Add 2.5 mL of sterile water for injection	Final volume 3 mL

Using the appropriate vial, how many milliliters should be added to each 50-mL piggyback?

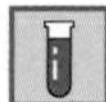

3. An order is received for a heparin drip 25,000 units in 500 mL.

How many milliliters of heparin sodium injection 10,000 units/mL should be added to the fluid?

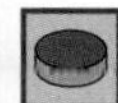

4. An order is received for 25 mEq of potassium chloride in 1 L of NS q8h.

The stock strength of KCl available is 20 mEq/10 mL vials.

How many milliliters of KCl should be added to each liter of fluid?

How many vials of KCl will be needed?

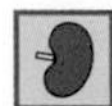

5. Medication order: furosemide drip 100 mg in 1,000 mL of fluid

   Stock strength: furosemide injection 40 mg/4 mL in 10 mL vials

   How many milliliters should be added to the 1-L IV?

   How many vials of furosemide will be needed?

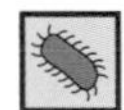

6. A 198-lb patient is ordered chloramphenicol 50 mg/kg/day in *divided doses* q4h placed in 500 mL D5NS for a *Salmonella typhi* infection.

   Stock medication: chloramphenicol 1-g vials 100 mg/mL

   How many milliliters should be added to each 500mL bag of fluids?

   How many milliliters are in one stock vial of chloramphenicol?

   *How many vials are needed to prepare a **24-hour** supply of IVs?*

CALCULATING INTRAVENOUS INFUSION RATES

A rate is a value per unit of time. An **infusion** or **flow rate** refers to the amount of IV fluid entering the body over a specific amount of time. It may be expressed in terms of milliliters per minute, milliliters per hour, an amount of drug (mcg, mg, g, units, or mEq) per minute or hour, or drops per minute. The reason for therapy dictates the type of fluid and rate of infusion ordered. Fluids given to keep a vein open (KVO) are given slowly, whereas replacement fluids are given at a rate that will provide the necessary fluids while preventing an overload on the vascular system. The pharmacy technician must be able to calculate how long a particular volume of fluid will run in order to calculate how much longer a currently hanging IV solution will last and when the next IV is due. This ultimately will determine the amount of IV solution to be prepared for a 24-hour period. Calculations with IV infusion rates can be used to determine the following:

1. The amount of medication delivered (mg, g, mEq, or units) over a specific period of time
2. The volume of medication delivered (gtt, mL, or L) over a specific period of time—**dose volume**
3. The volume of medication needed to last a specific amount of time
4. The length of time a medication dose will last—**dose time**

Each of these problems can be solved using dimensional analysis (DA) or ratio and proportion (R&P). The following examples are shown using the simplest method for solving each one.

EXAMPLE 15.3

How much fluid will a patient receive in 5 hours at an infusion rate of 125 mL/h?

$$\frac{125 \text{ mL}}{1 \text{ h}} = \frac{x}{5 \text{ h}}$$

$$x = 625 \text{ mL}$$

EXAMPLE 15.4

What is the infusion rate in milliliters per hour of a 1,000-mL IV to run over 8 hours?

This can be thought of as simply reducing the fraction $\frac{1{,}000 \text{ mL}}{8 \text{ h}}$ to 125 mL/h

EXAMPLE 15.5

What is the infusion rate in milliliters per minute of a 1,500-mL IV to run over 12 hours?

$$\frac{\text{mL}}{\text{min}} = \frac{1{,}500 \text{ mL}}{12 \text{ h}} \bullet \frac{1 \text{ h}}{60 \text{ min}} = 2 \text{ mL/min}$$

EXAMPLE 15.6

How long would a 1,000-mL IV last at 50 mL/h?

$$\frac{50 \text{ mL}}{1\text{h}} = \frac{1{,}000 \text{ mL}}{x}$$

$$x = 20 \text{ h}$$

Rates can also be presented as amount of medication delivered per hour or minute.

EXAMPLE 15.7

A physician orders heparin 10,000 units per liter for continuous infusion to run at 100 mL/h for a post–myocardial infarction patient.

How many units will be delivered per hour?

$$\text{units/h} = \frac{10{,}000 \text{ units}}{1 \text{ L}} \bullet \frac{1 \text{ L}}{1{,}000 \text{ mL}} \bullet \frac{100 \text{ mL}}{\text{h}} = \frac{1{,}000 \text{ units}}{\text{h}} = 1{,}000 \text{ units/h}$$

One more step is needed to get to units per minute.

$$\frac{\text{units}}{\text{min}} = \frac{10{,}000 \text{ units}}{1 \text{ L}} \bullet \frac{1 \text{ L}}{1{,}000 \text{ mL}} \bullet \frac{100 \text{ mL}}{\text{h}} \bullet \frac{1 \text{ h}}{60 \text{ min}} = 16.7 \text{ units/min}$$

This would be rounded to 17 units per minute.

Practice Problems B

Answer the following questions based on the previous examples. Show your work.

1. *What is the infusion rate in mL/h of 1 L (1,000 mL) D5W given over 10 hours?*

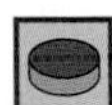

2. *What is the infusion rate in mL/h of 500 mL of NS administered over 10 hours?*

3. *How many milliliters of fluid will a patient receive in 3 hours at an infusion rate of 125 mL/h?*

4. *How much fluid will a patient receive in 10 hours if infusion rate is 50 mL/h?*

5. *How long will 500 mL of D5NS last at an infusion rate of 25 mL/h?*

6. *How long will a 50-mL piggyback last if the infusion rate is 100 mL/h?*

7. A physician orders an IV of 40 mEq of potassium chloride in 1,000 mL NS to run at 125 mL/h.

   How many milliequivalents will be delivered per hour?

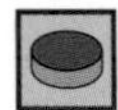

8. A 1,000-mL solution of NS runs over 24 hours.

   How many milliliters are delivered per minute?

9. A 1,500-mL IV is hung at 0830 at a rate of 100 mL/h.

   When will the next bag be due?

10. Calculate how many hours a 1-L IV will last at:

    50 mL/h

    100 mL/h

    125 mL/h

TECH NOTE

A large-volume IV bag can hang for a *maximum* of 24 h before it must be changed, according to the USP.

CALCULATIONS OF AMOUNTS OF MEDICATION RECEIVED

Calculations can also be made to determine how much medication a patient has received at a particular point in their therapy in case the IV is discontinued or infiltrates and must be stopped before it is completely finished.

EXAMPLE 15.8

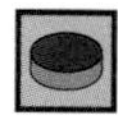
1 L IV of D5W with 80 mEq of KCl was discontinued after 650 mL of the fluid infused.

How many milliequivalents of KCl did the patient receive?

$$\frac{80 \text{ mEq KCl}}{1,000 \text{ mL}} = \frac{x}{650 \text{ mL}} \quad 1,000x = 52,000 \text{ mEq}$$

$$x = 52 \text{ mEq}$$

Practice Problems C

Calculate the amounts of medication received. Round to tenths if necessary. Show your work.

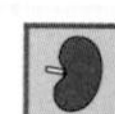
1. A 200-mL IV contains furosemide 100 mg. The patient received 150 mL.

   What amount of furosemide did the patient receive?

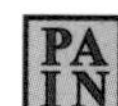
2. An IV contains Sublimaze (fentanyl) 50 mcg in D5W 500 mL. The patient received 400 mL.

   How many grams of dextrose did the patient receive?

   *How many **milligrams** of fentanyl did the patient receive?* (Do not round.)

3. A physician orders 1 L of 3% dextrose to be administered over 6 hours.

How many grams of dextrose are in 1 L?

After 5 hours, how many grams of dextrose has the patient received?

4. A physician writes a medication order for lidocaine 150 mg added to 200 mL of D5W. The available strength of medication to add is 1% lidocaine for injection.

How many milliliters of lidocaine 1% should be added to the 200 mL of D5W?

What is the total IV volume after adding the lidocaine?

How many milligrams of lidocaine are in each milliliter of fluid? (Use the total volume.)

The patient receives only 65 mL of the IV fluids.

How many milligrams of lidocaine did the patient receive?

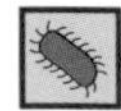

5. Order: 50mL NS with penicillin 1.5 million units (1,500,000 units), infuse over 30 min

The patient receives the medication for 25 minutes.

How many units of penicillin are delivered?

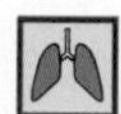

6. Order: aminophylline loading dose 5 mg/kg IVPB over 1 hour

The patient weighs 154 lb. The available medication is aminophylline 250 mg/10 mL.

How many milligrams of medication will the patient receive in 1 hour?

How many milligrams would the patient receive per hour if the IVPB was infused over 2 hours?

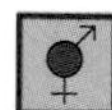

7. A physician orders Pitocin (oxytocin) 2 units in 1 L of D5W.

How many units are in 100 mL of the solution?

What is the dose of Pitocin if the patient only receives 750 mL of the IV fluids?

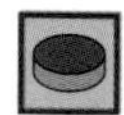

8. A physician orders magnesium sulfate 10 g added to 1 L of LR.

The available strength is 50% magnesium sulfate solution for injection.

What is the concentration of 50% magnesium sulfate in milligrams per milliliter?

How much magnesium sulfate solution should be added to the LR solution?

If this is infused over 5 hours, how many milligrams of magnesium sulfate will the patient receive per hour?

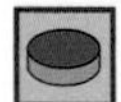

9. Order: 1,000 mL D5NS with 40 mEq KCL to infuse at 100 mL/hr

How many hours will the IV last?

How many mEq of KCl will the patient receive in 2 hours?

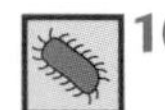

10. A physician orders Cefobid (cefoperazone) 1 g in D5NS with a total volume of 250 mL to run over 30 minutes q12h.

What is the flow rate in mL/h?

If the PB is pulled after 15 minutes, how much antibiotic did the patient receive?

CALCULATING INTRAVENOUS FLOW RATES IN DROPS PER MINUTE

A **drip rate** (DR), sometimes called a **drop rate**, represents the number of drops (gtt) administered over a specific time via IV infusion. It is a specific type of infusion or flow rate, measured in drops per minute. The calculation of drip rate is affected by the size of the tubing used to deliver the medication. A **drop factor** (gtt/mL) is found on each tubing package. Various drop factors are available: 10, 15, and 20 gtt/mL are **macrodrip tubing sets**, whereas 60 gtt/mL is considered a **microdrip tubing set** because the drops are much smaller (think of 1 mL divided into 60 drops) (Fig. 15.2).

TECH ALERT

The number of drops per milliliter for the infusion set is found on the tubing box. Tubing is not interchangeable! This information is essential for proper fluid administration time and calculation of IV flow rates.

Although it is very rare for a pharmacy technician to have to calculate drip rates, it is still an important skill to know. A physician's order provides the type and amount of fluids and usually a desired infusion rate or infusion time. The proper infusion set must be chosen to supply the fluids as ordered.

Four factors to be considered with administration are:

- The total amount of fluids to be administered in *milliliters (mL)*
- The calibration of the administration (infusion) set in *drops per milliliter (gtt/mL)*
- The flow rate of the fluids in *drops per minute (gtt/min)*
- The time for the fluids to infuse in *minutes (min)*

Calculating flow rates for IV fluids is accomplished most easily by using DA. You do not need a specific formula as long as you follow the rules for DA to achieve your desired answer. *Always* round drip rates measured in drops per milliliter to the nearest whole number.

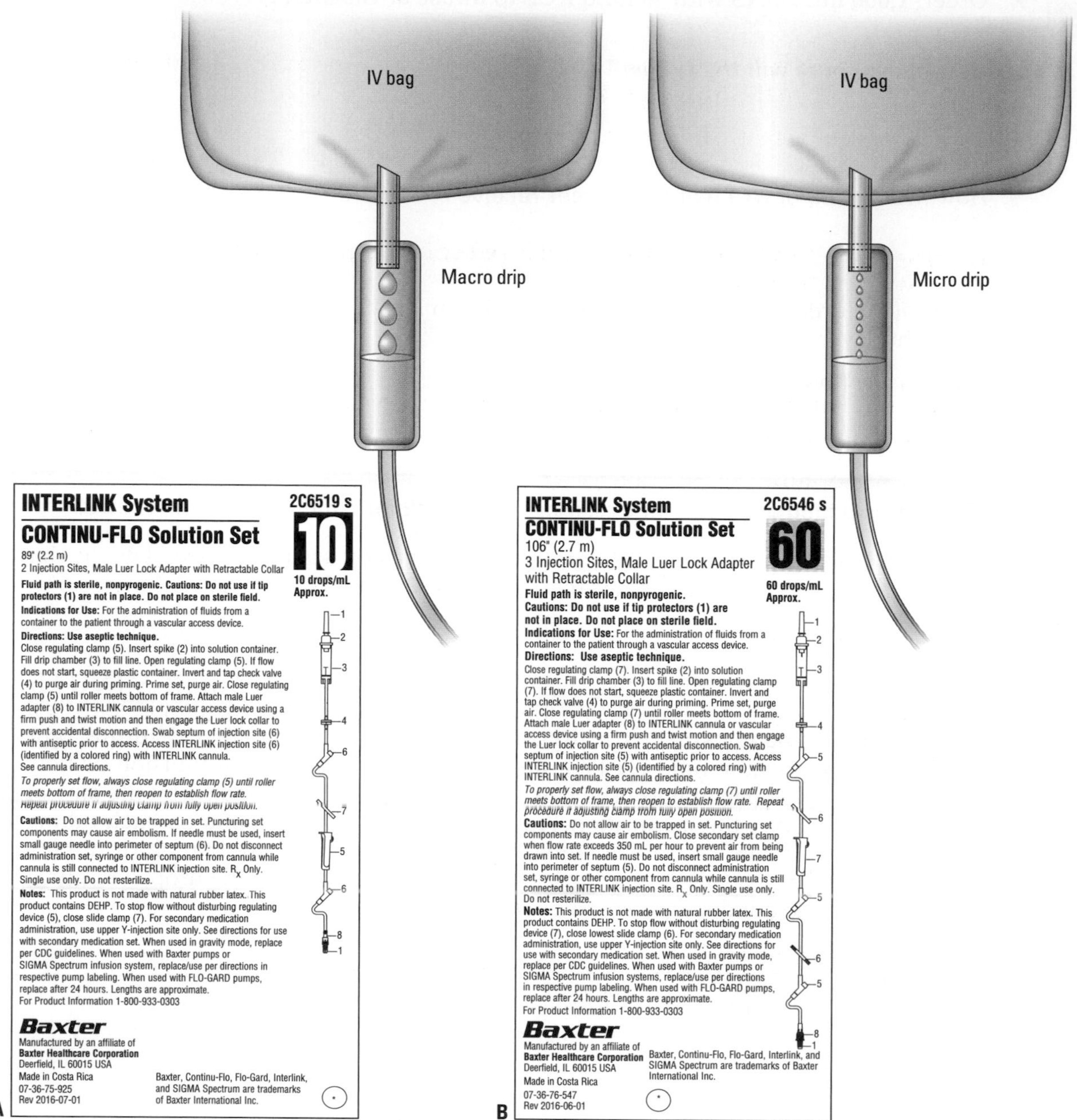

FIGURE 15.2 **Infusion Sets for Administration of Intravenous Fluids.** (A) Macrodrip set shows 10 gtt/mL. (B) Microdrip set shows 60 gtt/mL. (Labels courtesy of Baxter Healthcare Corporation. All rights reserved.)

EXAMPLE 15.9

A physician orders Pepcid (famotidine) 20 mg in a total of 50 mL NS to run over 25 minutes. Calculate the drops per minute if the drop factor is 20 gtt/mL.

First, start with the units of your desired answer followed by an equal sign:

$$\frac{\text{gtt}}{\text{min}} =$$

Next, place the information containing the desired unit of the numerator in the numerator position of the first fraction:

$$\frac{\text{gtt}}{\text{min}} = \frac{20\text{ gtt}}{\text{mL}}$$

Then place the information containing the unit you want to cancel with the first denominator in the numerator position of the next fraction:

$$\frac{\text{gtt}}{\text{min}} = \frac{20\text{ gtt}}{\text{mL}} \bullet \frac{50\text{ mL}}{25\text{min}}$$

Continue this process until you only have the units of the desired answer left. In this example, the desired unit is drops per minute, so the only step left is to solve the equation.

$$\frac{\text{gtt}}{\text{min}} = \frac{20\text{ gtt}}{\text{mL}} \bullet \frac{50\text{ mL}}{25\text{ min}} = \frac{40\text{ gtt}}{\text{min}}$$

This same pattern can be repeated for any infusion or drip rate problem. Sometimes these calculations will require the use of the conversion factor for volume, 1 L = 1,000 mL, and/or the conversion factor for time, 1 hour = 60 minutes.

EXAMPLE 15.10

A physician orders 3 L of D5W to run over 24 hours.

If the drop factor is 20 gtt/mL, what is the drip rate?

$$\frac{\text{gtt}}{\text{min}} = \frac{20\text{ gtt}}{\text{mL}} \bullet \frac{1{,}000\text{ mL}}{1\text{ L}} \bullet \frac{3\text{ L}}{24\text{ hr}} \bullet \frac{1\text{ hr}}{60\text{ min}} = 41.6 = 42\text{ gtt/min}$$

TECH NOTE

Remember that with DA, you are completing the entire problem in one step.

Practice Problems D

Calculate the flow rate in drops per minute. Round answers for medication weight/volume to the nearest tenth and for drops per minute to the nearest whole number.

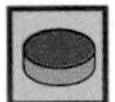

1. Order: 2 L of lactated Ringer's solution over 12 hours with a drop factor of 20 gtt/mL.

   How many drops per minute should be infused?

2. A physician orders D5W 100 mL IV over 2 hours. The drop factor is 50 gtt/mL.

How many drops per minute should be infused?

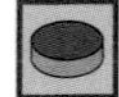

3. Order: 250 mL D5NS over 16 hours to keep a vein open. The drop factor is 60 gtt/mL.

How many drops per minute should be administered?

How many milliliters will be administered per hour?

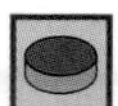

4. Order: 1,000 mL D5NS over 12 hours. The drop factor is 10 gtt/mL.

How many drops per minute should be infused?

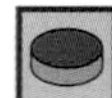

5. Order: 150 mL of D5NS to be infused over 40 minutes. The drop factor is 15 gtt/mL.

How many drops per minute should be infused?

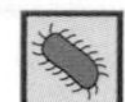

6. Order: IVPB ampicillin 250 mg in 75 mL NS over 1 hour. Use infusion set of 50 gtt/mL.

How many drops per minute will be infused?

What weight (in mg) of ampicillin will be infused in 45 minutes?

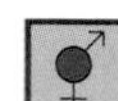

7. Order: oxytocin 10 units in 500 mL NS over 30 minutes. The drop factor is 20 gtt/mL.

How many drops per minute should be infused?

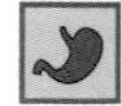

8. Order: ranitidine 50 mg in 100 mL NS over 15 minutes. The drop factor is 15 gtt/mL.

How many drops per minute should be infused?

How many milligrams of ranitidine will the patient receive in 12 minutes?

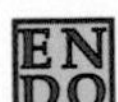

9. A physician orders Solu-Medrol (methylprednisolone sodium succinate) 500 mg in 150 mL NS to infuse over 2 hours with a drop factor of 20 gtt/mL.

   How many drops per minute should be infused?

   How many milligrams of methylprednisolone will the patient receive in 1 hour and 15 minutes?

10. Order: nafcillin 1 g in 100 mL D5W to run over 1 hour. The drop factor is 15 gtt/mL.

    How many drops per minute should be infused?

11. Order: Novolin R 60 units in 500 mL NS over 4 ½ hours with a drop factor of 15 gtt/mL.

    How many drops per minute will be infused?

    How many units of regular insulin will infuse in 1 hour?

12. A physician orders tobramycin 1 mg/kg in LR 50 mL IVPB to run over 50 minutes.

    The patient weighs 178 lb. The drop factor is 10 gtt/mL.

    What dose (in mg) of tobramycin should be prepared for the infusion?

    How many drops per minute should be set for the infusion to meet the physician's order?

    How many milligrams of tobramycin will be infused in 45 minutes?

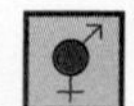

13. A physician orders Premarin (conjugated estrogens) 25 mg in 50 mL D5W to run over 15 minutes. The drop factor is 15 gtt/mL.

How many drops per minute should be infused?

How many milligrams of estrogens will be infused in 6 minutes?

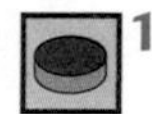

14. Order: 2 L of ½ NS over 16 hours. The drop factor is 50 gtt/mL.

How many drops per minute should be infused?

How many total grams of NaCl will the patient receive?

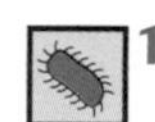

15. Order: Garamycin (gentamicin) 0.02 g in 50 mL NS for infusion over 45 minutes. The drop factor is 20 gtt/mL.

How many drops per minute should be infused?

How many milligrams of gentamicin would be added to the fluids?

CALCULATING INTRAVENOUS INFUSION TIMES

In some instances the physician will provide an order for the amount of fluids to be infused and the milliliters per hour without providing the specific infusion time. The problem then becomes a question of how long it will take for each volume of fluid to be infused using the rate ordered by the physician. As the pharmacy technician, you have a responsibility to ensure that fluids are available for the next dose as ordered. Therefore, when the time is not designated but the amount is designated, the necessary calculation may include deciding how long the ordered fluids will take to infuse when the infusion rate and/or drop factor is provided.

EXAMPLE 15.11

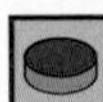

Order: 250 mL LR to be infused at 50 gtt/min with an infusion set of 10 gtt/mL.

What is the infusion time in minutes?

$$\text{min} = \frac{1\text{ min}}{50\text{ gtt}} \bullet \frac{10\text{ gtt}}{\text{mL}} \bullet \frac{250\text{ mL}}{1} = 50\text{ min}$$

EXAMPLE 15.12

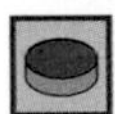

Order: 2,500 mL of D5NS to infuse at 30 gtt/min with an infusion set of 10 gtt/mL.

How many minutes will it take for these fluids to infuse?

$$\text{min} = \frac{1\text{ min}}{30\text{ gtt}} \bullet \frac{10\text{ gtt}}{\text{mL}} \bullet \frac{2{,}500\text{ mL}}{1} = 833\text{ min}$$

What is the infusion time in hours and minutes?

$$\text{h} = \frac{1\text{ h}}{60\text{ min}} \bullet \frac{1\text{ min}}{30\text{ gtt}} \bullet \frac{10\text{ gtt}}{\text{mL}} \bullet \frac{2{,}500\text{ mL}}{1} = 13.9\text{ h}$$

Because there are 60 minutes in 1 hour, multiply 0.9 × 60 to change to minutes.

$$\text{min} = \frac{60\text{ min}}{1\text{ h}} \bullet \frac{0.9\text{ h}}{1} = 54\text{ min}$$

The answer is 13 hours and 54 minutes.

EXAMPLE 15.13

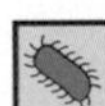

A physician orders amphotericin B 40 mg IVPB in D5W 250 mL infused at a rate of 20 gtt/min with a drop factor of 60 gtt/mL.

Amphotericin B is reconstituted to 50 mg/10 mL.

How many milliliters of amphotericin B should be added to the fluids?

$$\frac{50\text{ mg}}{10\text{ mL}} = \frac{40\text{ mg}}{x} \quad 50x = 400\text{ mL} \quad x = 8\text{ mL}$$

What is the total volume to be infused? 250 mL + 8 mL = 258 mL

How many minutes will the IV take to infuse?

$$\text{min} = \frac{1\text{ min}}{20\text{ gtt}} \bullet \frac{60\text{ gtt}}{\text{mL}} \bullet \frac{258\text{ mL}}{1} = 774\text{ min}$$

EXAMPLE 15.14

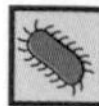 Order: Vancocin (vancomycin) IVPB 1 g in 100 mL D5W.

The drop factor is 20 gtt/mL and the infusion rate is 1.5 mL/min.

Vancomycin is reconstituted to 500 mg/10 mL.

How many milliliters of Vancocin solution should be added to the 100-mL piggyback fluid?

$$\text{mL} = \frac{10 \text{ mL}}{500 \text{ mg}} \bullet \frac{1{,}000 \text{ mg}}{1 \text{ g}} \bullet \frac{1 \text{ g}}{1} = 20 \text{ mL}$$

What is the total volume to be infused? 100 mL + 20 mL = 120 mL

How many minutes will it take for the Vancocin order to infuse?

$$\text{mL} = \frac{1 \text{ min}}{1.5 \text{ mL}} \bullet \frac{120 \text{ mL}}{1} = 80 \text{ min}$$

How many drops per minute would be infused?

$$\frac{\text{gtt}}{\text{min}} = \frac{20 \text{ gtt}}{\text{mL}} \bullet \frac{120 \text{ mL}}{80 \text{ min}} = 30 \text{ gtt/min}$$

TECH NOTE

When using DA, always start with the unit of the answer desired followed by an equal sign.

Practice Problems E

Complete the following problems. Round all answers to whole numbers. Show your work.

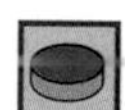

1. Order: 500 mL D5NS to be infused at 15 gtt/min. The drop factor is 10 gtt/mL.

   How many minutes will it take to infuse?

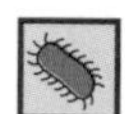

2. Order: Amikin (amikacin) 1 g in 100 mL D5W to infuse at 25 gtt/min using an infusion set delivering 60 gtt/mL.

   What is the running time for the infusion in minutes?

   What is the running time for the infusion in hours?

   The drug has a recommended infusion time of at least 1 hour. *Is this order safe?*

   ___

   How many milligrams of Amikin will the patient receive in 10 minutes?

3. A physician orders 2 L of D5W to be infused at 25 gtt/min. The drop factor is 10 gtt/mL.

   How many minutes will the infusion last?

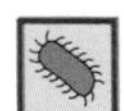

4. Order: gentamicin 1.5 mg/kg per dose q8h IVPB in 150 mL NS for a 148-lb patient

   How many milligrams of gentamicin should the patient receive per dose?

   The infusion rate is 25 gtt/min. The drop factor is 20 gtt/mL.

   How long will it take for this medication to be infused in hours?

   How many milligrams will the patient receive in 45 minutes?

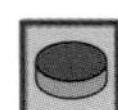

5. Order: 500 mL of D5 ½ NS at 30 gtt/min with a drop factor of 60 gtt/mL.

   How long will this infusion last in hours and minutes?

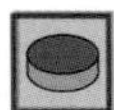

6. Order: 1.5 L of D5 ½ NS at 100 gtt/min with an administration set of 10 gtt/mL.

   How long will it take for these fluids to infuse in minutes?

   How long will it take in hours and minutes?

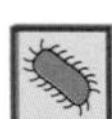

7. Order: ampicillin 250 mg in 50 mL NS IVPB at 30 gtt/min.

   The volume of ampicillin added to 50 mL of NS is 8 mL. The drop factor is 10 gtt/mL.

   How long will it take for the entire piggyback to infuse in minutes?

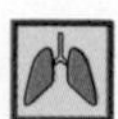

8. Order: aminophylline 750 mg in 100-mL of fluid

Aminophylline is available as 500 mg/25 mL.

What volume of aminophylline should be added to the IVPB?

The drop factor is 60 gtt/mL, and the rate of infusion is 10 gtt/min.

How long in minutes will it take for the entire bag of fluids to infuse?

How long is this in hours and minutes?

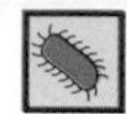

9. A physician orders erythromycin 200 mg in 250 mL D5W.

Erythromycin is available as 400 mg/5 mL after reconstitution.

How many milliliters of erythromycin should be added to the bag of fluids?

The drop factor is 30 gtt/mL, and the rate of infusion is 20 gtt/min.

How many minutes will it take for the piggyback to infuse?

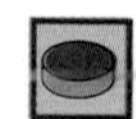

10. A physician orders 1 L of LR with 20 mEq KCl.

The drop factor is 10 gtt/mL. The infusion rate is 20 gtt/min.

How long will it take for this order to infuse in minutes?

How long will it take in hours and minutes?

11. A physician orders heparin sodium 3,500 units (from the following vial) to be added to 100 mL of NS for IV infusion.

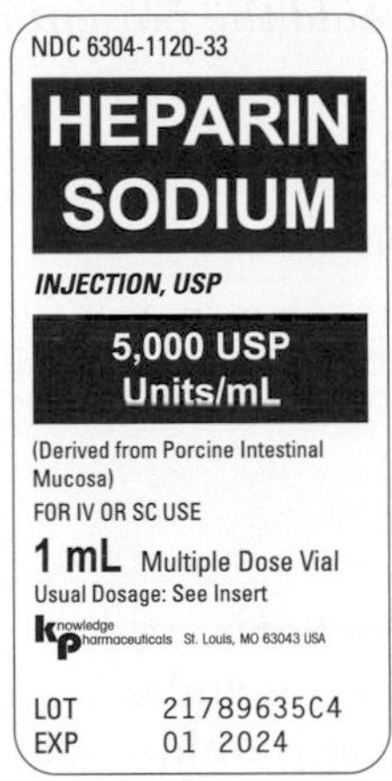

NDC 6304-1120-33
HEPARIN SODIUM
INJECTION, USP
5,000 USP Units/mL
(Derived from Porcine Intestinal Mucosa)
FOR IV OR SC USE
1 mL Multiple Dose Vial
Usual Dosage: See Insert
St. Louis, MO 63043 USA
LOT 21789635C4
EXP 01 2024

How many milliliters of heparin should be added to the fluids?

The drop factor is 60 gtt/mL, and the infusion rate is 20 gtt/min.

How many minutes will it take for these fluids to infuse?

12. Order: 150 mL D5W. The drop factor is 60 gtt/mL, and the infusion rate is 0.5 mL/min.

How long in hours will it take for the fluids to be infused?

How many drops per minute will be infused?

13. A physician orders 2 L of D5NS to infuse at 8 mL/min with a drop factor of 20 gtt/mL.

How many drops per minute should the patient receive?

How long will it take for the fluids to infuse in hours and minutes?

14. *How many hours will it take to infuse 500 mL D5W at 40 gtt/min with a drop factor of 15 gtt/mL?* (Round to nearest hour.)

15. A physician orders heparin sodium 6,000 units in 500 mL of D5LR to run at 1,000 units/h with a drop factor of 10 gtt/mL.

How many drops per minute should the patient receive?

How many hours will the IV run?

PARENTERAL NUTRITION

Traditional 2-in-1 PN supplementation includes **base solutions** of two essential macronutrients, dextrose (carbohydrates) and amino acids (protein), along with electrolytes, vitamins, trace elements, and water. A stable IV lipid (fat) emulsion, IVFE, is included in some formulations, resulting in what is called a 3-in-1 formulation, which includes three macronutrients: carbohydrates, protein, and fats. In addition, PN solutions can contain medications such as regular insulin and others as needed and indicated given the patient's clinical situation.

PN can be administered via either central or peripheral lines, with central lines often placed in the superior vena cava and peripheral lines inserted into the veins of the arm or hand. **Peripheral parental nutrition** (PPN) must be *lower* in strength than **total parenteral nutrition** (TPN). TPN is administered through larger central lines where the solution is diluted in the bloodstream quickly. Peripheral vessels are smaller so the solution is not diluted in the bloodstream as quickly. Chronic PN can even be administered and managed by patients in the ambulatory setting.

Parenteral Nutrition Calculations

Two types of calculations are used to determine the contents of a PN solution. The first involves determination of the amount of base solutions: dextrose, amino acids, and lipids. The second involves calculation of the amount of additives, such as electrolytes and medications, to be included. When calculating the amount of stock solutions to use to obtain the appropriate strength of base solution ordered, the dilution equation, SV • SS = DV • DS, may be used.

EXAMPLE 15.15

Order: 1 L of TPN solution containing 2.125% amino acids and 25% dextrose.

In stock are 8.5% amino acids, 50% dextrose, and sterile water for injection.

Calculate the volumes of each solution needed to prepare the desired concentration, then qs with sterile water for injection to 1,000 mL.

What volume of 8.5% amino acids injection is needed to prepare 1 L of 2.125% amino acids?

Identify the variables, remembering that the total amount needed, the **DV**, is 1,000 mL.

$$SV \bullet SS = DV \bullet DS$$

$$SV \bullet 8.5\% = 1{,}000\text{ mL} \bullet 2.125\%$$

$$SV \bullet 8.5 = 2{,}125\text{ mL}$$

$$SV = 250\text{ mL of }8.5\%\text{ amino acids needed}$$

What volume of 50% dextrose injection is needed to prepare 1 L of 25% dextrose?

$$SV \bullet SS = DV \bullet DS$$

$$SV \bullet 50\% = 1{,}000\ mL \bullet 25\%$$

$$SV \bullet 50 = 25{,}000\ mL$$

$$SV = 500\ mL\ of\ 50\%\ dextrose\ needed$$

To calculate the volume of sterile water for injection needed to bring the solution to a final volume of 1 L, subtract the volumes calculated above from the desired volume:

$$1{,}000\ mL\ (1\ L) - 250\ mL - 500\ mL = 250\ mL\ of\ sterile\ water\ for\ injection\ needed$$

TECH NOTE

If electrolytes and other medications are added before bringing the volume up to the total desired, their total volume will also be subtracted before determining the amount of sterile water needed.

EXAMPLE 15.16

An order calls for the following to be added to a standard 1-L TPN solution that contains 50% dextrose, 10% amino acids, and 20% fat. *Calculate the amount of each additive needed.*

TPN ADDITIVE ORDERS	ADDITIVE STOCK STRENGTHS
sodium chloride 30 mEq	50 mEq/20 mL vial
potassium acetate 15 mEq	40 mEq/20 mL vial
potassium chloride 25 mEq	30 mEq/15 mL vial
calcium gluconate 9.4 mEq	4.7 mEq/10 mL vial
regular insulin 10 units	U-100 (1,000 units/10 mL vial)

How much of each additive is required to be added to the 1-L solution?

Sodium chloride: When the stock strength is presented as the entire vial, it can be reduced before making calculations, so 50 mEq/20 mL can be reduced to 5 mEq/2 mL.

$$\frac{5\ mEq}{2\ mL} = \frac{30\ mEq}{x}$$

Cross-multiply and divide: $5x = 60\ mL \quad x = 12\ mL$

Potassium acetate: 40 mEq/20 mL can be reduced to 2 mEq/mL

$$\frac{2\ mEq}{1\ mL} = \frac{15\ mEq}{x} \quad 2x = 15\ mL \quad x = 7.5\ mL$$

Potassium chloride: 30 mEq/15 mL can be reduced to 2 mEq/mL

$$\frac{2\ mEq}{1\ mL} = \frac{25\ mEq}{x} \quad 2x = 25\ mL \quad x = 12.5\ mL$$

Calcium gluconate:

$$\frac{4.7\ \text{mEq}}{10\ \text{mL}} = \frac{9.4\ \text{mEq}}{x} \quad 4.7x = 94\ \text{mL} \quad x = 20\ \text{mL}$$

Regular insulin:

$$\frac{100\ \text{units}}{1\ \text{mL}} = \frac{10\ \text{units}}{x} \quad 100x = 10 \quad x = 0.1\ \text{mL}$$

What is the total amount of additives?

$$12\ \text{mL} + 7.5\ \text{mL} + 12.5\ \text{mL} + 20\ \text{mL} + 0.1\ \text{mL} = 52.1\ \text{mL}$$

If the TPN is hung at 0800 and is to run at 75 mL/h, when will the next bag be due?

$$\frac{75\ \text{mL}}{1\ \text{h}} = \frac{1{,}052.1\ \text{mL}}{x} \quad 75x = 1{,}052.1\ \text{h} \quad x = 14\ \text{h}$$

14 hours after 0800 is 2200.

Some additive strengths are labeled in more than one way. Use the one that is in the order or perform a conversion if needed.

EXAMPLE 15.17

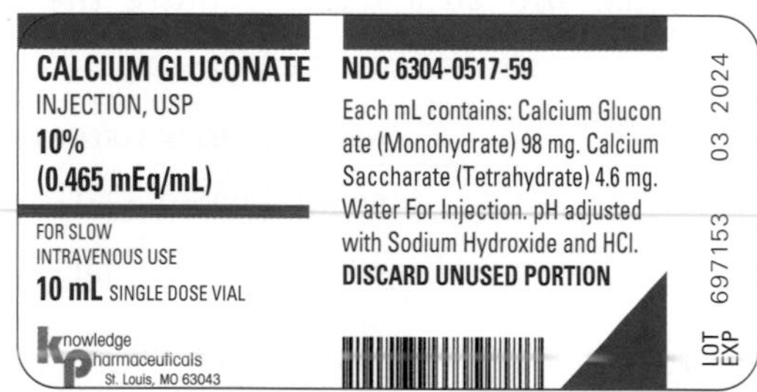

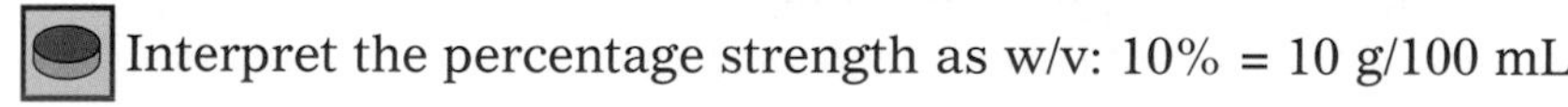
Interpret the percentage strength as w/v: 10% = 10 g/100 mL

How many grams are in the 10-mL vial?

$$\frac{10\ \text{g}}{100\ \text{mL}} = \frac{x}{10\ \text{mL}}$$

$$x = 1\ \text{g}$$

How many mEq are in the 10-mL vial?

$$\frac{0.465\ \text{mEq}}{1\ \text{mL}} = \frac{x}{10\ \text{mL}}$$

$$x = 4.65\ \text{mEq}$$

Practice Problems F

Perform the following calculations showing all of your work.

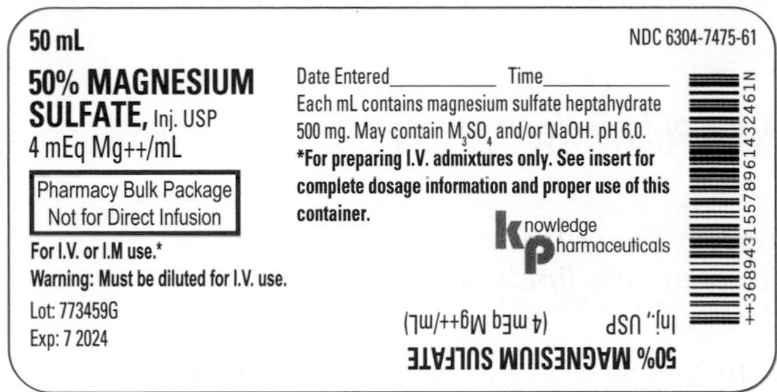

50 mL
NDC 6304-7475-61
50% MAGNESIUM SULFATE, Inj. USP
4 mEq Mg++/mL
Pharmacy Bulk Package
Not for Direct Infusion
For I.V. or I.M use.*
Warning: Must be diluted for I.V. use.
Lot: 773459G
Exp: 7 2024
Date Entered Time
Each mL contains magnesium sulfate heptahydrate 500 mg. May contain M_3SO_4 and/or NaOH. pH 6.0.
*For preparing I.V. admixtures only. See insert for complete dosage information and proper use of this container.
knowledge pharmaceuticals
50% MAGNESIUM SULFATE
Inj., USP (4 mEq Mg++/mL)
++368943155789614324 61N

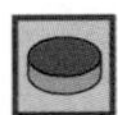

1. Interpret the percentage strength as w/v: ______________________________

   How many grams are available in the entire vial?

   How many mEq are available in the entire vial?

   What is the strength in mg/mL?

2. A physician writes an order for a 1-L TPN containing 4.25% amino acids and 20% dextrose. Available stock is 8.5% amino acids injection, 50% dextrose injection, and sterile water for injection.

   How many milliliters of 8.5% amino acids injection are needed?

   How many milliliters of 50% dextrose injection are needed?

   How many milliliters of sterile water for injection are needed to reach the desired volume?

3. Prepare a 1.5-L TPN solution containing 2.125% amino acids, 10% dextrose, and 3% lipids.

How many milliliters of 8.5% amino acids injection are needed?

How many milliliters of 50% dextrose injection are needed?

How many milliliters of 20% lipids are needed?

How many milliliters of sterile water for injection are needed to reach the desired volume?

4. An order is received for the following to be added to a standard TPN solution containing 10% amino acids, 50% dextrose, and 20% fat.

TPN ADDITIVE ORDERS	ADDITIVE STOCK STRENGTHS
sodium chloride 25 mEq	50 mEq/20 mL vial
potassium acetate 15 mEq	40 mEq/20 mL vial
calcium gluconate 4.7 mEq	4.7 mEq/10 mL vial
MVI-12 (multivitamin injection) 10 mL	10 mL (two-chambered single-dose vial)
regular insulin 25 units	U-100 vial

How much of each additive is needed?

Sodium chloride:

Potassium acetate:

Calcium gluconate:

MVI-12: 10 mL

Regular insulin:

What is the total of all of the additives?

5. A compounded TPN contains 400 mL of 8.8% Travasol (amino acid), 300 mL of 50% dextrose, 100 mL of lipids, and 200 mL of sterile water.

   What is the final concentration of Travasol?

   What is the final strength of the dextrose?

Use the following chart for the next four questions.

TPN ADDITIVES	ADDITIVE STOCK STRENGTHS AVAILABLE	
potassium chloride		2 mEq/ mL
sodium chloride	14.6%	2.5 mEq/ mL
calcium gluconate	10%	4.65 mEq/10 mL
magnesium sulfate[a]	50%	40.6 mEq/10 mL
sodium acetate		2 mEq/mL
sodium phosphates	45 mM/15 mL	60 mEq/15 mL
potassium acetate	19.6%	2 mEq/mL
potassium phosphate	15 mM/5 mL	4.4 mEq/mL
Humulin R insulin	100 units/mL	
vitamin C	250 mg/2 mL	
folic acid	5 mg/mL	

[a]50% magnesium sulfate means 50 g/100 mL.
TPN, Total parenteral nutrition.

6. Calculate the amounts needed for each of the following ordered additives.

   Potassium chloride 15 mEq:

   Sodium chloride 10 mEq:

   Magnesium sulfate 250 mg:

   Sodium acetate 4 mEq:

   Sodium phosphate 20 mEq:

   Humulin R insulin 50 units:

   Vitamin C 500 mg:

   Folic acid 10 mg:

   Trace elements: 5 mL

   MVI-12: 5 mL

   What is the total amount of all of the additives?

Base Solutions

Travasol (amino acids) 7.5%	400 mL
dextrose 50%	400 mL
sterile water for injection	qs ad, 1,000 mL

What is the final concentration of Travasol (amino acids)?

What is the final concentration of dextrose?

How much sterile water for injection is needed to reach 1,000 mL? (Be sure to account for the total amount of additives.)

How many grams of amino acids are in this TPN?

How many grams of dextrose are in this TPN?

If it is hung at 0600 and run at 75 mL/h, when will the next bag be due?

7. Calculate the amounts needed for each of the following ordered additives.

Potassium chloride (KCl) 80 mEq:

Sodium chloride (NaCl) 45 mEq:

Magnesium sulfate 24 mEq:

Trace elements:	3 mL
MVI:	10 mL

Humulin R insulin 60 units:

What is the total volume of the additives?

Base Solutions Ordered

10% Travasol	1,000 mL
50% dextrose	1,000 mL
sterile water for injection	500 mL

What is the total volume of the TPN?

How many grams of dextrose are in this TPN?

What is the final concentration of Travasol (amino acid)?

What is the final concentration of dextrose?

If it is hung at 0800 and runs at 125 mL/h, when will the next bag be due?

8. The following TPN to be run over 24 hours is for a 20-pound infant.

Calculate the amounts needed for each of the following ordered additives.

Potassium chloride 2.5 mEq/kg:

Sodium chloride 2.5 mEq/kg:

Magnesium sulfate 0.5 mEq/kg:

What is the total volume of the additives?

Base Solutions Ordered

5.5% Travasol	200 mL
20% dextrose	150 mL

What is the total volume of the TPN?

How many grams of amino acids are in this TPN?

How many grams of dextrose are in this TPN?

What is the final concentration of Travasol (amino acids)?

What is the final concentration of dextrose?

9. Calculate the amounts needed for each of the following ordered additives.

Potassium chloride 15 mEq:

Sodium chloride 10 mEq:

Magnesium sulfate 250 mg:

Sodium phosphates 20 mEq:

Vitamin C 500 mg:

Folic Acid 10 mg:

Trace elements:	5 mL
MVI-12:	10 mL

What is the total volume of the additives?

Base Solutions Ordered

Travasol (amino acids)	30 g
dextrose	200 g
Sterile water for injection	qs ad 1,000 mL

Base Solutions Available

Travasol	8.8%
dextrose	50%

Round the following two answers to whole numbers.

How many milliliters of 8.8% Travasol are needed to provide 30 grams of amino acids?

How many milliliters of 50% dextrose are needed to provide 200 g of dextrose?

How many milliliters of sterile water are needed?

Run at 100 mL/h.

If it is hung at 0600, when will the next IV be due?

REVIEW

The pharmacy is responsible for providing the medications and fluids to fill physicians' medication orders. In addition, the pharmacy is responsible for ensuring that adequate amounts of fluids are provided for the desired length of therapy. Furthermore, you may be asked to calculate the amount of time that a container of fluids will last, the necessary volume of fluids, or the rate of infusion per minute or hour to provide the medication as ordered. Patient safety is ensured when the correct fluids ordered by the physician are calculated for the correct infusion rate. Because of the immediate action of medications administered through an IV route, the pharmacy must take extreme care with the calculations and the sterility of preparation. As the pharmacy technician, you must be sure the correct fluids are chosen, along with the correct medications. Rechecking calculations always enhances patient safety.

Posttest

Calculate the following using the method most comfortable for you. Use total volume after addition of additives for calculations. Round to the nearest whole number for minutes and drip rates. Show your calculations.

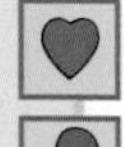

1. A physician orders furosemide 60 mg in 500 mL of D5W. The drop factor is 20 gtt/mL, and the drop rate is 60 gtt/min. Use the following label for your calculations.

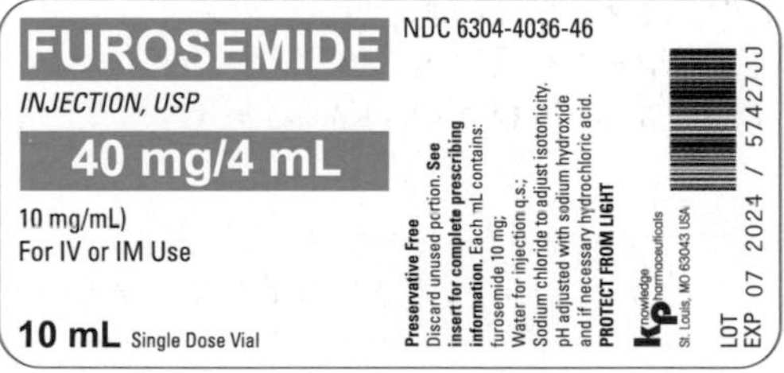

How much furosemide should be added to the fluids?

How long in minutes will the fluids take to infuse?

Continued

Posttest, cont.

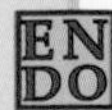

2. A physician orders Humulin R 60 units added to NS 100 mL as an IVPB. The drop factor is 60 gtt/mL. The physician wants the insulin to infuse at 2.5 units/h. Use the following label for your calculations.

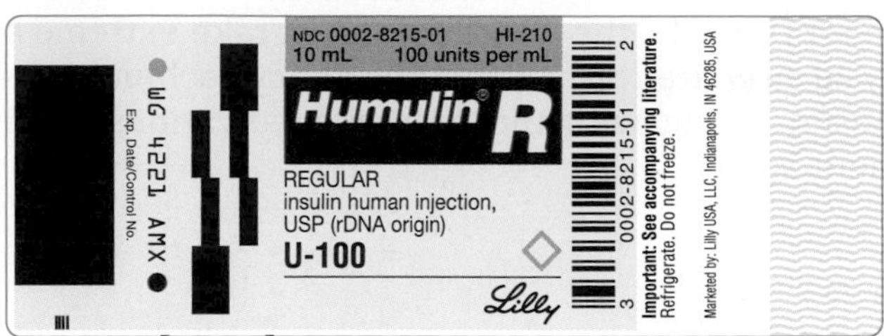

How many milliliters of insulin should be added to the fluids?

How many milliliters per hour will be infused?

How long will the fluids take to infuse?

Posttest, cont.

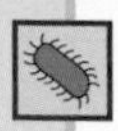

3. Order: ampicillin sodium 1 g in 100 mL LR over 2 hours. The drop factor is 60 gtt/mL. Use the directions on the following label for reconstitution with 1.8 mL of diluent.

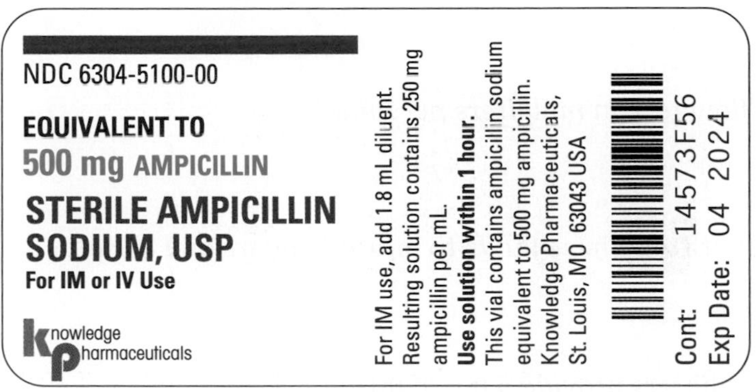

NDC 6304-5100-00
EQUIVALENT TO
500 mg AMPICILLIN
STERILE AMPICILLIN
SODIUM, USP
For IM or IV Use
knowledge pharmaceuticals
For IM use, add 1.8 mL diluent.
Resulting solution contains 250 mg
ampicillin per mL.
Use solution within 1 hour.
This vial contains ampicillin sodium
equivalent to 500 mg ampicillin.
Knowledge Pharmaceuticals,
St. Louis, MO 63043 USA
Cont: 14573F56
Exp Date: 04 2024

How many milliliters of ampicillin should be added to the fluids?

What is the flow rate in mL/min?

How many drops per minute will the patient receive?

How many milligrams of medication will be administered in 45 minutes?

If the order is for q6h, how many vials of medication will be used in 1 day?

What will be the total daily dose of medication in milligrams?

Continued

Posttest, cont.

4. Order: nitroglycerin 50 mg in D5W 250 mL at 50 mcg/min with a drop factor of 60 gtt/mL.

   How many micrograms are in 1 mL of solution?

   What is the flow rate in milliliters per minute?

   How long will it take these fluids to infuse in hours and minutes?

   How many milliliters provide 5 mg of nitroglycerin?

5. Order: 3 L D5NS over 24 hours. The drop factor is 15 gtt/mL.

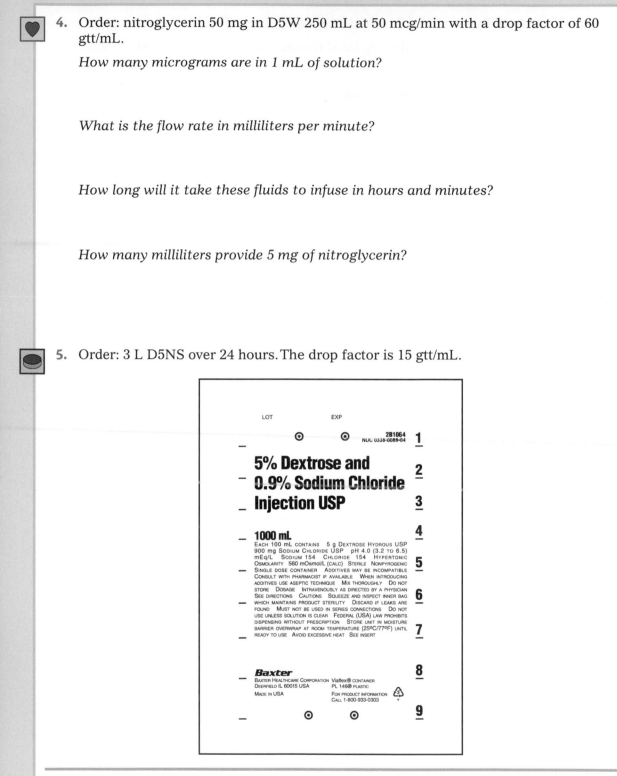

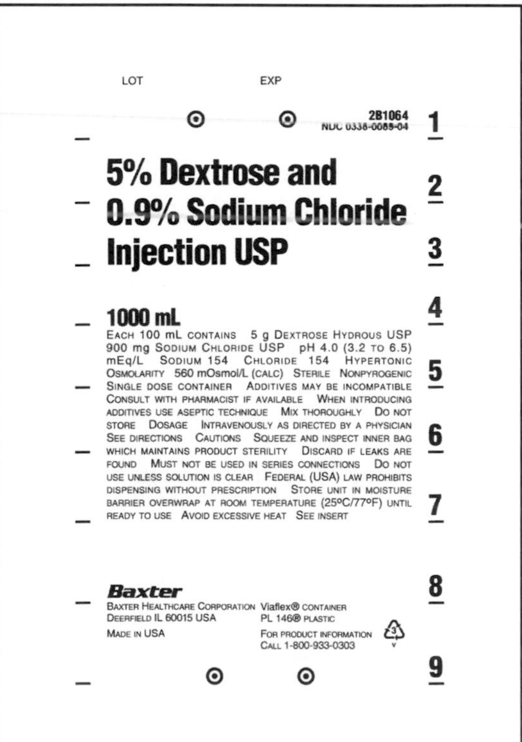
LOT
EXP
2B1064
NDC 0338-0089-04
5% Dextrose and 0.9% Sodium Chloride Injection USP
1000 mL
Each 100 mL contains 5 g Dextrose Hydrous USP 900 mg Sodium Chloride USP pH 4.0 (3.2 to 6.5) mEq/L Sodium 154 Chloride 154 Hypertonic Osmolarity 560 mOsmol/L (calc) Sterile Nonpyrogenic Single dose container Additives may be incompatible Consult with pharmacist if available When introducing additives use aseptic technique Mix thoroughly Do not store Dosage Intravenously as directed by a physician See directions Cautions Squeeze and inspect inner bag which maintains product sterility Discard if leaks are found Must not be used in series connections Do not use unless solution is clear Federal (USA) law prohibits dispensing without prescription Store unit in moisture barrier overwrap at room temperature (25°C/77°F) until ready to use Avoid excessive heat See insert
Baxter
Baxter Healthcare Corporation
Deerfield IL 60015 USA
Made in USA
Viaflex® container
PL 146® plastic
For product information
Call 1-800-933-0303
1
2
3
4
5
6
7
8
9

Posttest, cont.

How many milliliters of fluids should be supplied for each 8-hour shift?

How many 1-L bags of solution should be provided for the physician's order?

How many milliliters per hour should be infused?

How many milliliters will the patient receive in 5 hours?

How many grams of dextrose will the patient receive after 5 hours?

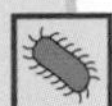

6. A physician orders Amikin 5 mg/kg q8h in 100 mL IVPB for a 176-lb patient.
How many milligrams of amikacin should be added to the fluids?

If amikacin is available as 50 mg/mL, how many milliliters should be added to the PB?

The drop factor is 20 gtt/mL. The time of infusion is 2 hours.
What is the flow rate in drops per minute?

Continued

Posttest, cont.

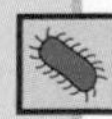

7. *How many minutes will it take to infuse 1 L of D5W at 3 mL/min?*

   How many total milliliters of fluids are required for 24 hours?

   How many grams of dextrose will the patient receive in a 24-hour period?

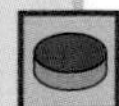

8. Order: 500 mL D5LR over 12 hours with a drop factor of 60 gtt/mL.
   What is the flow rate in milliliters per minute?

   How many milliliters of IV fluid will be infused in an hour?

   How many drops per minute should be infused?

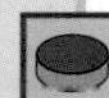

9. A physician orders D5NS 1,000 mL for a child who is dehydrated.
   He wants the patient to receive 90 mL the first hour and the remainder over 12 hours.
   The drop factor is 60 gtt/mL.
   What is the flow rate in milliliters per minute for the first hour?

   What is the flow rate in mL/min for the remaining 12 hours?

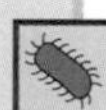

10. Order: Rocephin (ceftriaxone) 25 mg/kg IVPB in 100 mL NS to run over 1 hour q12h. The patient weighs 176 lb.
    How many grams of Rocephin are administered every 12 hours?

    The drop factor is 15 gtt/mL.
    What is the infusion rate in milliliters per minute?

Posttest, cont.

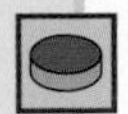

11. Order: KCl 30 mEq added to D5W 150 mL IVPB to infuse over 2 ½ hours with a drop factor of 20 gtt/mL.

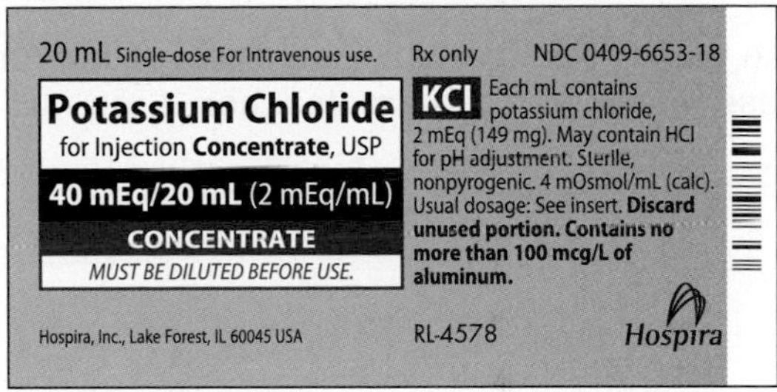

20 mL Single-dose For Intravenous use.
Rx only
NDC 0409-6653-18
Potassium Chloride
for Injection Concentrate, USP
40 mEq/20 mL (2 mEq/mL)
CONCENTRATE
MUST BE DILUTED BEFORE USE.
KCl
Each mL contains potassium chloride, 2 mEq (149 mg). May contain HCl for pH adjustment. Sterile, nonpyrogenic. 4 mOsmol/mL (calc). Usual dosage: See insert. Discard unused portion. Contains no more than 100 mcg/L of aluminum.
Hospira, Inc., Lake Forest, IL 60045 USA
RL-4578
Hospira

(© Pfizer. Used with permission.)

How many milliliters of KCl should be added to the IVPB fluids?

How many milliliters of fluids will be infused in a minute?

How many milliliters of fluids will be infused in an hour?

What is the infusion rate in drops per minute?

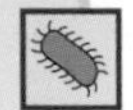

12. Order: doxycycline 150 mg IVPB in LR 85 mL to be administered over 1 ½ hours. Doxycycline is available as 100 mg/10 mL. The drop factor is 20 gtt/mL.

How many milliliters of doxycycline should be added to the fluids?

What is the flow rate in milliliters per minute for this order?

What would the flow rate be in mL/min if the fluids were infused over 1 hour?

Continued

Posttest, cont.

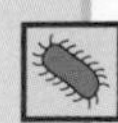

13. A physician orders Retrovir (zidovudine) 2 mg/kg/dose IVPB for a 165-lb patient. The dose is to be placed in 100 mL D5W and infused over 1 hour with a drop factor of 15 gtt/mL q4h × 24 hours.

The 20-mL single-use vial of Retrovir for IV infusion 10 mg/mL must be further diluted in 5% dextrose injection to no greater than 4 mg/mL before being infused.

How many milliliters of the reconstituted medication should be added to the D5W per dose?

What is the infusion rate in milliliters per minute?

How many milligrams of zidovudine will the patient receive in a 24-hour period?

How many drops per minute will the patient receive with each dose?

What is the final concentration of zidovudine in each bag?

Is this within the allowable concentration? ______________

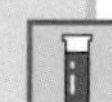

14. A physician orders heparin sodium 20,000 units in NS 500 mL to run over 24 hours. The administration set delivers 60 gtt/mL.

What is the flow rate in drops per minute?

How many units of heparin will the patient receive each hour?

Posttest, cont.

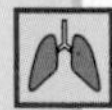

15. A physician orders epinephrine 3 mg added to D5W 250 mL to be infused at 10 mL/h. The administration set delivers 60 gtt/mL.

How many milligrams of epinephrine will the patient receive in an hour? (Do not round.)

How many micrograms will the patient receive in a minute?

What volume will infuse in 24 hours?

How many drops per minute will the patient receive?

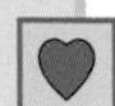

16. A physician orders lidocaine 100 mg in D5W 250 mL to be infused over an hour. The lidocaine is available in 10 mg/mL. The drop factor is 40 gtt/mL.

What volume of lidocaine should be added to the fluids?

What is the flow rate in milliliters per minute that the patient will receive?

How many milligrams of lidocaine will the patient receive per minute?

How many drops per minute will be administered?

Continued

Posttest, cont.

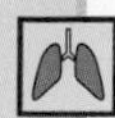

17. A physician orders epinephrine 50 mcg/min to be administered from fluids that contain epinephrine 5 mg in D5LR 500 mL. The drop factor is 20 gtt/mL.

How many minutes will it take for the fluids to infuse?

What is the rate of infusion in drops per minute?

What is the flow rate in milliliters per hour?

How many milligrams of epinephrine did the patient receive if the IV was stopped after 300 mL?

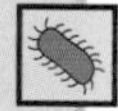

18. Order: amphotericin B 200 mg added to 500 mL D5W to infuse over 6 hours with a drop factor of 15 gtt/mL. Amphotericin is available in a 100 mg/20 mL vial.

How many milliliters of amphotericin should be added to the fluids?

How many vials of medication are needed to complete the order?

What is the flow rate in drops per minute?

What is the flow rate in milliliters per hour?

If the fluids infused for 4 hours, how many milligrams of amphotericin B were received?

Posttest, cont.

19. The following solutions are ordered for a TPN:

Travasol (amino acids) 7.5%	500 mL
dextrose 70%	300 mL
sterile water for injection	200 mL

What is the final concentration of Travasol?

What is the final concentration of dextrose?

If the TPN is hung at 0200 and run at 50 mL/h, when will the next bag be due?

20. A physician orders 1,000 mL of D5NS to infuse over 8 hours.

How many milliliters will be delivered per hour?

How much dextrose is in 1 L of D5NS?

How many grams of dextrose will the patient receive in 2 hours?

How many grams of NaCl will the patient receive in 2 hours?

If the drop factor is 20 gtt/mL, what is the drip rate?

21. Medication order: 500 mL D5-½-NS to infuse over 6 hours with a drop factor of 10 gtt/mL.

What is the weight of dextrose in the solution?

What is the weight of NaCl in the solution?

What is the flow rate in mL/h?

What is the drip rate in gtt/min?

Continued

Posttest, cont.

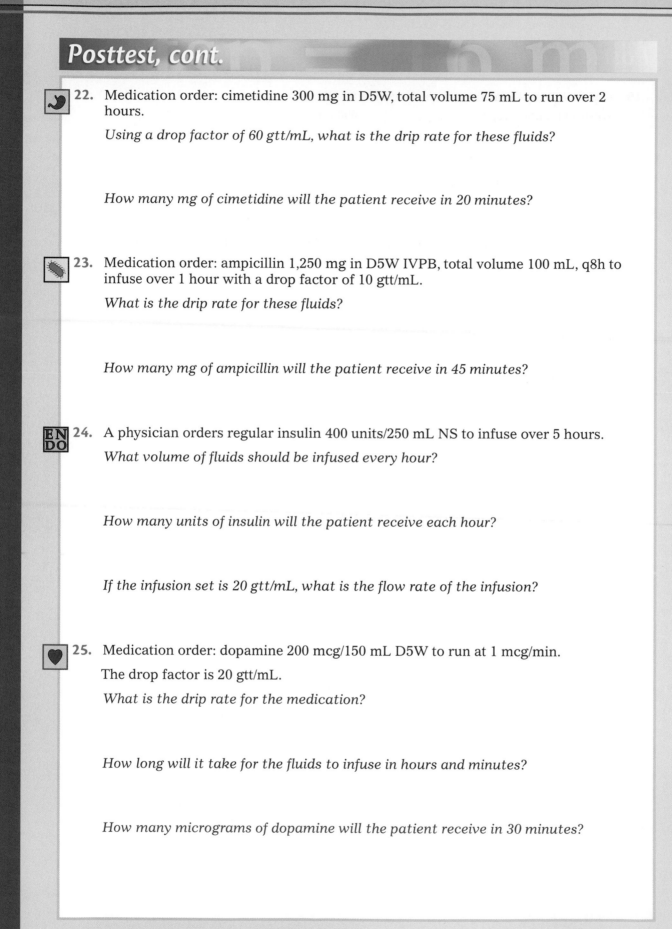

22. Medication order: cimetidine 300 mg in D5W, total volume 75 mL to run over 2 hours.

Using a drop factor of 60 gtt/mL, what is the drip rate for these fluids?

How many mg of cimetidine will the patient receive in 20 minutes?

23. Medication order: ampicillin 1,250 mg in D5W IVPB, total volume 100 mL, q8h to infuse over 1 hour with a drop factor of 10 gtt/mL.

What is the drip rate for these fluids?

How many mg of ampicillin will the patient receive in 45 minutes?

24. A physician orders regular insulin 400 units/250 mL NS to infuse over 5 hours.

What volume of fluids should be infused every hour?

How many units of insulin will the patient receive each hour?

If the infusion set is 20 gtt/mL, what is the flow rate of the infusion?

25. Medication order: dopamine 200 mcg/150 mL D5W to run at 1 mcg/min.

The drop factor is 20 gtt/mL.

What is the drip rate for the medication?

How long will it take for the fluids to infuse in hours and minutes?

How many micrograms of dopamine will the patient receive in 30 minutes?

Posttest, cont.

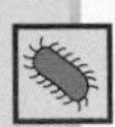

26. Order: vancomycin 400 mg/100 mL IVPB over 4 hours with an infusion set of 20 gtt/mL.

    What is the flow rate in mL/h?

    What is the drip rate in gtt/min?

27. Order: ampicillin 1 g/100 mL to run over 30 min q6h with a drop factor of 15 gtt/mL

    What is the drip rate?

28. Order: 1 L of DNS to be administered at 20 gtt/min with a drop factor of 30 gtt/mL.

    How many hours would this IV run?

    What volume should be left when it is time to change the IV?

29. A compounded TPN has 400 mL of 8.8% Travasol (amino acid), 300 mL of 50% dextrose, 100 mL of lipids, and 200 mL of sterile water.

    What is the final concentration of Travasol?

    What is the final strength of the dextrose?

Use the following chart for the last four questions.

TPN ADDITIVES	ADDITIVE STOCK STRENGTHS AVAILABLE	
potassium chloride		2 mEq/mL
sodium chloride	14.6%	2.5 mEq/mL
calcium gluconate	10%	4.65 mEq/10 mL
magnesium sulfate	50%	40.6 mEq/10 mL
sodium acetate		2 mEq/mL
sodium phosphates	45 mM/15 mL	60 mEq/15 mL
potassium acetate	19.6%	2 mEq/mL
potassium phosphate	15 mM/5 mL	4.4 mEq/mL
Humulin R insulin	100 units/mL	
vitamin C	250 mg/2 mL	
folic acid	5 mg/mL	

TPN, Total parenteral nutrition.

Continued

Posttest, cont.

30. Complete the following TPN order from the stock available. Calculate amounts needed for each additive. Show your work.

Potassium chloride 10 mEq:

Sodium chloride 15 mEq:

Calcium gluconate 7.5 mEq:

Magnesium sulfate 2 mEq:

Sodium acetate 3 mEq:

Sodium phosphate 12 mEq:

Humulin R insulin 41 units:

Vitamin C 500 mg:

Folic acid 10 mg:

MVI-12: 10 mL

What is the total amount of all of the additives?

Base Solutions

Travasol 10%	300 mL
dextrose 50%	400 mL
lipids 20%	100 mL
sterile water for injection	qs ad 1,000 mL

What is the final concentration of Travasol?

What is the final concentration of dextrose?

What is the final concentration of lipids?

How much sterile water for injection is needed to reach 1,000 mL? Be sure to account for the total amount of additives.

If it is hung at 0400 and run at 100 mL/h, when will the next bag be due?

Posttest, cont.

31. The following TPN to be run over 24 hours is for a 20-pound infant. Calculate the amounts needed for each ordered additive.

Potassium chloride 2.5 mEq/kg:

Sodium chloride 2.5 mEq/kg:

Magnesium sulfate 0.5 mEq/kg:

What is the total volume of the additives?

Base Solutions Ordered

5.5% Travasol	200 mL
20% dextrose	150 mL

What is the total volume of the TPN?

How many grams of amino acids are in this TPN?

How many grams of dextrose are in this TPN?

What is the final concentration of Travasol (amino acids)?

What is the final concentration of dextrose?

Continued

Posttest, cont.

32. Complete the following TPN order from the stock available.
Calculate the amounts needed for each of the following ordered additives.

Potassium chloride 15 mEq:

Sodium chloride 10 mEq:

Magnesium sulfate 250 mg:

Sodium phosphates 20 mEq:

Vitamin C 500 mg:

Folic acid 10 mg:

Trace elements:	5 mL
MVI-12:	10 mL

What is the total volume of the additives?

Base Solutions Ordered

Travasol (amino acids)	30 g
dextrose	200 g
sterile water for injection	qs ad 1,000 mL

Base Solutions Available

Travasol	8.8%
dextrose	50%

Round the following two answers to whole numbers.

How many milliliters of 8.8% Travasol are needed to provide 30 grams of amino acids?

How many milliliters of 50% dextrose are needed to provide 200 g of dextrose?

How many milliliters of sterile water are needed?

Run at 100 mL/h.

If it is hung at 0600, when will the next IV be due?

REVIEW OF RULES

IV calculations involve determination of the:

- amount of medication delivered (mg, g, mEq, or units) over a specific period of time
- volume of medication delivered (gtt, mL, or L) over a specific period of time—*dose volume*
- volume of medication needed to last a specific amount of time
- length of time a medication dose will last—*dose time*

Equations used:

Flow rate = dose volume/dose time

Specific type of flow rate:

Drip rate = gtt/min

Factors to be considered with IV administration are as follows:

- Total amount of fluids to be administered in *milliliters—dose volume (mL)*
- Calibration of the administration (infusion) set in *drops per milliliter—drop factor (gtt/mL)*
- Flow rate of the fluids in drops per minute—drip rate (*gtt/min*)
- Time for the fluids to infuse in *minutes (min)* or *hours (h or hr)*

IN SECTION V

16 Pharmacy Business Math

SECTION V
Business Math

CHAPTER 16

Pharmacy Business Math

OBJECTIVES

1. Manage inventory, including par levels and inventory turnover rate.
2. Calculate overhead expenses.
3. Calculate depreciation.
4. Calculate prescription markup.
5. Calculate discounts on merchandise.
6. Calculate net and gross income/profit.
7. Calculate insurance reimbursement using average wholesale prices, dispensing fees, and capitation.
8. Discuss a daily cash report.

KEY WORDS

Adjudication Electronic process by which insurance companies evaluate prescriptions to determine their validity and the price to charge the patient

Assets Any property owned by a business

Average wholesale price (AWP) Price that a pharmacy theoretically pays for medication; this price is theoretical because discounts, sales, and special deals may affect the actual wholesale price; this is the price basis used for insurance reimbursement

Capitation fee Set amount of third-party money paid monthly to the pharmacy for a specific patient regardless of the number of prescriptions filled

Cash flow Receipts and expenses for a business

Daily cash or sales report Report made at the end of each day that summarizes the sales, discounts, and amount of cash, checks, refunds, and credit card charges that have occurred during the day's operations

Depreciation Decrease in value of an asset based on total value of the asset, its estimated length of use, and its value at disposal; part of overhead

Discount Reduction in the price of an item; offered to customers by the pharmacy (**markdown**) or offered to the pharmacy from wholesalers when a bill is paid by a certain date

Discount percentage A percentage amount to be subtracted from the retail price of an item to lower the selling price

Dispensing fee Amount of money added to the cost of a prescription; intended to cover various aspects of preparing and dispensing; often a set price determined by insurance companies

Gross income/gross profit Sales price of merchandise minus its purchase cost; usually refers to total income for a business

Inventory All of the merchandise in stock

Markup Amount of money added to the purchase cost of a product to obtain the selling price

Markup percentage or gross margin A percentage amount added to the purchase cost of merchandise to ensure a profit

Net income/net profit Gross profit minus overhead; usually refers to total income for a business

Overhead Expenses of a business, *not including cost of inventory,* such as rent, wages, utilities, insurance, license fees, depreciation, taxes paid, and other costs of doing business

PAR level (periodic automatic replenishment) Predetermined point for automatic inventory reordering of items used in a pharmacy; **par level** is also used to indicate a specific quantity to be kept in stock

Purchase cost Price paid by a business to obtain items for sale; also referred to as **wholesale, acquisition**, or **inventory cost**

Selling price Price at which items are offered for sale to customers; also referred to as **retail price**

Turnover rate Rate at which the inventory is sold over a specified period of time

Pretest

If you are already comfortable with the subject matter, perform the following business math calculations to test your knowledge. If not, work your way through the chapter and return to them for extra practice. Round answers to the nearest tenth or dollars and cents as appropriate.

1. A pharmacy sells a prescription for $43.50. The medication costs the pharmacy $22.65.

   What is the markup?

2. A pharmacy buys a medication at a discount rate of $555 for 1,000 tablets. The selling price for the medication is $45.50 for 50 tablets.

   What is the markup on the prescription?

Pretest, cont.

3. A customer brings in a discount coupon for 25% off her first prescription and 10% off her second prescription. One prescription costs $15 and the other costs $24.50. The pharmacist tells you to take the 25% off the most expensive prescription.

   What will the first prescription cost the patient?

   What will the second prescription cost the patient?

   What is the total cost for both prescriptions?

4. A pharmacy has a monthly income of $535,356 with inventory purchases of $456,980, salaries and wages of $76,000, and maintenance costs of $1,567.50.

   What is the net income of the pharmacy for the month?

5. *What is the percentage markup of a prescription that has an inventory cost of $14.50 and is sold for $21?*

6. A pharmacy buys a new computer program for $9,500 in January. The expected time of use is 3 years, and it will be discarded at the end of 3 years.

   What is the amount of depreciation for this equipment for a year?

7. A pharmacy has a reorder level of 2,500 capsules for antibiotic during the winter. The pharmacy technician counts 950 capsules in inventory.

   How many capsules need to be ordered to maintain the par level?

   The wholesaler has a deal on 5,000 capsules for $1,500 with a 10% discount. The average use of the capsules in the winter is 3,000 capsules per week.

   Would it be appropriate for the pharmacy technician to ask the pharmacist if she desires to take advantage of the discounted medication? ____________ Explain your answer. ____

   What is the discounted price for 5,000 capsules?

Continued

Pretest, cont.

8. A pharmacy is contracted with an insurance company for a reimbursement of AWP plus 15% and a dispensing fee. The AWP for the prescription is $12.50. The dispensing fee is $7.50.

   What is the amount to be charged to the insurance company?

9. A pharmacy is contracted with an insurance company for reimbursement based on a capitation fee of $55 per month for a patient. The patient received prescriptions for $16.50 and $12.00.

   What is the balance available for additional prescriptions?

   The patient brings in other prescriptions totaling $27.50 before the end of the month.

   What will the pharmacy lose from capitation reimbursement?

PA IN 10. A pharmacy purchases aspirin at an AWP of $3.00 for 100 tablets.

   Mark the price up by 45% and then offer a 25% discount.

   What is the price of the medication after the 45% markup?

   What is the selling price after the 25% discount?

   What profit would the pharmacy make on 10 bottles of 100?

INTRODUCTION

Pharmacy technicians in retail settings, as well as in hospital settings, may be involved with business calculations. For a business to remain profitable, the **net income**, or **net profit**, from the sales of medications must exceed the cost of doing business. Mathematical calculations include using percentages to determine **discounts** and **markups**, as well as addition and subtraction to maintain the necessary inventory **par levels**. An adequate markup must be in place so the receipts of the business are in excess of the expenses, and the supply of **inventory** must be adequate to cover demand but not so excessive that it ties up the **cash flow** of the business. Monitoring of pricing and inventory, as well as obtaining necessary inventory levels, may be a task of the pharmacy technician. The cash flow of the pharmacy is directly related to the mathematical calculations performed for inventory and **profit** (or loss) that are calculated routinely. Therefore costs of new inventory must be carefully checked each time new stock arrives to be sure they have not changed since the last order. If inventory prices change and the prices for sales are not changed simultaneously, profits will be affected. A pharmacy technician may have a major role in inventory control and reordering, which affects **turnover rate** and **gross and net income or profit**.

INVENTORY MANAGEMENT

Inventory includes all stock *available for sale* by a business. Pharmacies take inventory by making a list of all merchandise on hand at a specific time. Controlled drugs are normally inventoried more often than other medications, depending on the protocol of the particular business and state and federal regulations.

Par Level

A **par** or reorder level is determined by sales history. For seasonal medications, such as antihistamines and flu vaccines, the par level may need to be increased at certain times of the year. To maintain the inventory flow and minimize the need for extra shelf space, replacements for medications should be ordered shortly before they are needed for use.

$$\text{Amount to reorder} = \text{Par or reorder level} - \text{Amount in stock}$$

With certain inexpensive or fast-moving items, it may be advantageous to order slightly above par, especially if a deal is being offered on a particular size. With other slower-moving or very expensive items, ordering close to par or waiting to order may be the best idea. This will also depend on how quickly the medication can be delivered to the pharmacy once it is ordered.

In many pharmacies, a perpetual inventory is automatically maintained using a computer program. As medication is sold it is subtracted from inventory, and when medication is received it is added to the inventory. With **PAR** (periodic automatic replenishment), restocking occurs on a continual basis because the computer submits the order to the wholesaler electronically as stock is used or purchased by customers.

TECH NOTE

A **PAR** (periodic automatic replenishing) level is set in some pharmacies that have the capability of reordering medications automatically as they are used.

EXAMPLE 16.1

The par level or reorder point for amoxicillin during the winter is 1,500 capsules. Prescriptions for 1 day show dispensing 750 capsules. The bottle of 1,000 capsules has been opened and appears to be about half full.

How many capsules should be ordered?

Amount to reorder = 1,500 − 500 = 1,000 capsules

The pharmacy can purchase 100 caps for $25, 500 caps for $95, and 1,000 caps for $156.

What is the cost per capsule for each size container?

$$\frac{\$25}{100} = \frac{x}{1} \quad \text{so, } 1 \times \$25 \div 100 = \$0.25/\text{cap}$$

$$\frac{\$95}{500} = \frac{x}{1} \quad \text{so, } 1 \times \$95 \div 500 = \$0.19/\text{cap}$$

$$\frac{\$156}{1,000} = \frac{x}{1} \quad \text{so, } 1 \times \$156 \div 1,000 = \$0.16/\text{cap}$$

Which combination of bottles should be ordered to ensure the lowest cost?

The order should be one bottle of 1,000 capsules because the cost is less with this size and fewer larger containers require less storage space.

The original par level would suggest ordering one bottle of 1,000 capsules; however, with what seems to be the increased seasonal use of the medication, the technician may want to consult with the pharmacist about increasing the par level temporarily and ordering an additional 1,000 at the lowest price.

Practice Problems A

Calculate the amount of product to reorder, using the lowest cost.

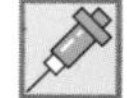

1. The par level for Enbrel (etanercept) pre-filled autojector 50 mg/mL is 12.

   The pharmacy currently has 7 in stock.

   How many are needed to reach par?

   The wholesaler sells these in sets of 4 for $5,174.00.

   Why might you want to check with the pharmacist before ordering above par?

   ____

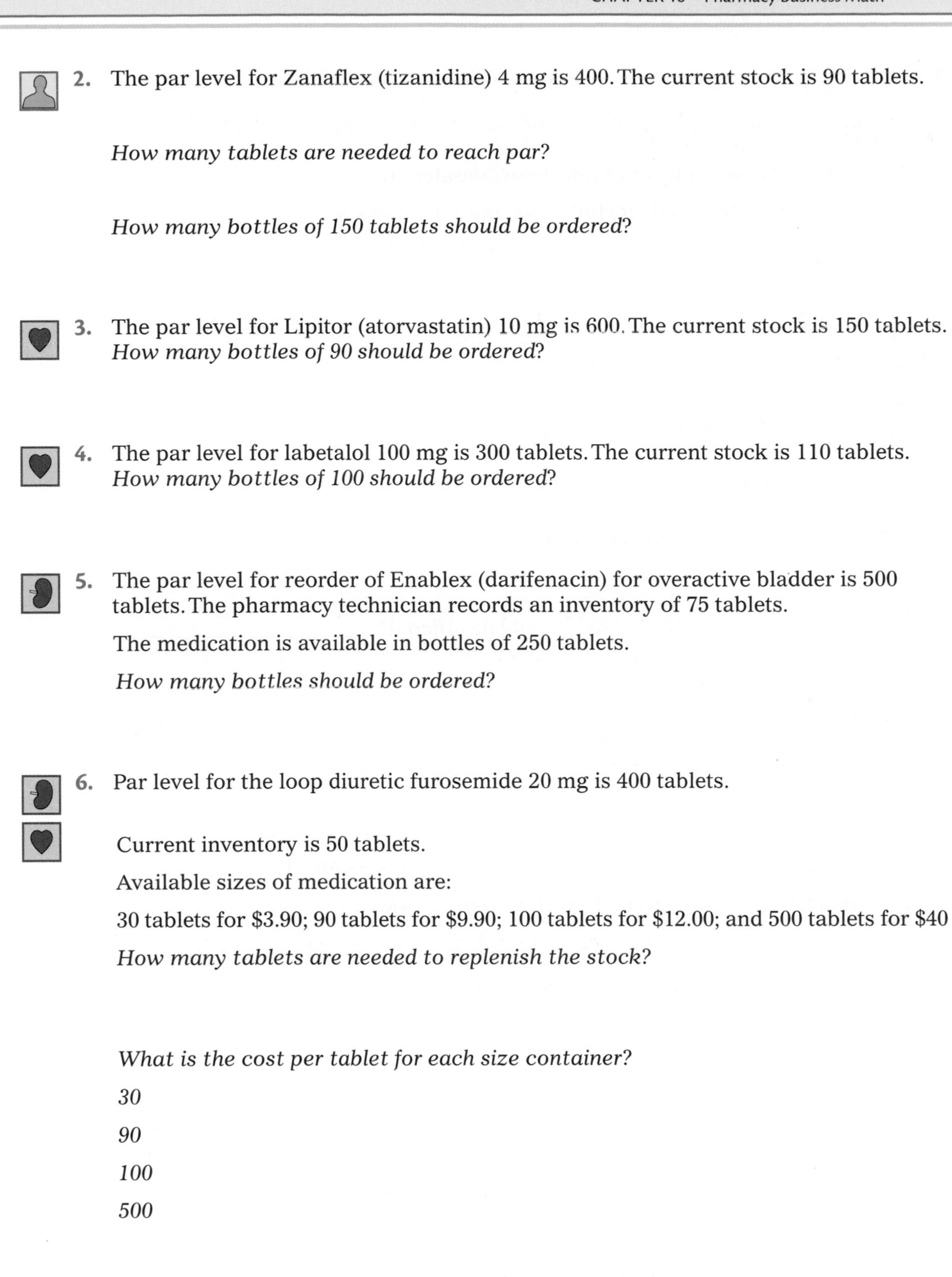

2. The par level for Zanaflex (tizanidine) 4 mg is 400. The current stock is 90 tablets.

How many tablets are needed to reach par?

How many bottles of 150 tablets should be ordered?

3. The par level for Lipitor (atorvastatin) 10 mg is 600. The current stock is 150 tablets. *How many bottles of 90 should be ordered?*

4. The par level for labetalol 100 mg is 300 tablets. The current stock is 110 tablets. *How many bottles of 100 should be ordered?*

5. The par level for reorder of Enablex (darifenacin) for overactive bladder is 500 tablets. The pharmacy technician records an inventory of 75 tablets.

The medication is available in bottles of 250 tablets.

How many bottles should be ordered?

6. Par level for the loop diuretic furosemide 20 mg is 400 tablets.

Current inventory is 50 tablets.

Available sizes of medication are:

30 tablets for $3.90; 90 tablets for $9.90; 100 tablets for $12.00; and 500 tablets for $40

How many tablets are needed to replenish the stock?

What is the cost per tablet for each size container?

30

90

100

500

What is the most appropriate size to order considering cost? ______________________

How many containers of this size should be ordered? ______________________________

7. Par level for the inotropic agent digoxin 0.25 mg is 200 tablets.

Current inventory is 25 tablets.

The available sizes and costs from the wholesaler are:

25 tablets for $6.50; 50 tablets for $7.50; and 100 tablets for $14.00

How many tablets are needed to replenish the stock?

What is the cost per tablet for each size container?

25

50

100

What is the most cost-efficient stock medication size? ____________

How many containers of this size should be ordered? ____________

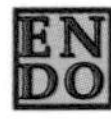

8. Par level for the thyroid hormone levothyroxine 0.1 mg is 225 tablets.

The current inventory is 75 tablets.

Available sizes of medications and the wholesale cost for each are as follows:

50 tablets for $4.75; 100 tablets for $8.50; and 250 tablets for $12.50

How many tablets are needed to replenish the stock?

What is the cost per unit for each size container?

50

100

250

What is the most cost-efficient stock medication size? ____________

How many containers of this size should be ordered? ____________

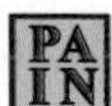

9. Par level for the nonsteroidal anti-inflammatory ibuprofen, 800 mg, is 1,500 tablets.

The inventory on hand is 250 tablets.

The available sizes from the wholesaler are:

100 tablets for $7.50; 200 tablets for $13.75; and 500 tablets for $27.45

How many tablets are needed to replenish the stock?

What is the cost per unit for each size container?

100

200

500

Which is the most cost-efficient stock medication size? ____________________

How many containers of this size should be ordered? ____________________

10. Par level for the antidepressant Paxil (paroxetine) 20 mg is 400 tablets.

The current inventory is 180 tablets.

Available sizes of medications are:

40 tablets for $9.20; 90 tablets for $17.10; 150 tablets for $24.00; and 250 tablets for $37.50

How many tablets are needed to replenish the stock?

What is the cost per unit for each size container?

40

90

150

250

What is the most cost-efficient stock medication size? ____________________

How many containers should be ordered? ____________________

Inventory Turnover Rate

Inventory turnover rate is the frequency at which inventory is sold and replaced over a specified time period. The turnover rate is important for setting par levels of medications. This number helps the pharmacy determine whether inventory should be increased or decreased, thus controlling the amount of cash that is tied up in inventory. The turnover rate is the total value of inventory ordered over a specific time period, such as 1 month, 6 months, or 1 year, divided by the average value of inventory on hand. The formula for turnover rate is as follows:

$$\text{Inventory turnover rate} = \text{Total purchases over a given time} \div \text{Average inventory value}$$

EXAMPLE 16.2

A pharmacy spends \$2,450,000 per year for inventory. The average inventory value is \$350,000.

$$\text{Turnover rate} = \$2,450,000/\text{year} \div \$350,000$$
$$\text{Turnover rate} = 7 \text{ times per year}$$

Practice Problems B

Calculate the inventory turnover rate in the following situations. Round all answers to tenths. Show your work.

1. A pharmacy has an average inventory value of \$500,000 at any given time. The total amount spent on inventory in a year is \$2,000,000.

   What is the inventory turnover rate for the year?

2. A pharmacy has an average inventory of \$225,000. The purchases for 6 months are \$1,237,500.

   What is the turnover rate for this pharmacy for 6 months?

3. A pharmacy has an average inventory of \$125,000. The purchases for 6 months are \$2,250,000.

   What is the turnover rate for this pharmacy for 6 months?

4. A hospital has an average inventory of \$70,000. The purchases for the past 2 months are \$270,000.

   What is the turnover rate for 2 months?

5. A pharmacy has an average inventory of $22,500. The purchases for the year are $775,200.

   What is the turnover rate for this pharmacy for the year?

6. A pharmacy maintains an average inventory of $120,000. The pharmacist is concerned that he keeps too much stock. He spends $870,000 per year for medications. He likes a turnover rate of 2.5 every 2 months or less.

   What is his approximate turnover rate every 2 months?

   Is he maintaining the turnover rate that he desires? ______________

   What is his turnover rate per year?

   How can the pharmacist increase his turnover rate?

   ____

OVERHEAD EXPENSES

Overhead is the actual cost of doing business. It includes all costs for the pharmacy, such as salaries, licenses, equipment purchases and repairs, depreciation, utilities, telephone, insurance, taxes paid (e.g., employer's payroll taxes), and rent. *Overhead does not include the cost of inventory!*

To calculate overhead, total all business expenses (*excluding* inventory).

Depreciation is a rate representing the decrease in value of an **asset** (equipment, building, computer, printer) over time.

$$\text{Annual depreciation} = \text{Cost} \div \text{Estimated time of use in years}$$

EXAMPLE 16.3

A pharmacy purchased a computer for $1,000, which is intended to be useful for 5 years.

$$\text{Annual depreciation} = \$1,000/5\text{ years} = \$200/\text{year}$$

If the depreciation is taken equally over 5 years, the amount is $200 per year.

EXAMPLE 16.4

A pharmacy spends $12,585 for inventory per week; the salaries for all employees are $12,500 per week. Rent is $1,600 per month and utilities cost $800 per month. In addition, the cost for insurance is $1,000 per month and depreciation on equipment is $2,500 per month. Taxes are $2,400 per month. *What is the overhead for 1 week?*

Salaries	$12,500
Rent	400 ($1,600 ÷ 4 weeks/month)
Utilities	200 ($800 ÷ 4 weeks/month)
Insurance	250 ($1,000 ÷ 4 weeks/month)
Depreciation	625 ($2,500 ÷ 4 weeks/month)
Taxes	400 ($2,400 ÷ 4 weeks/month)
Total overhead	$14,375/week

TECH NOTE

Remember that overhead does not include the cost of inventory.

Practice Problems C

Calculate depreciation or overhead in the following problems. Remember not to include the cost of inventory when calculating overhead. Show your calculations. All final answers should be shown in dollars and cents.

1. The pharmacy buys a new computer for $9,000. The expected time of use is 4 years.

   What is the amount of depreciation for the computer for 1 year?

2. A pharmacy has a monthly cost for medication inventory of $46,725, salaries of $58,000, utilities of $2,534, rent of $770, insurance of $1,575, taxes of $7,844, depreciation of equipment of $965, and business supplies and postage of $650.

   What is the overhead cost for the pharmacy for a month?

   What is the approximate overhead cost for a year?

3. A hospital pharmacy is asked to calculate the overhead necessary to maintain safety for the patients when medications are dispensed. The following amounts would be necessary per year: salaries for pharmacists—$264,000; four pharmacy technician salaries—$22,500 each; medication inventory—$56,525 each month; utilities—$750 per month; salaries for relief pharmacists—$12,500/year; computers and software updates—$56,000 yearly; yearly liability insurance for pharmacists and pharmacy technicians—$3,500; and use of hospital space—$3,600/year.

   What is the total overhead for this hospital pharmacy for a year?

   What is the overhead for a month?

4. A pharmacist needs to know how much income each month is necessary to meet the overhead for the business he owns. The expenses are salaries of $72,000 per year for the pharmacist, $27,500 per year each for two pharmacy technicians, $560,430 per year for inventory costs, $5,600 per year for utilities and rent, $27,500 per year for equipment replacement, and taxes and other business expenses of $1,560 per month.

   What is the overhead for this pharmacy per month?

   What is the overhead for the pharmacy for a year?

5. A retail pharmacy wants to ensure that sufficient income is being obtained for a new branch that has just opened. The monthly expenses are $6,500 for the pharmacist's salary, total of $1,250 for two pharmacy technicians who both work part-time while in school, $25,340 for inventory, $560 for taxes, business expenses of $980, utilities and rent of $11,500, and payment for equipment of $4,500 per month.

   What is the total amount of overhead for a month?

   What is the overhead for a year?

6. A pharmacy needs to compute the amount of overhead the store has in a year. The salaries are $54,000 per month, rent is $1,250 per month, utilities are $22,500 per year, inventory is $86,950 per month, equipment costs $60,000 per year in replacements, supplies are $1,250 per month, and miscellaneous expenses are $1,550 per month. The depreciation rate is $950 per month.

   What is the overhead for a year?

   What is the overhead for a month?

SELLING PRICE AND MARKUP

The **selling** or **retail price** is the price at which an item is offered for sale to a customer, once a **markup** is added to the **purchase cost** (wholesale, acquisition, or inventory cost). The selling price is calculated by adding a **markup percentage**, a percentage of the original purchase cost of the item, which increases the base price to the customer in order to make a profit in business. The amount of the markup is *always* based on the purchase cost to the pharmacy. The formulas are as follows:

$$\text{Selling (retail) price} = \text{Purchase cost} + \text{markup}$$

$$\text{Markup} = \text{Purchase cost} \times \text{Markup percentage (as a decimal)}$$

Or, if you know the selling price and purchase cost:

Markup = Selling price − Purchase cost

EXAMPLE 16.5

A pharmacy marks up private-pay prescriptions by 35%.

What will be charged for a prescription that costs the pharmacy $14.98?

Markup = $14.98 × 0.35 = $5.24

Selling (retail) price = $14.98 + $5.24 = $20.22

An alternative to finding the markup and then adding it to the purchase cost is to consider that the customer will pay the purchase cost plus the purchase cost times the markup percentage as a decimal. The equation can be set up as:

Selling price = Purchase cost + (Purchase cost × Markup percentage)

By factoring out purchase cost:

Selling price = Purchase cost × (1+ Markup percentage)

Using Example 16.5:

Selling price = $14.98 × 1.35 = $20.22

Markup on brand name drugs is generally lower than markup on generic drugs. For instance, if a brand name antibiotic, such as Keflex, costs $100 and has a 6% markup ($100 × 0.06 = $6), the cost to the customer is $106. A generic for the same drug, cephalexin, may cost $40 with a 25% markup ($40 × 0.25 = $10), so the cost to the customer is $50. Pharmacies have higher profit margins available with generics than they do with brand name drugs.

EXAMPLE 16.6

A prescription sells for $35.60, and the cost is $29.90. *What is the markup?*

Markup = $35.60 – $29.90

Markup = $5.70

Practice Problems D

Calculate the selling price or markup.

1. A pharmacy pays $36 for 30 tablets and marks the prescription up 20%.

   What is the selling price?

2. The purchase cost of a bottle of 100 acetaminophen is $1.21. The pharmacy wants to mark it up 86%.

   What is the retail price?

3. A patient brings in a prescription for 6 tablets of an antibiotic. The purchase cost of the brand is $42. The pharmacy marks up brand-name drugs 15%.
   What is the selling price?

4. The customer from question 3 asks how much this would be in the generic version. The purchase cost of 6 tablets of the generic is $10.14. The pharmacy marks up the generic 65%.

   What is the retail price of the generic prescription?

5. A medication has a selling price of $56 and a cost of $45.

   What is the markup?

6. A medication has a selling price of $34.50 and a cost of $15.60.

   What is the markup?

7. A medication has a selling price of $43.50 and a cost of $39.90.

   What is the markup?

8. A medication has a selling price of $10.20 and a cost of $9.20.

   What is the markup?

9. A medication has a selling price of $125 and a cost of $93.50.

   What is the markup?

10. A very expensive prescription costs the pharmacy $973.21 for a 1-month supply. To help out the customer it is only marked up 3.5%.

    What is the retail price?

    What is the markup?

Markup Percentage

The **markup percentage** or **gross margin** is calculated by dividing the markup by the cost and then multiplying by 100. Markup percentages provide information about which prescription medications have the greatest profit. The formula is as follows:

$$\text{Markup percentage} = \frac{\text{Markup}}{\text{Purchase cost}} \times 100$$

Since markup is selling price – purchase cost, the equation can also be written as:

$$\text{Markup percentage} = \frac{\text{Selling price} - \text{Purchase cost}}{\text{Purchase cost}} \times 100$$

EXAMPLE 16.7

A medication costs the pharmacy $29.90 and is sold for $35.60. What is the markup percentage?

$$\text{Markup} = \$35.60 - \$29.90 = \$5.70$$

$$\text{Markup percentage} = (\$5.70 \div \$29.90) \times 100 = 19\%$$

Alternately:

$$\text{Markup percentage} = \frac{\$35.60 - \$29.90}{\$29.90} \times 100 = 19\%$$

TECH NOTE

If the selling price is more than twice the purchase cost, the markup percentage will always be over 100%.

Practice Problems E

Calculate the percentage of markup in the following problems. Show your calculations. Round all final answers to tenths.

1. A medication has a selling price of $56 and a purchase cost of $45.

   What is the markup percentage?

2. A medication has a selling price of $34.50 and a cost of $15.60.

   What is the markup percentage?

3. A medication has a selling price of $43.50 and a cost of $39.90.

   What is the markup percentage?

4. A medication has a selling price of $10.20 and a cost of $9.20.

   What is the markup percentage?

5. A medication has a selling price of $125 and a cost of $93.50.

   What is the markup percentage?

6. A medication has a selling price of $45 and a cost of $42.

   What is the markup percentage?

7. A medication has a selling price of $27.90 and a cost of $23.60.

   What is the markup percentage?

8. A medication has a selling price of $33.75 and a cost of $30.

   What is the markup percentage?

9. A medication has a selling price of $12.90 and a cost of $9.20.

   What is the markup percentage?

10. A prescription for 60 tablets has a cost of $0.55 per tablet. This medication sells for $55.00.

    What is the markup on this prescription?

    What is the markup percentage on this prescription?

DISCOUNTS

A **discount or markdown** may be applied to prescriptions, over-the-counter (OTC) drugs, or other merchandise. The markdown price is calculated by subtracting a **discount percentage**, a percentage of the original selling price of the item, which lowers the price the customer pays. Discounts and markdowns are used as an incentive to encourage customers to purchase items by realizing a savings on the original selling or retail price. Markdowns and discounts may be in the form of manufacturers' coupons or special discounts for reasons such as senior citizens' initiatives. The amount of the discount is *always* based on the selling (retail) price, not on the purchase cost of the item. The item must be marked up for sale first, and then a discount can be applied. A discount *decreases* the selling price; markup is based on the pharmacy's purchase cost. The formulas for discounts are as follows:

$$\text{Discount amount} = \text{Selling price} \times \text{Discount percentage}$$

$$\text{Discounted price} = \text{Selling price} - \text{Discount amount}$$

When discounts are given based on manufacturers' or other coupons, the amount of the coupon should be subtracted from the selling price and the coupon placed in the cash drawer to be used at the end of the day to balance the cash drawer.

EXAMPLE 16.8

A customer has a 15% coupon for a medication that sells for $45.00.

What is the cost to the patient after the use of the discount coupon?

Hint: Change percentage to a decimal number for each calculation.

$$\text{Discount amount} = \$45.00 \times 0.15 = \$6.75$$

$$\text{Discount price} = \$45{:}00 - \$6{:}75 = \$38{:}25$$

An alternative to finding the discount amount and then subtracting it from the original price is to consider the percentage of the total price the customer will need to pay and multiply by that decimal. In Example 16.8, with a 15% discount, the customer will pay the remaining 85% of the cost (100% – 15% = 85%).

The customer will pay $45.00 times 0.85, which equals $38.25.

Discounts may also be offered to a pharmacy from the wholesaler for timely payment of an invoice. For example, the invoice may offer an 8% discount if paid by the 15th of the month. The supplier may also discount certain medications or provide a discount for bulk purchases. These discounts provide a way for pharmacies to increase their profits.

TECH NOTE

The customer discount is always calculated and subtracted from the selling or retail price, not the pharmacy's purchase cost, or the pharmacy will lose money.

Practice Problems F

Calculate the discounted prices in the following problems. Show your work. Remember that the discounted price must always be lower.

1. The pharmacy offers a 10% senior citizen discount on all prescriptions.

   What is the cost to a senior citizen for a $54.00 prescription?

2. The wholesaler offers a 7% discount if the invoice is paid within 10 days of delivery.

   How much could be saved on a $22,643 invoice?

3. A patient has a manufacturer's discount coupon in the amount of 25% for a new prescription. The selling price is $42.50.

   What is the discount amount?

   What is the price of the prescription after the discount?

4. An ad in the local paper offers ⅓ off a medication that is taken regularly by one of your customers. *Hint: Multiply by the fraction ⅓ as opposed to changing it to a decimal.* The patient brings in the coupon for the medicine that costs $33.

   What is the discount amount?

   What is the price of the medication after the discount?

5. A drug supplier offers a deal that will provide a 25% discount for 10 tubes of a new dermatologic preparation. The cost for the 10 tubes is $525.

   What is the discount amount?

   What is the discounted price for these tubes of medication?

6. An older patient on a fixed income comes to the pharmacy with a new prescription. The pharmacist tells the patient that he will provide a 12% discount for the medication, which costs $65.

   What is the discount amount?

   What is the price of the prescription after the discount?

7. An insurance company has a contract with the pharmacy to provide a 5% discount for any prescription for its members. A prescription has a retail price of $75.40.

   What is the discount amount?

   What discounted price should be charged to the insured?

8. A retail pharmacy has advertised a 35%-off sale on all pain relievers during the first 2 weeks of April. Tylenol's regular price is $7.59 and Aleve's price is $8.29.

   What is the discounted price for each of these OTC products? Perform these calculations by multiplying by 0.65 (the 65% balance that the customer will have to pay) to go directly to the discounted price. Verify your answers by determining the discount amount and subtracting from the selling price.

   Tylenol:

   Aleve:

9. An ad in the local paper offers 30% off an antacid with a regular price of $4.54.

   What is the discounted price for the product?

10. A manufacturer's coupon offers a 20% discount on cough syrup. The retail price is $5.79.

    What is the discounted price for the cough syrup?

11. A manufacturer offers a discount of 40% on the first prescription of a hypolipidemic agent that sells for $75 retail.

    What is the price of the prescription after the discount?

12. A pharmacy bought an OTC medication at 30% less than the usual wholesale price of $12.00 for 100 tablets.

    What is the discounted price?

    The usual retail price is $22 for 100 tablets and the pharmacist wants to offer a 25% discount to the patients as a means to bring in more customers.

    What is the discounted price of 100 tablets for the patient?

    How much would the pharmacy make on one 100-tablet bottle in this situation?

INCOME

Gross Income

The **gross income** (sometimes referred to as **gross profit**) is the difference in the sales price and the cost of the inventory with no other expenses of the business considered. This usually is calculated for the total income of the business.

$$\text{Gross income} = \text{Sales} - \text{Cost of inventory}$$

EXAMPLE 16.9

Calculate the gross profit if a pharmacy's sales were $200,000 and purchases were $175,000.

$$\text{Gross income} = \$200,000 - \$175,000 = \$25,000$$

Practice Problems G

Calculate the following problems. A month should be considered 4 weeks.

1. A pharmacy has sales of $1,253,000 with a cost of inventory of $1,125,566.

   What is the gross profit?

2. A pharmacy sells $25,420 a week with a monthly cost of inventory of $19,986.

   What is the gross profit?

3. A pharmacy has sales of $31,567 for the month of June.

   If this monthly income remains constant for a year, and the inventory costs for that year are $299,599, what is the year's gross profit?

4. A pharmacy that is open 7 days a week has sales amounting to $6,500/day with inventory costs of $5,990/day.

   What is the weekly gross profit?

5. The bank requests the gross profit of a store for a quarter. The sales are $65,432/month and inventory costs are $64,120/month.

   What is the gross profit for the quarter?

Net Income

Net income (sometimes referred to as the bottom line or **net profit**) is the gross profit minus the overhead. It is the difference between the sales and *all* of the costs related to the business (inventory and overhead). A positive net income is necessary to remain in business.

$$\text{Net income} = \text{Sales} - (\text{Inventory} + \text{Overhead})$$

Because sales minus inventory is gross profit, this can be simplified to:

$$\text{Net income} = \text{Gross income} - \text{Overhead}$$

EXAMPLE 16.10

If the overhead for the store from Example 16.9 is $18,000 for the month, what is the net income?

$$\text{Net income} = \$25{,}000 - \$18{,}000 = \$7{,}000$$

EXAMPLE 16.11

A pharmacy has monthly sales of $425,000, inventory purchases of $310,000, salaries and wages of $60,000, utilities of $2,500, insurance of $1,100, and maintenance costs of $775.

What is the gross income (sales – inventory cost)?

$$\$425{,}000 - \$310{,}000 = \$115{,}000$$

What is the overhead for the month (all expenses excluding inventory)?

$$\$60{,}000 + \$2{,}500 + \$1{,}100 + \$775 = \$64{,}375$$

What is the net income (gross income – overhead)?

$$\$115{,}000 - \$64{,}375 = \$50{,}625$$

Practice Problems H

Calculate the gross income, overhead, and net income in the following examples.

1. A retail pharmacy has monthly sales of $204,300. Inventory purchases were $177,700, salaries and wages were $21,350, utilities were $1,750, rent was $1,800, insurance was $750, and repairs were $900.

   What is the gross income for the month?

   What is the total overhead for the month?

   What is the net income?

2. A retail chain location has monthly sales of $354,740. Inventory purchases were $317,600, salaries and wages were $27,000, utilities were $2,400, rent was $3,800, insurance was $1,200, and repairs were $80.

   What is the gross income for the month?

   What is the total overhead for the month?

   What is the net income?

3. A hospital pharmacy's charges to patients are $454,000 for a month. Inventory purchases were $377,400, salaries and wages were $26,000, utilities allocated to the pharmacy were $850, licenses were $450, and supplies were $1,900.

   What is the gross income for the month?

   What is the total overhead for the month?

   What is the net income?

4. A retail pharmacy has monthly sales of $174,080. Inventory purchases were $146,220, salaries and wages were $16,200, utilities were $1,950, rent was $1,400, insurance was $800, and repairs were $270.

   What is the gross income for the month?

   What would be the total overhead for the month?

   What would be the net income?

5. A retail pharmacy has monthly sales of $379,300. Inventory purchases were $317,300, salaries and wages were $31,400, utilities were $2,675, rent was $3,500, insurance was $1,400, and supplies were $775.

   What is the gross income for the month?

   What is the total overhead for the month?

   What is the net income?

INSURANCE REIMBURSEMENT

Insurance or third-party reimbursement plays a major role in a pharmacy's income. The pharmacy signs contracts with insurance carriers for predetermined reimbursement amounts that may be specific to a medication or calculated based on the average wholesale price (AWP). To receive reimbursement, a pharmacy submits a claim electronically. The insurance company processes it according to the terms of the contract, supplies the pharmacy with the proper amount to charge the customer, and submits reimbursement, a process called **adjudication**. Most third-party reimbursements are based on AWP, markup or markdown rates, and a **dispensing fee**.

Average Wholesale Price

AWP is based on the national average cost of medication purchased from a wholesale market. A pharmacy may not actually pay AWP for medications because discounts are provided to pharmacies that order large quantities of drugs or for payment of invoices within a specified time. Fast-selling medications are often ordered in large quantities to obtain these discounts, thus increasing the profit on prescriptions. Today most patients have third-party payers (insurance companies) that reimburse the pharmacy for their prescriptions.

Applying a Markup or Markdown

In many instances, insurance companies provide reimbursement based on AWP plus a percentage of AWP, which is noted as AWP + %AWP. In other instances, reimbursement is based on AWP less a percentage of AWP, which is noted as AWP – %AWP. Applying a markdown to a prescription uses the same process as offering a discount. Applying a markup is the opposite. To apply a discount, multiply the discount percent (in decimal form) by the AWP and *subtract* this discount amount from the AWP. To apply a markup, multiply the markup percentage (in decimal form) by the AWP and *add* this markup amount to the AWP.

Dispensing Fees

Dispensing fees may vary by insurance companies and medications prescribed depending on the contract. The fees are a means of providing reimbursement for overhead expenses.

The following formula is used to determine insurance reimbursement:

$$\text{Reimbursement of prescription} = \text{AWP} \pm \text{Percentage of AWP allowed} + \text{Dispensing fee}$$

$$\text{Reimbursement of prescription} = \text{AWP} \pm (\%\text{AWP}) + \text{Dispensing fee}$$

EXAMPLE 16.12

The AWP for a drug is $64 for a 30-day supply.

Insurance will pay a 15% markup and the pharmacy charges a $3 dispensing fee.

What is the total charge for reimbursement?

$$\text{Reimbursement} = \$64 + (\$64 \times 0.15) + \$3 = \$76.60$$

The profit will be: $76.60 – $64.00 = $12.60.

If the pharmacy is able to purchase this medication for less than the AWP due to discounts, the profit will be greater, since reimbursement is based on AWP.

EXAMPLE 16.13

A pharmacy orders 1,000 tablets of medication at the AWP of $112 and takes advantage of the 10% discount offered on invoices paid within 10 days.

The AWP for this medication is $140.00/1,000 tablets.

Insurance reimbursement is AWP *less* (minus) 5% plus a $5 dispensing fee.

A prescription is written for 60 tablets.

What is the AWP for 60 tablets?

$$\frac{\$140}{1{,}000 \text{ tabs}} = \frac{x}{60 \text{ tabs}} \quad x = \$8.40$$

What is the discounted wholesale cost for 1,000 tablets?

$$\$112 - (\$112 \times 0.10) = \$112 - \$11.20 = \$100.80$$

Alternately, the pharmacy pays 90% of the AWP: $112 × 0.9 = $100.80

What is the cost for 60 tablets at the discounted wholesale cost?

$$\frac{\$108}{1{,}000\text{ tabs}} = \frac{x}{60\text{ tabs}} \quad x = \$6.53$$

What amount should be billed to insurance?

$\$8.40 - (5\% \times \$8.40) + \$5$

$\$8.40 - (0.05 \times \$8.40) + \$5$

$\$8.40 - (\$0.42) + \$5 = \$12.98$

What is the profit or loss on the prescription after insurance reimbursement?

$\$12.98 - \$6.53 = \$6.45$

TECH NOTE

Remember that when changing a percentage into a decimal, anything less than 10% will have a zero in the tenths place. For example, 5% is 0.05, whereas 50% is 0.5.

Practice Problems I

Calculate the following problems indicating the formula used.

1. A prescription has an AWP of $25.60. The insurance percentage is +18% AWP. The professional dispensing fee is $3.50.

   Total reimbursement:

   Profit:

2. A compounded prescription has a total AWP of $35.65. The insurance percentage is +9% AWP. The professional dispensing fee is $7.50.

   Total reimbursement:

   Profit:

3. A prescription has an AWP of $7.90. The insurance percentage is +12% AWP. The professional dispensing fee is $5.

Total reimbursement:

Profit:

4. An antibiotic prescription for 10 days has an AWP of $46.50. The insurance percentage is +7.5% AWP. The professional dispensing fee is $12.50.

Total reimbursement:

Profit:

5. A prescription for a month's supply of medication has an AWP of $120. The insurance percentage is –2% AWP on monthly prescriptions. The dispensing fee is $15.

Total reimbursement:

Profit:

Using the same AWP, change the insurance percentage to +3% AWP with a professional dispensing fee of $7.75.

Total reimbursement:

Profit:

Which of these two means of reimbursement would be most advantageous to the pharmacy?

___

6. A maintenance drug prescription has an AWP of $15.20. The insurance percentage is +9% AWP. The professional dispensing fee is $5.23.

   Total reimbursement:

7. A compounded prescription has a total AWP of $49.90. The insurance percentage is +7% AWP. The professional dispensing fee is $13.

   Total reimbursement:

8. A 7-day prescription of a medication taken three times daily has an AWP of $14.45. The insurance percentage is –5% AWP. The professional dispensing fee is $6.

   Total reimbursement:

9. A topical ointment prescription for 14 days has an AWP of $32.40. The insurance percentage is +12.25% AWP. The professional dispensing fee is $9.

   Total reimbursement:

10. A prescription for a 90-day supply of medication has an AWP of $190. The insurance percentage is +6% AWP. The professional dispensing fee is $18.

    Total reimbursement:

    Using the same AWP, change the insurance percentage to –1.5% AWP with a professional dispensing fee of $21.

    Total reimbursement:

    Which of these two means of reimbursement would be most advantageous to the pharmacy?

    ____

Capitation

Capitation refers to a contract between the pharmacy and the third-party payer to provide medications to the insured patient. **Capitation fees**, usually paid on a monthly basis, are a set amount of money paid to the pharmacy by a third party for a person whether the person receives a single prescription, multiple prescriptions, or no prescriptions. All prescriptions presented must be filled even if the cost exceeds the fee provided to the pharmacy. This type of reimbursement may provide the pharmacy with a loss during a 1-month period but can provide a profit over several months depending on the individual's prescription costs.

$$\text{Profit/(Loss)} = \text{Capitation fee} - \text{Prescription costs}$$

TECH NOTE

On financial statements, amounts that signify losses are often placed within parentheses.

EXAMPLE 16.14

A pharmacy accepts a capitation fee of $225 for a senior citizen who has four monthly maintenance prescriptions, most of which are available as generic drugs.

The cost for monthly maintenance medication is:

$$\$9.50 + \$27.00 + \$65.00 + \$42.00 = \$143.50.$$

What is the pharmacy's profit or (loss) for a typical month?

$$\$225.00 - \$143.50 = \$81.50 \text{ (profit)}$$

The next month the customer has a severe sinus infection requiring additional prescriptions of $45.00 and $55.00 for antibiotics, $15.00 for a decongestant, and $26.50 for pain medication. This is in addition to the maintenance medications.

What is the profit or loss for the second month?

$$\text{Additional prescription costs} = \$45.00 + \$55.00 + \$15.00 + \$26.50 = \$141.50$$

$$\text{Profit (or loss)} = \$225.00 - (\$143.50 + \$141.50) = \$225.00 - \$285.00 = -\$60.00$$

Or ($60.00), indicating a loss for the second month

What is the profit or loss over the 2-month time period?

Total capitation fee:	$450.00	($225.00 × 2)
Total cost of medications:	–428.50	($143.30 + $285.00)
Profit or (loss)	$21.50	

Practice Problems J

Calculate the profit or loss using the capitation fee supplied. Show your work.

1. A pharmacy agrees to a monthly capitation fee of $175 for a patient who has standing prescriptions of $43 and $27. This month, the person had two other prescriptions for $35 and $18.

   What is this month's profit or loss?

2. The pharmacy agrees to a capitation fee of $425 for a family of four. Prescriptions for the family in 1 month are $12.50, $25, $30, and $62.50.

   What is this month's profit or loss?

3. A capitation fee for a year for a patient is $1,800. Prescriptions for this person for routine medications cost $25, $30, and $15 per month.

   What would be the profit or loss for these medications for the year?

   If this patient had additional prescriptions for acute conditions for $56 twice, $75 twice, and $85 once, what would be the annual profit or loss?

4. The capitation fee accepted by the pharmacy for a child is $125 per month. The child has a total of $1,650 in prescriptions for the year.

   Did the pharmacy have a profit or loss? ______________

   What is the profit or loss?

   *Would it be advantageous for the business to recalculate the capitation fee for this child if the expected costs for prescriptions were to remain the same?*______________

5. A pharmacy is asked to accept a capitation fee of $350/month for an elderly patient who had six routine prescriptions of $25, $40, $35, $15, $80, and $75 monthly. Additional medications for acute conditions this month were $120, $25, and $160.

   What is the monthly profit or loss?

6. The pharmacy is under contract with an insurance company for a customer based on a capitation fee of $255 per month.

   The customer had three prescriptions filled today for $10.50, $65.00, and $45.00.

   If the customer already had prescriptions filled this month for $25.00, $46.00, and $32.50, what is the amount of profit or loss for the pharmacy?

DAILY CASH REPORT

Retail pharmacies may require technicians to prepare a daily **cash flow** report to verify that the payments received during the day balance with the amount of money in the cash drawer. This procedure varies for different pharmacies depending on how the store accounts for coupons, credit card payments, and discounts.

Posttest

Answer the following questions, rounding to dollars and cents. When calculating for a month use 4 weeks as the typical month and 28 days as the typical number of days per month.

1. The pharmacy spends $10,587.43 a week for medications. Salaries for the two registered pharmacists total $12,360 for the 4-week period. Rent is $1,825 per month, utilities are $1,450 per month, telephone is $576.08 per month, liability insurance on the building is $254 per month, professional malpractice insurance is $243 per month per pharmacist, and taxes paid are $3,856 per month. The total for pharmacy technicians is $2,650 per week. Depreciation on equipment is $4,320 per month.

   What is the overhead each month?

   If the pharmacy has an average income of $3,460 per day, what is the gross profit or loss for 1 month?

   If the pharmacy has an average income of $3,460 per day, what is the net profit or loss for 1 month?

2. A pharmacy buys new shelving costing $34,000 to be depreciated over 5 years; $2,500 for installation of the shelves should be added to the cost.

   What is the annual depreciation for the shelving?

Continued

Posttest, cont.

3. A pharmacy received an order of 1,000 tablets for $560.

   What is the cost of 50 tablets with a markup of 45%?

   What is the selling price per tablet with this markup?

   What is the selling price based on price per tablet for a prescription of 75 tablets?

4. During the past year, the pharmacy spent $1,600,000 for inventory supplies. The average inventory value during the past year was $250,000.

   What is the inventory turnover rate?

5. The pharmacy has announced a 25%-off sale on all generic medications for the last Friday of the month. A customer arrives and wants to buy the following generic OTC medications with a retail cost as shown:

   acetaminophen $7.99

   multiple vitamins $10.75

   docusate sodium $9.99

   neomycin cream $6.50

   What is the discounted price for acetaminophen?

   What is the discounted price for multiple vitamins?

   What is the discounted price for docusate sodium?

   What is the discounted price for neomycin cream?

   What are the customer's savings on the entire purchase?

Posttest, cont.

6. A medication has an AWP of $75.60 for 50 tablets. The contract with the third-party payer is AWP + 15% AWP + $7.85 dispensing fee for a prescription for 50 tablets.

   What is the total that should be billed to the insurance company?

   100 tablets of the medication were purchased for $152.50 with a 15% discount for payment made within 10 days.

   What is the cost to the pharmacy for the above prescription?

   What is the profit from insurance reimbursement in this case?

7. A pharmacy has a capitation contract with an insurance company to receive $250 a month for an elderly patient who fills 4 maintenance medications monthly. The patient takes prescriptions costing the pharmacy $7.68, $15.98, $46.32, and $48.21.

   For a routine month, what is the profit from the prescriptions for this patient?

   If the patient adds prescriptions costing $24.89, $50.65, and $12.50 to be taken on a regular basis, what is the profit or loss per month?

8. A pharmacy technician is responsible for inventory in the pharmacy department. The following medication is needed:

   Cogentin (benztropine): Inventory is 75 tablets. Par is 750 tablets.

   How many tablets are needed to reach par?

   The available stock bottles from the wholesaler are 1,000 tablets for $1,250.00, 500 tablets for $650.00, and 100 tablets for $140.00.

   What purchase would come closest to meeting the par level (within a 10% margin)?

   How much would this order cost the pharmacy if they took advantage of a 7% discount for paying the invoice within 10 days?

Continued

Posttest, cont.

9. Joseph is on an insurance plan that pays AWP + 12.5% AWP with a dispensing fee of $12.75. He brings prescriptions to the pharmacy for medications with an AWP of $34.50, $12.35, and $5.35.

What is the amount to be charged to the third-party payer for the prescription with an AWP of $34.50?

What is the profit on this prescription if it cost the pharmacy $29.50?

What is the amount to be charged for the prescription with an AWP of $12.35?

What is the profit if this prescription cost the pharmacy $15.45?

What is the amount to be charged for the prescription with an AWP of $5.35?

What would be the profit on this prescription if the medication costs the pharmacy $5.69?

Which prescription provides the highest gross profit?

10. A pharmacy has depreciation of $4,325/month, inventory costs of $2,678.36 for an average week, utilities of $1,025.25 per month, telephone bill of $568 per month, and salaries of $4,500 a week for the pharmacist and $1,500 a week for two pharmacy technicians. The income for the month is $65,342.

What is the total overhead expense for the month?

What is the net profit or loss for the month?

What is the discount amount for 1 week if the pharmacy uses a 20% markup on inventory and then offers it to the customers with a 5% discount?

Posttest, cont.

11. A pharmacy accidently ordered 100 bottles of mouthwash at $4.49 each instead of 10. In order to reduce inventory, they offered a 20% discount after marking the bottles up 40%.

What is the sale price for one bottle of mouthwash after the discount?

How much profit will be made on all 100 bottles?

12. A customer buys 2 bars of soap, aspirin, and a box of tissue. He has a coupon for the soap for $0.50 off two bars that sell for $2.50 each. The aspirin sells for $8.99 for 250 tablets. The tissue is on sale for 15% off the usual price of $1.89 a box.

What is the customer's price for all three items?

The customer reminds you that today is senior citizen discount day and he qualifies for the 10% discount.

What is the total that should now be charged to the customer?

You have already entered the original amount without the discount in the cash drawer before the person reminds you of the senior citizen discount.

How much should you refund to the person from the cash drawer?

Continued

Posttest, cont.

13. The pharmacist asks you to compute the overhead for the pharmacy for the month.

The salary for the pharmacist is $3,700.00 twice a month.

The two pharmacy technicians are each paid $3,400 per month.

Inventory costs per week average approximately $12,000.00 for medications while front end merchandise averages about twice that much.

Rent for the building is $950.00 per month; professional malpractice insurance is $255.00 per month; utilities average about $1,450.00 per month; supplies are about $672.00 per month; and miscellaneous expenses average about $565.00 per month.

What is the overhead for a month?

14. The pharmacy purchases a medication for $86.00 for 100 tablets. The pharmacy must have a 45% markup on these tablets because the medication is not ordered on a regular basis.

What is the cost for a prescription for 60 tablets for a customer who has no insurance?

The pharmacist approves a 20% discount for this customer to help with the cost.

What is the amount of the discount?

What is cost to the customer after the discount has been applied?

The pharmacy took advantage of the wholesaler's 8% discount by paying the invoice in 10 days, but did not pass this on to the customer.

What is the profit on this prescription?

Posttest, cont.

15. An insurance company allows AWP minus 10% AWP plus a $15.00 dispensing fee. The customer brings in a prescription for 60 tablets with an AWP of $5/tablet.

What should be charged to the insurance company?

16. A patient brings the following prescriptions to the pharmacy:

(A) The first prescription is for 75 tablcts at $0.70 per tablet.

(B) The second prescription is for 90 tablets that cost $1.10 per tablet.

(C) The third prescription is for 25 capsules at $2.50 per capsule.

The markup on each of the prescriptions is 25%. Because this person does not have insurance the pharmacist offers a 15% discount on the most expensive prescription and 10% on the other two prescriptions.

What is the cost to the pharmacy for prescription A?

What is the cost to the pharmacy for prescription B?

What is the cost to the pharmacy for prescription C?

What is the cost to the patient for prescription A prior to discount?

What is the cost to the patient for prescription B prior to discount?

What is the cost to the patient for prescription C prior to discount?

What is the final cost of prescription A with the allowable discount?

What is the final cost of prescription B with the allowable discount?

What is the final cost of prescription C with the allowable discount?

Continued

Posttest, cont.

17. *What is the percentage markup on a prescription based on a wholesale cost of $16.75 and a selling price of $31.50?*

18. A compounded prescription has a wholesale price of $21.28.

    The insurance company will pay AWP + 15% with a $9.00 dispensing fee.

    How much will the pharmacy be reimbursed from the insurance company?

    What is the pharmacy's profit on the compounded prescription?

19. A pharmacy had a monthly income of $132,987. The inventory for the month was 42,033; salaries and wages were 26,577; and rent, utilities, and insurance costs were $4,200.

    What was the net income (or loss) for this month?

20. An insurance company reimburses the pharmacy AWP – 5% with a dispensing fee of $14.00.

    A patient brings in a prescription for 60 capsules with an AWP of $0.75 each.

    What is the total amount to be billed to the insurance company?

    What is the profit for the pharmacy?

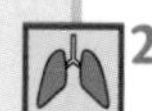

21. The retail prices of Flonase (fluticasone) nasal spray are $13.99 for 60 sprays and $41.99 for 288 sprays.

    How much is each bottle per spray?

    Which is the better choice for your customer if they use it routinely?

Posttest, cont.

22. A pharmacy is under contract with an insurance company for AWP plus 10% with a $7.00 dispensing fee.

A prescription for 30 tablets has an AWP of $1.05 per tablet.

The pharmacy buys this medication at AWP less 10% for payment within 10 days of invoice.

How much does the pharmacy pay for 30 tablets with the discount?

What is the amount that should be billed to the insurance company?

What is the profit on this medication for the pharmacy based on AWP?

REVIEW OF RULES—EQUATION REVIEW

Par Levels

- Needed inventory = Par level – Amount on shelf

Inventory Turnover Rate

- Inventory turnover rate = Total purchases over a given time ÷ Average inventory value

Overhead

- All expenses required for doing business *except the cost of inventory.*

Annual Depreciation

- Annual depreciation = Cost ÷ Estimated time of use in years

Markup

- Markup = Selling price – Purchase cost
  Markup = Purchase cost × Markup percentage (written as a decimal)

Selling/Retail Price

- Selling price = Purchase cost + Markup

Markup Percentage

- Markup percentage = (Markup ÷ Cost) × 100

Discounts

- Discount = Selling price × Discount percentage (written as a decimal)
- Discounted price = Selling price − Discount amount

Profit/Income or Loss (Typically Income Includes Total of All Business Transactions)

- Gross profit (or loss) = Sale price of merchandise − Purchase cost of inventory
- Net profit (or loss) = Gross profit − Overhead

Insurance Reimbursement

- Reimbursement of prescription = AWP ± Percentage of AWP + Dispensing fee
- Insurance profit (or loss) = Reimbursement amount − Purchase cost
- Capitation profit or loss = Capitation fee − Medication costs

Chapter 1

Practice Problems A

1. pound
3. nothing by mouth
6. four times a day
9. bedtime
12. microgram
15. grain
18. every hour
21. intramuscular
24. prescription; take
27. sufficient quantity
30. ointment
33. elixir
36. dram
39. by mouth
42. every afternoon or evening
45. daily
48. every

Basic Math Skills Proficiency Self-Test

1. 85
3. 1.59
6. $13.11
9. 8 5/8
12. XXX
15. 2 2/9
18. 2/5
21. 5 1/12
24. 1/150
27. 3.5
30. 3 7/8
33. 21
36. 60
39. 5,500 mg
42. 24.2
45. 20
48. $26.10

Chapter 2

Pretest

1. 1,618
3. 11,008
6. 308.9
9. 2 1/8
12. 21/40
15. 10
18. 1 4/15
21. 12
24. 6.13
27. 1.75
30. 1/3
33. 24
36. $\frac{44}{100} = \frac{11}{25}$
39. 0.33
42. 37.5 mL
45. 42.5%
48. $6.52

Practice Problems A

1. 81
3. 150 g
6. 8,500 mL
9. 75 mL
12. 225 mg
15. 40 mL
18. $30

Practice Problems B

1. 560
3. 8,700
6. 85,250
9. 74
12. 40
15. 2,500 mg
18. 2 mg

Practice Problems C

1. 5; 7
3. 7; 15

Practice Problems D

1. 5 1/3
3. 8 3/4
6. 3
9. 1 1/2tablets
12. 23/8
15. 33/7
18. 9/2 tablet
21. 1 1/4
24. 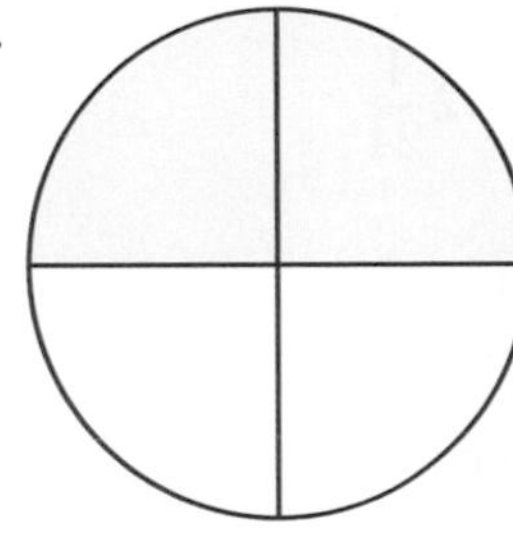

Practice Problems E

1. 1/2
3. 2/3
6. 1/4
9. 1/2

Practice Problems F

1. 2/3
3. 5/7
6. 3/15 = 1/5
9. 1 7/9
12. 65/77
15. 1/2 tsp
18. 1
21. 1 5/24 tsp
24. 9/16 oz

Practice Problems G

1. 2/5
3. 3/8
6. 4/15
9. 8 13/15
12. 10 61/72
15. 8/15
18. 1 5/16
21. 2 1/12
24. 125 tablets

Practice Problems H

1. four and thirty-four hundredths
3. six and seven hundred fifty-one thousandths
6. thirty-five ten thousandths
9. seventy-eight hundredths

Practice Problems I

1. 2.36
3. 36.45
6. 8.24
9. 3.6
12. 3.1
15. 2.5 mL
18. 14

Practice Problems J

1. 10.13
3. 1,363.08
6. $153.59
9. 2.81
12. $10.10
15. 2 mg
18. $76.10; $3.90

Practice Problems K

1. 653
3. 42.5
6. 8.25
9. 95.13

12. 162 mg
15. 5 mg
18. 25 mg

Practice Problems L

1. 67.1
3. 5
6. 0.25
9. 12
12. 2.5
15. $31.20
18. 20.25 mL

Practice Problems M

1. 125/1,000
3. 33/100
6. 5/100; 1/20
9. 1,244/10,000; 311/2,500

Practice Problems N

1. 0.5
3. 0.8
6. 0.83
9. 0.63

Practice Problems O

1. 50/100; ½
3. 76/100; 19/25
6. 12/100; 3/25
9. 33/100
12. 0.25/100; 1/400
15. 0.66/100; 33/5, 000
18. 2/3 × 1/100; 2/300; 1/150

Practice Problems P

1. 100/6; 16.67
3. 200/5; 40
6. 700/3; 233.33
9. 300/4; 75
12. 400/5; 80
15. 300/10; 30

Practice Problems Q

1. 0.6
3. 0.78
6. 3.25
9. 0.32
12. 12.45
15. 0.0006
18. 0.0013

Practice Problems R

1. 25
3. 2.5
6. 550
9. 1,040
12. 15
15. 46.7
18. 1

Practice Problems S

1. 2:7
3. 5:25; 1:5
6. 95:100; 19:20
9. 325:10,000; 13:400
12. 36:100; 9:25
15. 6:48; 1:8
18. 2:50; 1:25

Practice Problems T

1. yes
3. yes
6. yes
9. no

Practice Problems U

1. 4
3. 25
6. $5
9. 21 capsules
12. 3 tablets
15. 25 mg
18. 10 mL

Practice Problems V

1. 33.3%
3. 45
6. 81
9. 5.12 oz
12. $3.75
15. 24.5 tablets
18. 8%

Posttest

1. 81
3. 375 mg
6. $\frac{49}{24}$; $2\frac{1}{24}$
9. $\frac{3}{40}$
12. $\frac{24}{12}$; 2
15. 10.67
18. 100
21. 720.99
24. 2
27. 0.64
30. 1 64/100; 1 16/25
33. 8/10; 4/5
36. 1
39. $\frac{1}{2}$
42. $\frac{19}{25}$
45. 30%
48. 100%
51. 12.5%
54. 3:5
57. 250 mg:5 mL; 50 mg:1 mL
60. 3
63. 3.3%
66. 25%
69. 2.5 mL

Chapter 3

Pretest

1. xxi
3. liv
6. xcv
9. 8
12. 97
15. 37 ½
18. 44 ½
21. 0001
24. 0146
27. 11:02 AM
30. 11:57 PM
33. 4:45 PM
36. 40.3°C
39. 38°C
42. 39.2°C
45. −12.2°C
48. 33.6°C

Practice Problems A

1. vi
3. xxi
6. ix
9. lxxv
12. xxxv
15. xxxiii $\overline{\text{ss}}$
18. LIX

Practice Problems B

1. 8
3. 19
6. 66
9. 95
12. 37 ½
15. 99
18. 129

Practice Problems C

1. 0035
3. 0615
6. 0345
9. 0655
12. 2020
15. 2359
18. 12:01 PM
21. 4:15 PM
24. 7:05 AM
27. 8:20 PM
30. 9:45 AM

Practice Problems D

1. −17.2°C
3. 1.7°C
6. 93.2°F
9. 37°C
12. 37.9°C
15. 118.8°F
18. 37.9°C; yes

Posttest

1. 27 1⁄2
3. 93 1⁄2
6. xxxvi $\overline{\text{ss}}$
9. lxxv
12. 125
15. clxv
18. 4:25 PM
21. 12:45 AM
24. 1210
27. 1526
30. 6:35 AM
33. 82.2°C
36. 212°F
39. 35.6°F
42. 95.4°F; yes
45. 0600; 1200; 1800; 2400
48. 1630

Chapter 4

Pretest

1. milligram
3. gram
6. inch
9. milliequivalent
12. teaspoon
15. pound
18. 1 1⁄2 tsp
21. 1,000 units
24. 1,000
27. viii (8)
30. 4

Practice Problems A

1. 8
3. 2
6. 2
9. tablespoon
12. gallon
15. 200 lb or 200 #
18. 2 ½ c

Practice Problems B

1. mcg
3. mL
6. gram
9. milliliter
12. 3.5 L
15. 100 g
18. 0.8 mg

Practice Problems C

1. viii
3. minim
6. grain
9. fl℥ viii
12. ♏ ix
15. gr x
18. gr xx

Posttest

1. 36 kg
3. 3 tsp
6. fl℥ x
9. 12.5 mg
12. 2 1⁄2 qt
15. 4 c
18. 110 # or 110 lb
21. 40 mEq
24. 8
27. Tbsp
30. mg

Chapter 5

Pretest

1. 1⁄4
3. 5
6. i
9. 1 1⁄2
12. 1,560 mg
15. 2,500
18. 5,000,000,000
21. 18
24. 32

Practice Problems A

1. 3
3. 1 1⁄2
6. 5
9. 1 1⁄4
12. 1 1⁄2
15. 180
18. 80
21. ½ Tbsp
24. 4 c

Practice Problems B

1. 2,000
3. 4,000
6. 500
9. 0.05
12. 6,540,000
15. 50,600
18. 3.5
21. 0.005
24. 300,000
27. 0.25 mg
30. 1.5 g

Practice Problems C

1. 3⁄4
3. 1⁄15
6. xl (40)
9. $\overline{\text{ss}}$

Posttest

1. 36,000
3. 120
6. 1 1⁄4
9. 0.0125
12. 1⁄2
15. 2
18. 1⁄2
21. 0.0405
24. 3
27. 0.075
30. 4
33. 4
36. 32
39. 0.6
42. 2 1⁄2
45. 2,500
48. fl℥ 64
51. 0.025 g
54. 3 tsp
57. fl℥ 32
60. 1.5 L
63. 250 mcg
66. 75"
69. 1⁄2 gal

Chapter 6

Pretest

1. 30
3. 4.4
6. 10
9. iv
12. ii
15. v
18. 0.4
21. ½
24. 15.2
27. 60
30. 2

Practice Problems A

1. 30
3. 5
6. 15
9. 2.2
12. 20

Practice Problems B

1. ii
3. xvi; xii
6. 5
9. 3
12. 7.5; 10
15. 1 cup or 8 ounces

Practice Problems C

1. 480
3. 15
6. 720
9. 2 ½
12. ¾
15. 30
18. 152.4

Practice Problems D

1. 325
3. ¼
6. 0.5
9. 30
12. 45,000
15. no; 15 mg

Posttest

1. $\overline{ss}$
3. 45
6. 1⁄100
9. 3.8
12. viii
15. 1⁄600
18. ix
21. ii $\overline{ss}$
24. 7
27. 5.2
30. 50 kg
33. 5 mL
36. 76.4 kg
39. 100 kg
42. gr v
45. 30 mL
48. 0.4 mg
51. 30.9 kg
54. 3 oz
57. 2,500 g
60. gr 1/150

Chapter 7

Pretest

1. Take 1 tablet by mouth 4 times a day for 10 days
3. Take 1 tablet by mouth every morning as needed for swelling
6. Take 2 tablets by mouth now, then take 1 tablet by mouth daily on days 2 through 5
9. Take 1 tablet by mouth 3 times a day
12. Take 1 tablet by mouth daily with evening meal or at bedtime with a snack for hyperlipidemia
15. Take ½ to 1 tablet by mouth every 4 to 6 hours as needed for anxiety or muscle spasms
18. metoprolol 50 mg by mouth 2 times a day

Practice Problems A

1. atorvastatin 10 mg, 30 tablets, one tablet by mouth nightly at bedtime; Take 1 tablet by mouth nightly at bedtime
3. Zoloft 50 mg, 30 tablets, one tablet by mouth daily with morning meal; Take 1 tablet by mouth daily with morning meal
6. ibuprofen 800 mg, 100 tablets, one tablet by mouth every 8 hours; Take 1 tablet by mouth every 8 hours
9. Fosamax 70 mg, 4 tablets, one tablet by mouth on same day every week; Take 1 tablet by mouth once a week on the same day every week
12. Glucotrol XL 10 mg, 30 tablets, one tablet by mouth with morning meal; Take 1 tablet by mouth daily with morning meal
15. Take 1 tablet by mouth 2 times a day
18. Take 1 tablet by mouth every morning before eating with a full glass of water

Practice Problems B

1. discontinue Zocor; add Lipitor 10 mg, one tablet by mouth at bedtime
3. cephalexin 500 mg by mouth every 8 hours for 3 days
6. albuterol sulfate two puffs every 4 hours for shortness of breath
9. Levothroid 100 micrograms by mouth every day with morning meal
12. hydrocodone/ acetaminophen 7.5/325 by mouth every 6 hours as needed for pain
15. furosemide 40 mg by mouth every morning as needed for swelling
18. cephalexin suspension 500 mg by mouth every 12 hours

Practice Problems C

1. Pfizer; 0009-5013-01; Glyset; miglitol; 50 mg/ tablet; 100
3. Unit dose blisterpaks; 100; 250 mcg; 0.25 mg; Store at 25°C (77°F) in a dry place; tablets

Posttest

1. Take 1 tablet by mouth at bedtime
3. Dilantin 100-mg capsules, 120 capsules, four capsules by mouth now, then one capsule by mouth four times a day; Take 4 capsules by mouth now; then take 1 capsule by mouth 4 times a day
6. Take 1 tablet by mouth every 4 to 6 hours as needed
9. Take 1 tablet 4 times a day (before meals and at bedtime)
12. Apply to affected area 2 times a day
15. Inject 15 units subcutaneously 3 times a day before meals
18. Humulin 70/30 25 units subcutaneously every morning before breakfast and before supper
21. warfarin 5 mg by mouth on even days and 2.5 mg by mouth on odd days
24. Maalox 20 mL by mouth 1 hour after meals as needed for gastric distress
27. cefazolin 500 mg intramuscularly every 8 hours
30. Reglan 10 mg by mouth 4 times a day 30 minutes before meals and at bedtime
33. Narcan 0.2 mg intravenously immediately and may repeat until desired response up to 0.8 mg total
36. 40 mEq; 20 mL; Hospira; injection; MUST BE DILUTED BEFORE USE

Chapter 8

Pretest

1. ½ tablet
3. 1 tablet
6. ½ tablet
9. 2 capsules
12. 1 tablet
15. 1 tablet
18. 2 capsules

Practice Problems A

1. 2 capsules
3. 2 capsules
6. ½ tablet
9. 3 tablets
12. 2 tablets
15. 2 tablets
18. 2 tablets

Practice Problems B

1. 2 tablets
3. 3 capsules
6. 2 tablets
9. 4 tablets
12. 2 tablets
15. 3 tablets
18. 3 tablets

Posttest

1. 2 tablets
3. 2 tablets
6. 1 capsule
9. 1 capsule
12. 2 capsules
15. Take 4 tablets at bedtime
18. Take 1 tablet by mouth at bedtime on day 1, take 2 tablets by mouth at bedtime on day 2, take 4 tablets by mouth at bedtime on day 3, and then take 6 tablets by mouth at bedtime

Chapter 9

Pretest

1. 10 mL; 2 tsp
3. 10 mL
6. 7.5 mL; 1 ½ tsp
9. 2.5 mL; ½ tsp

Practice Problems A

1. 15 mL
3. 2.5 mL; ½ tsp
6. 2.5 mL; ½ tsp; 5-mL dose spoon, 3-mL or 5-mL oral syringe
9. 10 mL; 5 mL; 3.3 mL
12. 0.6 mL,

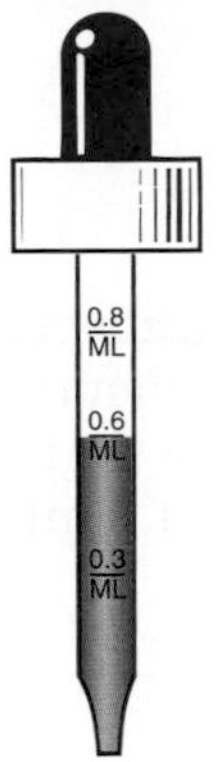

15. 3.8 mL
18. 3 mL

Practice Problems B

1. 35 mL; distilled water or purified water, USP; 24 mL; 11 mL; tap bottle lightly to loosen powder before adding 24 mL diluent; 10 mg/mL; 5 mL; 3 mL
3. 150 mL; water; 90 mL; 60 mL; add water in two portions, shake well; 125 mg/5 mL; store in refrigerator, shake well, discard after 14 days; 14 days; 15 mL

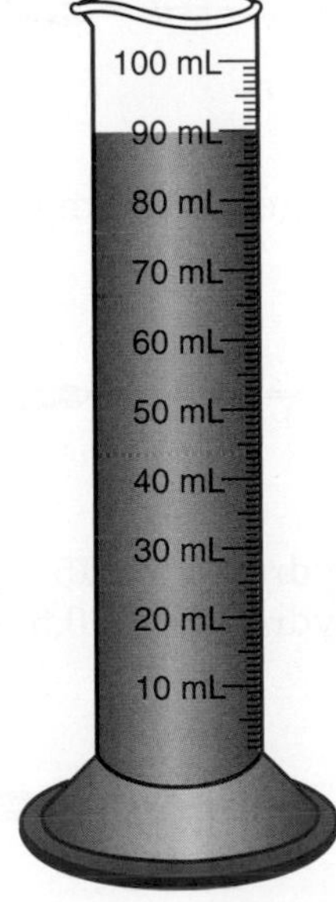

Posttest

1. 20 mL
3. 7.5 mL
6. 15 mL
9. 4 mL
12. 2.5 mL; ½ tsp
15. 3 mL; 1.5 mL
18. Take 3 mL by mouth 2 times a day 30 minutes before a meal
21. Place 2 mL in each side of the mouth 4 times a day, swish as long as possible, then swallow
24. Take 20 mL by mouth every 12 hours with a high fat snack for 6 months for nail fungus

Chapter 10

Pretest

1. Zofran 2 mg intramuscularly 30 minutes before chemotherapy treatment; 1 mL
3. Dilaudid 1.3 mg subcutaneously every 6 hours for pain; 0.65 mL
6. codeine phosphate ½ grain subcutaneously every 4 hours; 1 mL
9. 500,000 units/mL; 1.6 mL; 0.5 mL

Practice Problems A

1. 1.5 mL
3. 1.8 mL
6.

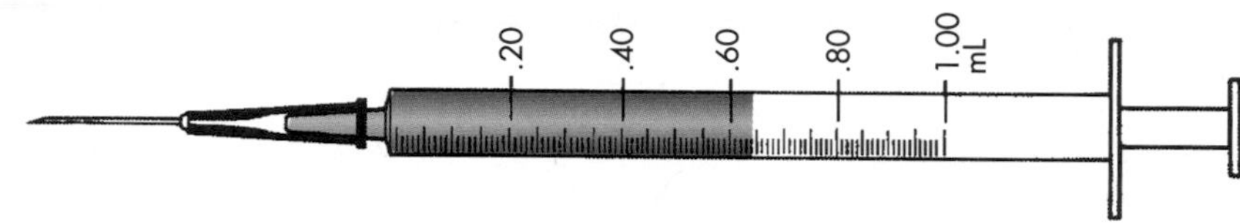

9.

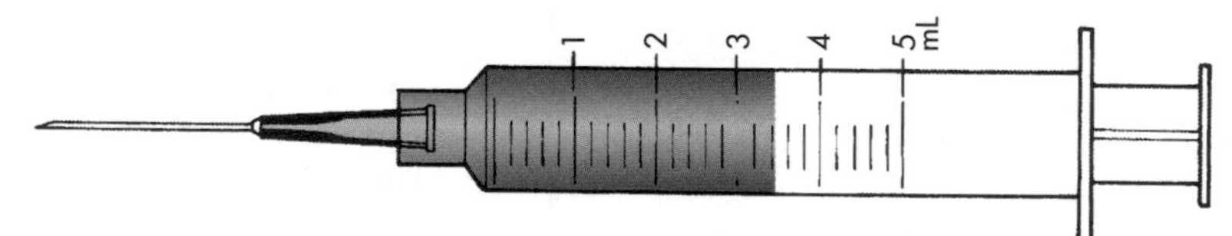

Practice Problems B

1. morphine sulfate 15 mg intramuscularly every 4 hours as needed for pain; 0.6 mL
3. tobramycin (Nebcin) 60 mg intramuscularly every 8 hours; 1.5 mL

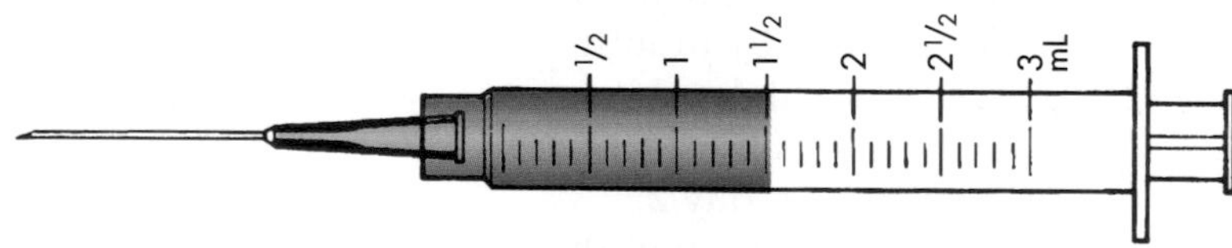

6. Cogentin 1.5 mg intramuscularly daily; 1.5 mL

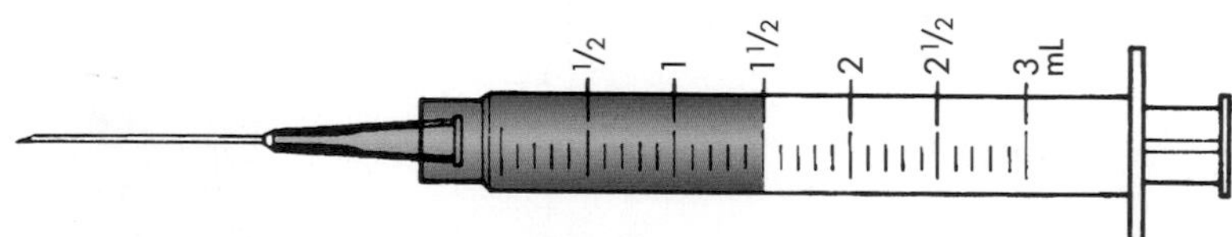

9. hydroxyzine 75 mg and meperidine 50 mg intramuscularly immediately; 1.5 mL hydroxyzine; 0.5 mL meperidine

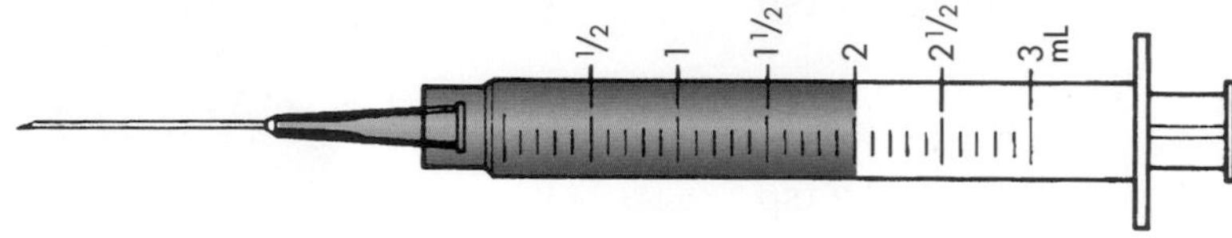

12. 50 mg/mL; 2 mL
15. 2.6 mL; 3-mL syringe
18. 0.5 mL; 1-mL TB syringe

Practice Problems C

1. C; B
3. D; B

Practice Problems D

1. 0.5 mL

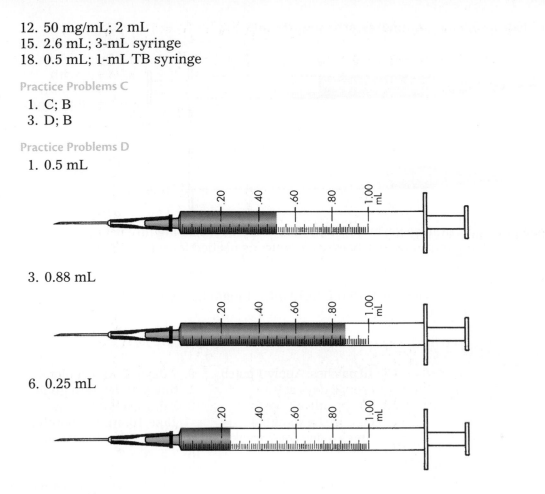

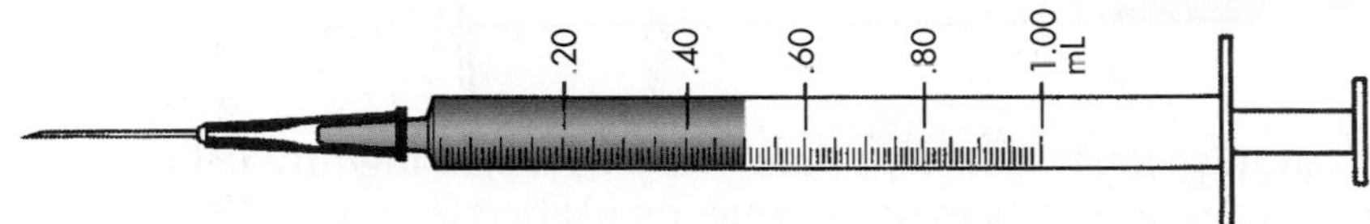

3. 0.88 mL

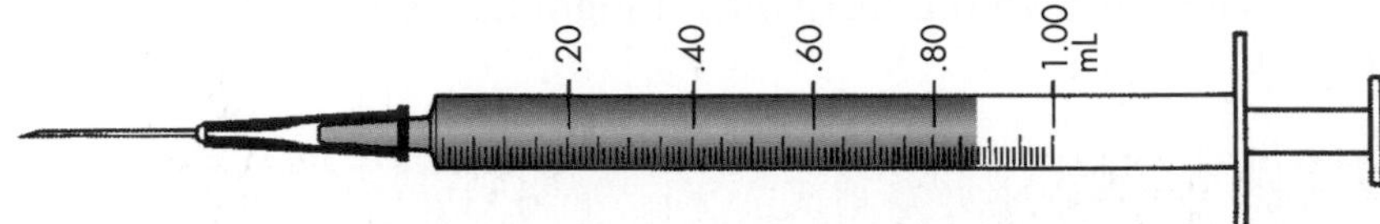

6. 0.25 mL

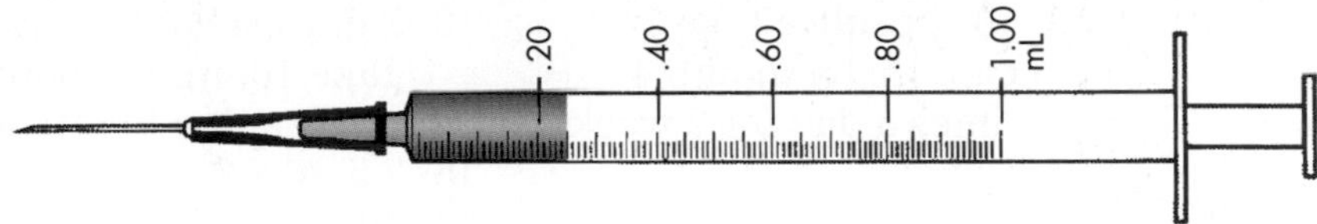

Practice Problems E

1. Solu-Cortef 125 mg intramuscularly immediately; 250 mg/2 mL; 3 days; Protect from light; 1 mL; 2
3. sterile water for injection; 4.8 mL; 100 mg/mL; 5 mL; IV infusion only; must be further diluted before use; 5 mL; 3 mL

Posttest

1. butorphanol 1 mg intramuscularly immediately for pain; 0.5 mL

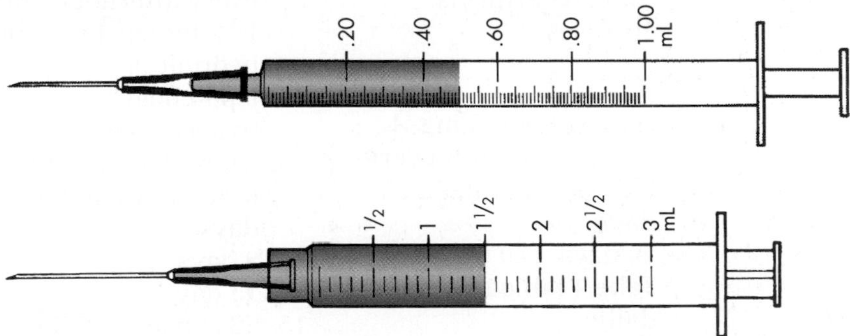

3. Solu-Medrol 37.5 mg intramuscularly now; 0.6 mL

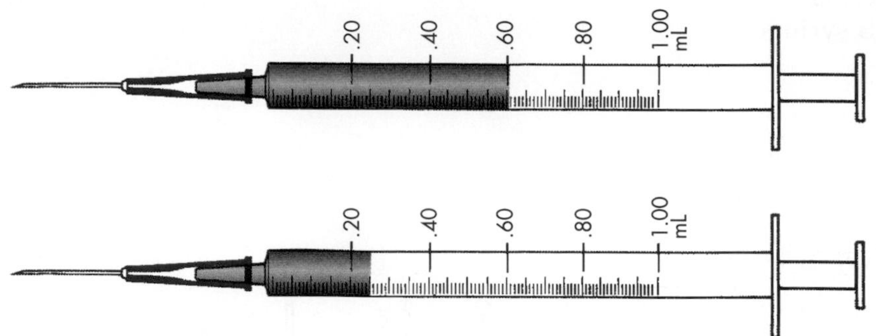

6. digoxin 0.1 mg intramuscularly now and then every day; 0.25 mg/mL; 0.4 mL
9. meperidine 50 mg intramuscularly every 4 hours as needed for pain; 0.67 mL; 0.5 mL; meperidine 100 mg/mL
10. 1.6 mL; 0.8 mL; 0.4 mL
13. 0.75 mL; 0.375 mL (3.8 mL); 0.1875 mL (0.19 mL); 1 mg/mL; 760 mcg
16. 0.25 mL; 1-mL TB syringe
19. 0.35 mL

Chapter 11

Pretest

1. 30 days
3. 90 days
6. 10 days
9. 11 tablets; Take 2 tablets by mouth at once and repeat in 12 hours, then take 1 tablet daily for 1 week
12. Strattera 40 mg, 2 capsules by mouth every evening; 28 capsules
15. 25 days; 50 days; 5 mL
18. 12 days

Practice Problems A

1. 30 tablets
3. 180 tablets
6. 196 mL
9. 90 tablets; Take 1 tablet by mouth 3 times a day with meals or snacks
12. Trileptal 150 mg per tablet, 3 tablets by mouth 2 times a day, 1 month supply; 180 tablets
15. 10 patches; Apply 1 patch every 3 days at 9 AM
18. 56 capsules; Take 1 capsule by mouth 4 times a day for 2 weeks

Practice Problems B

1. 24 doses; 6 days; 2; Take 2.5 mL by mouth 4 times a day for 10 days for bronchitis
3. 7 doses; Take 4 capsules daily, 1 hour before a meal for tuberculosis
6. 50; Take 2 tablets 3 times a day after meals for osteoarthritis
9. 10 doses

Practice Problems C

1. Zaroxolyn 2.5 mg, 1 tablet by mouth every 3 days, 30 tablets; 90 days
3. 10 days; 120 tablets; Take 4 tablets by mouth daily
6. 31 days; Altace 5 mg #62, one tablet twice a day for blood pressure
9. 7 days; Take 1 tablet 4 times a day until gone
12. 2 days; 4 containers; Take 10 mL by mouth 2 times a day for 10 days
15. 7.5 mL; 16 doses; 4 days
18. 90 days; 45 tablets; Take 1 tablet every morning and 1/2 tablet every evening

Posttest

1. trazodone 100 mg, 1 month supply, 1/2 tablet by mouth every morning, 1/2 tablet every afternoon, and 1 1/2 tablets by mouth at bedtime; 75 tablets
3. 9 patches; Apply 1 patch twice a week
6. Cipro 500 mg #20, one tablet twice a day; 10 days
9. 8 days
12. 15 days
15. 56 capsules; Take 2 capsules by mouth 2 times a day for 14 days
18. 240 mL

Chapter 12

Pretest

1. 71.4 mg
3. 25 mg; 25 mg tid
6. 12 mg; 3 mL

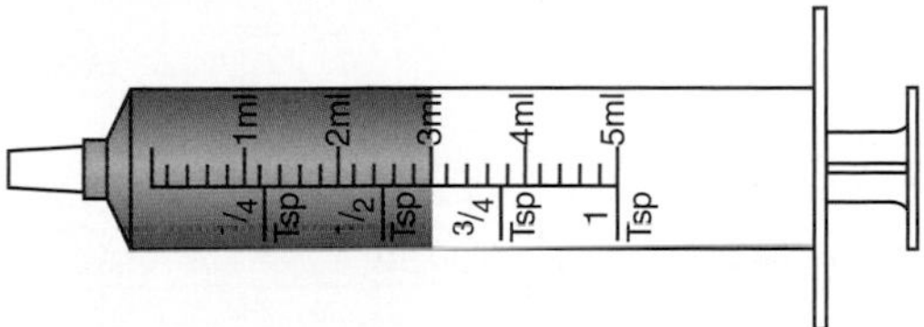

9. 227.3 mg bid; 9.1 mL
12. 0.88 m^2; 51.8 mg; 2.1 mL; 37.3 mg; 45.5 mg; no
15. 40 mg; 8 mL

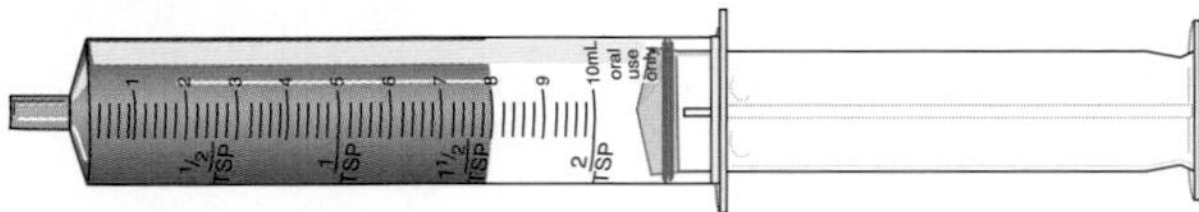

18. 7.8 mL

Practice Problems A

1. 29.55 kg
3. 34.09 kg

Practice Problems B

1. 5 mL; 250 mg; 750 mg

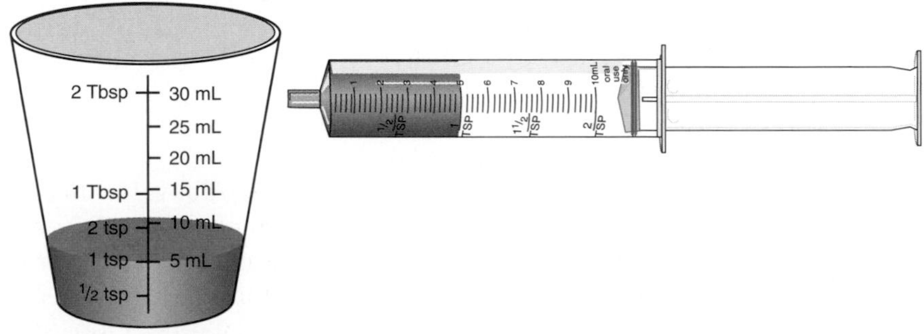

3. 2.5 mL; 1/2 tsp

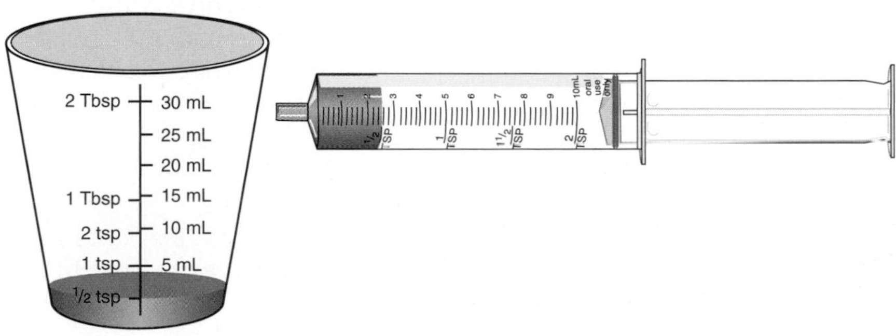

6. 4 mL
9. 9.8 mg; one tablet
12. 45.5 mg; 2.5 mL; ½ tsp
15. 25 mg; 0.5 mL
18. 300 mg; 60 tablets; Chew 1 ½ tablets every 6 hours for 10 days; 150 mL; 3.8 mL

Practice Problems C

1. 25.6 mg
3. 4 mg; 1.3 mL; ¼ tsp

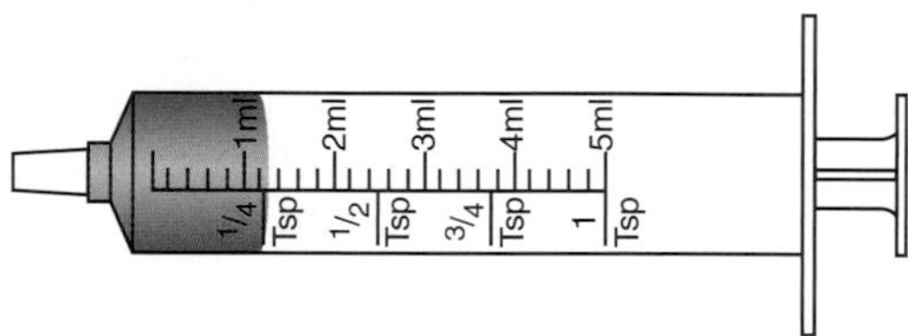

Practice Problems D

1. 0.36 m^2
3. 0.29 m^2

Practice Problems E

1. 0.36 m^2; 0.05 mg; 1 mL
3. 1.34 m^2; 3.94 mg; 3.9 mL
6. 1.4 mL
9. 810 mg; two tablets

Practice Problems F

1. 6 mL
3. 100 mg; 200 mg; 4 mL

Posttest

1. Clark's Rule; 10 mg
3. Body weight; 12 mg; 4.8 mL; 1 tsp
6. Clark's Rule for BSA; 3.2 mL
9. Young's Rule; 20 mg; 2 tablets
12. Clark's Rule; 1.71 mg; 17 mL
15. 10.64 mg; one 10-mg tablet; 10.6 mL; 2.1 mL
18. 254.55 mg; 6.4 mL; 127.27 mg; 3.2 mL

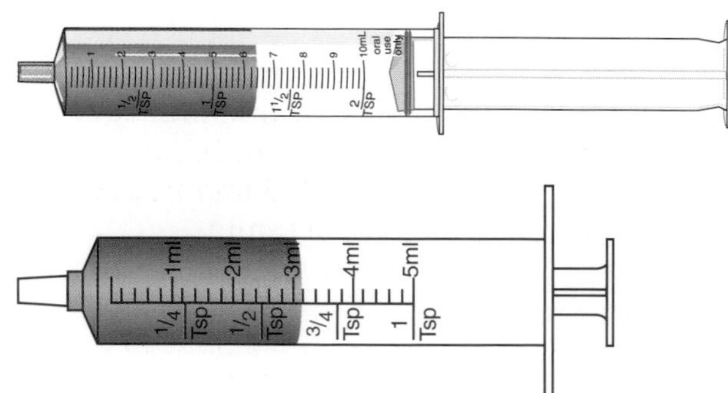

21. 13.5 mg; 4.5 mL; yes
24. 1.1 mL/dose

Chapter 13

Pretest

1. 4.5 g
3. 12%
6. 5%
9. 9 g
12. 25 g; 2.25 g
15. 10 g sodium hypochlorite in 100 mL of total solution; 24 g
18. 0.8 mL

Practice Problems A

1. 25 g
3. 3 g; 25 g
6. 2.5 g
9. 16.5 g

Practice Problems B

1. 7.5 g magnesium sulfate in 100 mL of solution; 75 mg/mL
3. 0.5 g glycerol in 100 mL of solution: 5 mg/mL
6. 0.3 g ciprofloxacin in 100 mL of solution; 7.5 mg
9. 100 g
12. 1 g; 5%
15. 0.6 mL
18. 1.5 mL

Practice Problems C

1. 1 g of epinephrine in 10,000 mL of solution; 0.01 g
3. 1 g of lidocaine in 50,000 mL of solution; 0.0004 g; 400 mcg; 0.02 mg/mL
6. 0.001 g; 1 mg/mL
9. 4 mL
12. 25 mL
15. 1:200
18. 2 g

Practice Problems D

1. 1%
3. 0.1%
6. 0.2%; 500 mg

Practice Problems E

1. 1:20
3. 1:100
6. 1:400

Posttest

1. 9 g; 50 g; 20 g
3. 12.5 g
6. 12%
9. 0.015%
12. 2.5 mL; 0.5%
15. 2,000 mg
18. 5 g
21. 9.6 mL; 2 tsp
24. 250 mL
27. 60 mg
30. 25 g

Chapter 14

Pretest

1. 1.5 g of 10% ointment; 28.5 g of petrolatum
3. 3 g of 2.5% ointment; 12 g of petrolatum
6. 50 mL; 950 mL
9. 100 mL; 0 (no solvent necessary; the solution is 50% as described)
12. 10 mL; 990 mL
15. 500 mL of 0.9% NaCl; 250 mL of 0.45% NaCl
18. 450 mL

Practice Problems A

1. 300 mL; 700 mL
3. 375 mL; 1,125 mL
6. 90 mL; 150 mL
9. 48 mL; 192 mL
12. 1,600 mL; 2,400 mL
15. 180 mL
18. 20 mL; 60 mL

Practice Problems B

1. 222.2 mL of 15%; 277.8 mL of 6%
3. 4.6 g of 25%; 15.4 g of 12%
6. 107.1 mL of 15%; 642.9 mL of 1%
9. 20 g of 15%; 30 g of 2.5%
12. 150 mL of D10W; 100 mL of D5W
15. 11 mL of 5% sodium chloride; 39 mL of 0.9% sodium chloride
18. 33.3 mL of 1:10; 66.7 mL of 1:100

Practice Problems C

1. 15 g of 0.1% triamcinolone; 15 g of petrolatum
3. 0.15 g of menthol; 0.18 g of phenol; 29.67 g

Practice Problems D

1. 3 g drug B; 3 g lanolin; 24 g petrolatum
3. 10 mg/mL
6. 22 g mupirocin; 0.022 g betamethasone dipropionate; 0.88 g miconazole

Practice Problems E

1. 300 mg tetracycline; 15 mL nystatin; 22.5 mL diphenhydramine; qs ad 90 mL with dexamethasone elixir
3. 108 g glycerin; 10.8 g sodium stearate; 5.4 mL water
6. 6 g

Posttest

1. 50 mL
3. 120 mL
6. 225 mL; 75 mL
9. 62.5 mL; 187.5 mL; seven vials
12. 62.5 mL; 187.5 mL
15. 83.3 mL of D50W; 416.7 mL of D5W
18. 50 mg
21. 2 mL 5% suspension; 3 mL sterile normal saline solution

Chapter 15

Pretest

1. 2 mEq/mL; 20 mL; 40 mEq; 10 mL
3. 125 mL/hr; 2 mL/min; 42 gtt/min
6. 111 gtt/min
9. 1,200 mL
12. 125 min; 160 gtt/min
15. 180 mL/hr
18. 6 mL; 253 mL/hr; 42 gtt/min

Practice Problems A

1. 0.8 mL
3. 2.5 mL
6. 7.5 mL; 10 mL; 5 vials

Practice Problems B

1. 100 mL/hr
3. 375 mL
6. ½ hr
9. 2330

Practice Problems C

1. 75 mg
3. 30 g; 25 g
6. 350 mg; 175 mg
9. 10 hr; 8 mEq

Practice Problems D

1. 56 gtt/min
3. 16 gtt/min; 15.6 mL/hr
6. 63 gtt/min; 187.5 mg
9. 25 gtt/min; 312.5 mg
12. 80.9 mg; 10 gtt/min; 72.8 mg
15. 22 gtt/min; 20 mg

Practice Problems E

1. 333 min
3. 800 min
6. 150 min; 2 hr and 30 min
9. 2.5 mL; 379 min
12. 5 hours; 30 gtt/min
15. 14 gtt/min; 6 hours

Practice Problems F

1. 50 g of magnesium sulfate in 100 mL of solution; 25 g; 200 mEq; 500 mg/mL
3. 375 mL of 8.5% amino acids injection; 300 mL of D50W; 225 mL of 20% lipids; 600 mL of sterile water for injection
6. 7.5 mL potassium chloride; 4 mL sodium chloride; 0.5 mL magnesium sulfate; 2 mL sodium acetate; 5 mL sodium phosphates; 0.5 mL Humulin R insulin; 4 mL vitamin C; 2 mL folic acid; 5 mL trace elements; 5 mL MVI-12; 35.5 mL; 3% Travesol; 20% dextrose; 164.5 mL; 30 g; 200 g; 1920
9. 7.5 mL KCl; 4 mL NaCl; 0.5 mL $MgSO_4$; 5 mL sodium phosphates; 4 mL vitamin C; 2 mL folic acid; 5 mL trace elements; 10 mL MVI-12; 38 mL; 341 mL of Travesol; 400 mL of 50% dextrose; 221 mL sterile water for injection; 1600

Posttest

1. 6 mL; 169 min
3. 4 mL; 0.9 mL/min; 52 gtt/min; 375 mg; 8 vials; 4,000 mg
6. 400 mg; 8 mL; 18 gtt/min
9. 1.5 mL/min; 1.3 mL/min
12. 15 mL; 1.1 mL/min; 1.7 mL/min
15. 0.12 mg/hr; 2 mcg/min; 240 mL; 10 gtt/min
18. 40 mL; two vials; 23 gtt/min; 90 mL/hr; 133.3 mg
21. 25 g dextrose; 2.25 g NaCl; 83.3 mL/hr; 14 gtt/min
24. 50 mL/hr; 80 units of insulin per hour; 17 gtt/min
27. 50 gtt/mL
30. potassium chloride 5 mL; sodium chloride 6 mL; calcium gluconate 16.1 mL; magnesium sulfate 0.49 mL; sodium acetate 1.5 mL; sodium phosphates 3 mL; Humulin R insulin 0.41 mL; vitamin C 4 mL; folic acid 2 mL; MVI-12 10 mL; 48.5 mL; amino acids 3%; dextrose 20%; lipids 2%; 151.5 mL sterile water for injection; 1400
32. 7.5 mL KCl; 4 mL NaCl; 0.5 mL $MgSO_4$; 5 mL sodium phosphates; 4 mL vitamin C; 2 mL folic acid; 5 mL trace elements; 10 mL MVI-12; 38 mL; 341 mL of Travesol; 400 mL of 50% dextrose; 221 mL sterile water for injection; 1,600

Chapter 16

Note: Losses are shown in parentheses ( ).

Pretest

1. $20.85
3. $18.37; $13.50; $31.87
6. $3,166.67
9. $26.50; ($1.00)

Practice Problems A

1. 5; The difference in purchasing 4 or 8 is quite costly.
3. 5
6. 350 tablets;13¢; 11¢; 12¢; 8¢; 500 tablets/container; 1
9. 1,250 tablets; 7.5¢; 6.9¢; 5.5¢ 500 tablets/container; 3

Practice Problems B

1. 4 turnovers/year
3. 18 turnovers/6 months
6. 1.2 turnovers/2 months: no; 7.3 turnovers/year: decrease his average inventory

Practice Problems C

1. $2,250
3. $438,600; $36,550
6. $790,500; $65,875

Practice Problems D

1. $43.20
3. $48.30
6. $18.90
9. $31.50

Practice Problems E

1. 24.4%
3. 9%
6. 7.1%
9. 40.2%

Practice Problems F

1. $48.60
3. $10.63; $31.87
6. $7.80; $57.20
9. $3.18
12. $8.40; $16.50; $8.10

Practice Problems G

1. $127,434
3. $79,205

Practice Problems H

1. $26,600; $26,550; $50
3. $76,600; $29,200; $47,400

Practice Problems I

1. $33.71; $8.11
3. $13.85; $5.95
6. $21.80
9. $45.37

Practice Problems J

1. $52 profit
3. $960 annual profit; $613 annual profit
6. $31.00 profit

Posttest

1. $35,727.08; $54,530.28; $18,803.20
3. $40.60; $0.81; $60.75
6. $94.79; $64.81; $29.98
9. $51.56; $22.06; $26.64; $11.19; $18.77; $13.08; prescription for $34.50
12. $15.10; $13.59; $1.51
15. $285.00
18. $33.47; $12.19
21. $0.23/spray; $0.15/spray; The 288 spray bottle

A

Active ingredients The ingredient in a medication that has the desired effect on the body

Additives Medications to be added to IV infusions including total parenteral nutrition (TPN) solutions and peripheral parenteral nutrition (PPN) solutions; electrolytes, multiple vitamins, trace elements, regular insulin, and other medications

Adjudication Electronic process by which insurance companies evaluate prescriptions to determine their validity and the price to charge the patient

Adolescent 12 through 21 years of age[a]

Alligation alternate Mathematical method for determining the amount of *two* preparations of different strengths needed to prepare a required strength in between the two; aka **tic-tac-toe**

Alligation medial Calculation method by which the weighted average strength of a mixture of *two or more* preparations of known quantity and concentration may be determined

Ampule Sealed glass container that holds a single dose of medication, usually for injection

Anticoagulant Substance that stops or delays the clotting of blood

Apothecary system One of the oldest measurement systems used to calculate drug orders using measurements such as grains and minims

Arabic numerals The numbers 1, 2, 3, etc.

Assets Any property owned by the business

Auxiliary label Label added to prescriptions to provide supplementary instructions

Average wholesale price (AWP) Price that a pharmacy theoretically pays for medication; this price is theoretical because discounts, sales, and special deals may affect the actual wholesale price; this is the price basis used for insurance reimbursement

B

Base solution Solution for a TPN or PPN that contains carbohydrates (dextrose), protein (amino acids), and sometimes lipids (fatty acids)

Beyond use date (BUD) Date assigned by the pharmacy to a reconstituted or repackaged medication beyond which the preparation is no longer considered usable

Biologics Substances made from natural sources such as humans, animals, or microorganisms that are used as drug treatments or to prevent or diagnose diseases; tested for potency in a biologic system

Body surface area (BSA) Measurement of total body area exposed to the environment; calculated from weight and height and expressed in square meters (m^2); used as a basis for calculating some medication doses

Buccal Between the gum and cheek; medications dissolved between the gum and cheek

C

Capitation fee Set amount of third-party money paid monthly to the pharmacy for a specific patient regardless of the number of prescriptions filled

Cash flow Receipts and expenses for a business

Celsius (Centigrade) System of measuring temperature; 0° is the freezing point and 100° is the boiling point of water

Child 2 to less than 12 years of age[a]

Clark's rule Means of calculating a dose of medication for a child from an adult dose using weight in pounds

Complex fraction Fractions in which the numerator, denominator, or both are fractional units

Compounding Preparing a product in the pharmacy that is not commercially available in the ordered dose or dosage form

Compounding formulation Similar to a recipe; a list of all components needed for a particular compound

Continuous infusion Introduction of IV fluids without interruption of therapy

Conversion factor A ratio equal to 1 that is used to change one unit to another without changing the value of the answer

Convert Change from one form to another

D

Daily cash or sales report Report made at the end of each day that summarizes the sales, discounts, and amount of cash, checks, refunds, and credit card charges that have occurred during the day's operations

Days' supply Number of days a prescription will last; important to input for insurance reimbursement

Decimal Representation of a fraction where the denominator is a power of 10 and the numerator is a number placed to the right of a decimal point

Decimal place Place values found to the right of the decimal point

Denominator The bottom number of a fraction

Depreciation Decrease in value of an asset based on the total value of the asset, its estimated length of use, and its value at disposal; part of overhead

Diluent An agent that dilutes a substance; in pharmacy, the liquid added to a powder to change the powder to a liquid or the liquid used to dilute another liquid; aka solvent; in compounding, an inert component in which other components (such as the active ingredient) are mixed or dissolved (e.g., water, elixir, cream, or ointment bases); aka base or solvent

Dilution Process of making a more concentrated preparation less concentrated by adding a diluent containing no active ingredient such as water or white petrolatum

Dimensional analysis (DA) A method used for converting between units and calculating medication doses and dosages that involves multiplying a series of fractions in an order whereby all unnecessary units

[a] According to the U.S. FDA (https://www.fda.gov/medical-devices/products-and-medical-procedures/pediatric-medical-devices)

are sequentially canceled until the desired unit is reached

Discount Reduction in the price of an item; offered to customers by the pharmacy (markdown) or offered to the pharmacy from wholesalers when a bill is paid by a certain date

Discount percentage A percentage amount to be subtracted from the retail price of an item to lower the selling price

Dispensing fee Amount of money added to the cost of a prescription; intended to cover various aspects of preparing and dispensing; often a set price determined by insurance companies

Dividend The number being divided in division

Divisor Number by which another number is divided

Dosage Size, frequency, and number of doses of medication prescribed

Dosage form The physical structure of a dose; for example: capsule, tablet, solution

Dosage strength Weight of medication in a dose

Dose Amount of a medication to be administered at one time

Dose time Amount of time needed to administer medication

Dose volume Volume of medication administered at a given time

Drip rate The specific type of flow rate calculated in drops per minute; gtt/min

Drop factor Size of a drop from the drip chamber; found on IV tubing (drops/mL)

E

Electrolytes Elements such as sodium (Na), potassium (K), magnesium (Mg), and calcium (Ca) that are necessary for normal body functions

Elixir Sweetened, flavored medication dissolved in a mixture of alcohol and water

Enteric-coated tablet Dosage form that allows medication to pass through the stomach unchanged; to prevent stomach irritation or prevent degradation of the active ingredient by stomach acid

Excipients Medicinally inactive substances that are added to medication formulations; fillers, binders, coloring agents, flavorings, preservatives

Expiration date Date assigned by the manufacturer of a medication beyond which it is not considered usable (no longer valid once a medication is repackaged or reconstituted)

F

Fahrenheit System of measuring temperature; 32° is the freezing point and 212° is the boiling point of water

Flow rate The speed at which IV medications are infused into the body; aka infusion rate

Fraction (Proper fraction) Part of a whole number containing a numerator and denominator

Fried's rule Means of calculating a dose of medication for an infant from an adult dose using age in months

G

Generic name Official nonproprietary name given to a drug by the U.S. Food and Drug Administration (FDA)

Graduates Containers, calibrated in the metric system, that are used to measure liquid

Gross income/gross profit The sales price of merchandise minus its purchase cost; usually refers to total income for a business

H

High-alert medications Medications that have a higher risk of causing significant harm to a patient if dosed or used incorrectly

I

Improper fraction Fraction in which the numerator is equal to or greater than the denominator; a fraction that is equal to or greater than 1

Indication Reason to prescribe a medication

Infant 29 days to less than 2 years of age[a]

Infusion Slow administration of fluids, other than blood, into a vein

Inhaler A device used to deliver medicine by breathing it in through the mouth or nose

Injection A dose of medication administered with a needle and syringe

Inscription Part of prescription indicating medication name, dosage form, strength, and quantity

International System of Units (metric system) Internationally accepted system of measurement of mass, length, and time

International unit/unit A specific unit of measurement used for biologicals; describes a standard amount of an individual drug that can produce a given biological effect; a measurement of a medication's action as opposed to its weight (as with the units mcg, mg, g); units of one substance are not equivalent to the same number of units of another substance (specific to each particular medication)

Intradermal Into or within the dermis of the skin (ID)

Intramuscular Into or within a muscle (IM)

Intravenous Into or within a vein (IV)

Inventory List of the quantity and respective cost of the merchandise in stock

Invert To turn upside down or switch positions

L

Large-volume parenteral (LVP) IV bag sized over 250 mL up to 3 L for infusion

Leading zero A zero placed before the decimal point in a number that is less than 1; necessary in pharmacy to reduce possible dosing errors

[a]According to the U.S. FDA (https://www.fda.gov/medical-devices/products-and-medical-procedures/pediatric-medical-devices)

Least common denominator (LCD) The smallest whole number that can be divided evenly by all denominators of fractions within a problem; necessary for addition and subtraction of fractions; also known as least common multiple (LCM)
Lowest term Form of a fraction in which no common number will divide into both the numerator and denominator evenly

M

Macrodrip infusion sets Infusion sets used for measuring the rate of IV fluids; macrodrip sets provide large drops (10 to 20 drops/mL) of fluid called macrodrops
Markup Amount of money added to the purchase cost of a product to obtain the selling price
Markup percentage or gross margin A percentage amount added to the purchase cost of merchandise to ensure a profit; markup amount divided by the cost times 100
Measurable amount The quantity of medication that can be most accurately measured on the device available
Medication order Physician's written or verbal direction for the administration of medication in an inpatient health care setting
Medication strength The concentration of an active ingredient in a medication
Meniscus The curved line that develops on the upper surface of a liquid when poured into a container: always read at the bottom of the curve
Microdrip infusion sets Infusion sets used for measuring the rate of IV fluids; microdrip sets supply small drops (e.g., 60 drops/mL) called microdrops
Military time (International Standard Time) System of time that recognizes a 24-hour notation of hours and minutes
Milliequivalent (mEq) A type of unit used to express the concentration of electrolytes
Mixed number Number containing a whole number and a fraction

N

National Drug Code (NDC) The unique number on the drug label that identifies the manufacturer, product, and size of the container
Nebulizer A device used to produce a fine spray of medication for inhalation
Neonate From birth through the first 28 days of life[a]
Net income/net profit Gross profit minus overhead; usually refers to total income for a business
Nomogram A chart on which height and weight are plotted to determine BSA
Nonsterile compounding The mixing of two or more components that do not require a sterile environment
Numerator Top number found in a fraction

O

Oral medications Medications taken by mouth (PO)
Overhead Expenses of a business, not including the cost of inventory, such as rent, wages, utilities, insurance, license fees, depreciation, taxes paid, and other costs of doing business

P

PAR (periodic automatic replenishment) level Predetermined point for automatic inventory reordering of items used in a pharmacy; par level is also used to indicate a specific quantity to be kept in stock
Parenteral Administration outside the gastrointestinal tract; mostly considered to be by injection or infusion
Parenteral nutrition IV solution used to provide nutrition to a patient; aka hyperalimentation
Patent Open and unobstructed as in IV lines or blood vessels
Percent Means of expressing a portion of 100 parts
Percentage strength An amount of active ingredient per 100 parts total: $x/100 = x\%$
Peripheral parenteral nutrition (PPN) IV containing a low concentration of amino acids, dextrose, electrolytes, and sometimes lipids, which is administered through a peripheral vessel
Pharmacokinetics Movement of drugs through the body; absorption, distribution, metabolism, and excretion (ADME)
Pharmacology Study of drugs, their uses, and their interactions with living systems
Pharmacotherapeutics Effects of drugs in the treatment of conditions and diseases in the body
Piggyback A small-volume parenteral; IV sized 50 to 250 mL with added medication that is administered through an established IV line
Powder volume Space occupied by the powdered active ingredient relative to the total volume of medication following reconstitution; aka displacement value; a measurement of the amount of active substance that displaces (takes the place of) some of the liquid diluent added for reconstitution
Prescription A written order by a licensed health care professional for dispensing medications
Product The number obtained by multiplying two numbers together

[a]According to the US FDA (https://www.fda.gov/medical-devices/products-and-medical-procedures/pediatric-medical-devices)

Profit See *Gross income/gross profit* and *Net income/net profit*
Proper fraction Fraction in which the numerator is less than the denominator; value is less than 1
Proportion Comparative relationship between the parts; one or more ratios that are compared
Purchase cost Price paid by a business to obtain items for sale; also referred to as wholesale, acquisition, or *inventory cost*

Q

qs Quantity sufficient or required
qs ad Quantity sufficient to make
Quotient Answer to a division problem

R

Ratio Means of describing the relationship between two numbers; for example, 1:2
Ratio and proportion (R&P) A method used for single-step conversions between units and calculating medication doses and dosages; involves solving for two equivalent fractions using cross-multiplication and division
Ratio strength The expression of strength of weak solutions or liquid preparations; one part active ingredient in x parts total: (1: x)
Reconstitution Process of adding fluid, such as water or saline, to the powdered or crystalline form of medication to make a specific liquid dosage strength
Remainder The amount left over after division
Roman numerals Letters from the Roman alphabet that are used to represent numbers, such as I for 1, V for 5, X for 10, etc.
Round To express a number to its nearest place value such as ones, tenths, hundredths, etc.

S

Scheduled medications Classification of medications with potential for abuse and misuse: CII, CIII, CIV, and CV
Scored tablet Tablet containing an indention for ease of breaking into equal parts
Selling price Price at which items are offered for sale to customers; aka retail price
Signa (Sig) Part of prescription; directions for the patient—how, how much, when, how long
Small-Volume Parenteral (SVP) IV bag 250 mL or less
Solute A substance that is dissolved in a solution or semisolid
Solution The dosage form in which the medication is completely dissolved in the liquid
Solvent Substance doing the dissolving; aka diluent
Specific gravity The ratio of the density of a substance to the density of water when dealing with liquids in pharmacy
Standard An exact quantity agreed on for use in comparing measurements
Stock medication Medication provided by a manufacturer and kept on hand for use in preparing medication orders or prescriptions
Stock strength Strength or weight of medication available for doses
Subcutaneous Beneath the skin; medications injected into the subcutaneous tissue (Subcut)
Sublingual medications Medications placed under the tongue to dissolve (SL)
Subscription Part of a prescription that contains instructions for the pharmacist on how to compound if necessary
Superscription Part of a prescription designated with the symbol ℞, meaning, "take this drug"
Suspension The dosage form in which small particles of medication are dispersed throughout the liquid; most require shaking before dispensing and administering
Syrup Aqueous solution sweetened with sugar or a sugar substitute to disguise taste

T

Therapeutic range A dosage or blood concentration range that normally produces desired results; too much may be toxic, and too little may not achieve the desired effect
Total parenteral nutrition (TPN) IV containing a high concentration of amino acids, dextrose, and sometimes lipids with electrolytes and other medications, which is administered through a large central vessel
Toxicology Study of adverse toxic reactions or toxic levels of chemicals and drugs
Trade/Brand name A proprietary name given to a medication by the manufacturer
Trailing zero A zero in the farthest right place of a number following the decimal; not used in medication dosing due to the increased potential for dosing errors
Turnover rate Rate at which the inventory is sold over a specified period of time

U

Unit A *general term* covering any quantity chosen as a standard; for a measurement to make sense, it must include a number and a unit; examples of units: mg, mL, tsp
U.S. customary system (Household system) System of measurement based on U.S. common kitchen measuring devices

V

Vaccination Act of introducing a vaccine into the body to produce immunity
Vaccine A substance causing the immune system to respond better when it is exposed to

a disease-causing agent; prepared from the disease-causing agent or a synthetic (man-made) substitute

Vial Glass or plastic container with metal-enclosed rubber seal for injectable medications; may contain single or multiple doses

Viscosity Thickness of substance

W

Whole number Numeral consisting of one or more digits; number that is not followed by a fraction or decimal

Y

Young's rule Means of calculating a dose of medication for a child from an adult dose based on age in years

Index

Page numbers followed by "f" indicate figures, "t" indicate tables, and "b" indicate boxes.